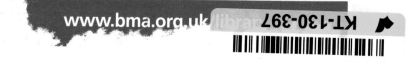

Public health response to biological and chemical weapons

WHO guidance

Second edition of
Health aspects of chemical and biological weapons:
report of a WHO Group of Consultants,
Geneva, World Health Organization, 1970

World Health Organizati
Geneva, 2004

WHO Library Cataloguing-in-Publication Data

World Health Organization.
Public health response to biological and chemical weapons : WHO guidance —
2nd ed.

1.Chemical warfare agents 2.Biological warfare 3.Bioterrorism
4.Environmental monitoring 5.Environmental pollution 6.Disease outbreaks
7.Disaster planning 8.Risk assessment 9.Risk management 10.Guidelines
I.Title.

ISBN 92 4 154615 8   (LC/NLM Classification: QV 663)

First edition, 1970
Second edition, 2004

Publications of the World Health Organization can be obtained from Marketing and Dissemination, World Health Organization, 20 Avenue Appia, 1211 Geneva 27, Switzerland (tel: +41 22 791 2476; fax: +41 22 791 4857; email: *bookorders@who.int*). Requests for permission to reproduce WHO publications, in part or in whole, or to translate them – whether for sale or for noncommercial distribution – should be addressed to Publications, at the above address (fax: +41 22 791 4806; email: *permissions@who.int*).

Layout: WHO/CME/A. Guilloux – Bruno Duret, France
Cover based on photographs: NASA/Hubble, NASA/Goddard
Printed in China

CONTENTS

FOREWORD

The message contained in this publication is clear: countries need a public health system that can respond to the deliberate release of chemical and biological agents. Regrettable though this message may be, the use of poison gas in the war between Iraq and the Islamic Republic of Iran in the 1980s, the recent anthrax incidents in the United States, and the attack with sarin nerve agent, six years earlier, on the Tokyo underground, illustrate why it is necessary to prepare.

Recognizing this need, the Fifty-fifth World Health Assembly in May 2002 adopted resolution WHA55.16 calling on Member States to "treat any deliberate use, including local, of biological and chemical agents and radionuclear attack to cause harm also as a global public health threat, and to respond to such a threat in other countries by sharing expertise, supplies and resources in order rapidly to contain the event and mitigate its effects." This is but the first step. The need has been identified. What is now required are national and international procedures to meet it, suitably resourced.

This manual describes these procedures. Written 30 years after WHO published its first report on the subject, the new volume could not be more timely. Lessons learned about the consequences following deliberate use of chemical and biological agents in a range of wars and in other crimes, serve as the foundation for its recommendations.

One consistent theme is evident throughout. It is the importance of using existing systems to protect public health and to augment these where appropriate. For example, better disease surveillance locally, nationally, and internationally will provide a surer way of detecting and responding to unusual disease outbreaks than a system geared only to detect deliberate release of candidate biological warfare agents. Similar principles apply for the provision of health care; management of health emergencies, delivery of clean water or protecting food supplies.

For those charged with protecting the health of the public and who now have also to be concerned about the deliberate use of chemical and biological warfare agents, this manual will prove invaluable. As the former Executive Director of WHO Communicable Diseases, I am glad to have been associated with this publication and welcome and support what it has to say.

Dr David L. Heymann

ACKNOWLEDGEMENTS

WHO wishes to acknowledge the Swiss Humanitarian Aid Unit of the Federal Department of Foreign Affairs, Switzerland, for its financial contribution to this project; the Harvard Sussex Program on Chemical and Biological Warfare Armament and Arms Limitation for supporting the work of the Executive Editor; and the Pugwash Conferences on Science and World Affairs for technical and other assistance. The continued technical support to this project from the Organisation for the Prohibition of Chemical Weapons is also appreciated.

EXECUTIVE SUMMARY

The development, production and use of biological and chemical weapons are prohibited by international treaties to which most WHO Member States have subscribed, namely the 1925 Geneva Protocol, the 1972 Biological and Toxin Weapons Convention, and the 1993 Chemical Weapons Convention. Not all have done so, however, and valid concerns remain that some may yet use such weapons. Moreover, non-state entities may try to obtain them for terrorist or other criminal purposes.

In fact, biological and chemical weapons have only rarely been used. Their development, production and use entail numerous difficulties and pose serious hazards to those who would seek to use them. This applies particularly to biological weapons. Even so, the magnitude of the possible effects on civilian populations of their use or threatened use obliges governments both to seek to prevent such use and to prepare response plans, which can and should be developed as an integral part of existing national-emergency and public-health plans.

New technology can contribute substantially to such plans, as is evident, for example, from the increasing availability of robust and relatively simple methods of rapid and specific laboratory diagnosis by DNA-based and other molecular methods. Such methods are widely used in the surveillance, prevention and treatment of natural disease.

The extent to which specialist personnel, equipment and medical stockpiles may be needed for protective preparation is a matter for national judgement in the light of the prevailing circumstances, including national assessments of the likelihood of attacks using biological or chemical weapons and consideration of existing demands on health and emergency services generally.

The danger should not be disregarded that overoptimistic evaluation of protective preparation may distract attention from the continuing importance of prevention, e.g. by the full implementation of the 1972 and 1993 Conventions.

The two Conventions include provision for assistance in the event of attack or threat of attack. The Organisation for the Prohibition of Chemical Weapons (OPCW), which is the international authority for the 1993 Convention, is making practical arrangements for providing such assistance if chemical weapons are used or threatened. As yet, however, there is no similar organization for biological weapons, but WHO, among others, can provide some assistance to its Member States.

Each of these matters is discussed in detail in the main body of the present report, which makes the following practical recommendations.

1) Public health authorities, in close cooperation with other government bodies, should draw up contingency plans for dealing with a deliberate release of biological or chemical agents intended to harm civilian populations. These plans should be consistent or integral with existing plans for outbreaks of disease, natural disasters, large-scale industrial or transportation accidents, and terrorist incidents. In accordance with World Health Assembly resolution WHA55.16 adopted in May 2002, technical support is available to Member States from WHO in developing or strengthening preparedness for, and response to, the deliberate use of biological and chemical agents to cause harm.

2) Preparedness for deliberate releases of biological or chemical agents should be based on standard risk-analysis principles, starting with risk and threat assessment in order to determine the relative priority that should be accorded to such releases in comparison with other dangers to public health in the country concerned. Considerations for deliberate releases should be incorporated into existing public health infrastructures, rather than developing separate infrastructures.

3) Preparedness for deliberate releases of biological or chemical agents can be markedly increased in most countries by strengthening the

public health infrastructure, and particularly public health surveillance and response, and measures should be taken to this end.

4) Managing the consequences of a deliberate release of biological or chemical agents may demand more resources than are available, and international assistance would then be essential. Sources of such assistance are available and should be identified.

5) Attention is drawn to the international assistance and support available to all countries that are Member States of specialized organizations such as OPCW (e.g. in cases of the use or threat of use of chemical weapons, and for preparedness planning), and to States Parties to the 1972 Biological and Toxin Weapons Convention (e.g. in cases of violation of the treaty). Countries should actively participate in these multilateral regimes.

6) With the entry into force of the 1972 and 1993 Conventions and the increasing number of states that have joined them, great strides have been made towards "outlawing the development and use in all circumstances of chemical and biological agents as weapons of war", as called for in the 1970 edition of the present report. However, as the world advances still further into the new age of biotechnology, Member States are reminded that every major new technology of the past has come to be intensively exploited, not only for peaceful purposes, but also for hostile ones. Prevention of the hostile exploitation of biotechnology therefore rises above the security interests of individual states and poses a challenge to humanity generally. All Member States should therefore implement the two Conventions fully and transparently; propagate in education and professional training the ethical principles that underlie the Conventions; and support measures that would build on their implementation.

The statement by the World Health Assembly in resolution WHA20.54 of 25 May 1967 that "scientific achievements, and particularly in the field of biology and medicine – that most humane science – should be used only for mankind's benefit, but never to do it any harm" remains as valid today as it was then.

ABBREVIATIONS AND ACRONYMS

ABC	American Broadcasting Company
AMI	American Media Incorporated
BSE	bovine spongiform encephalopathy
BWC	Biological and Toxin Weapons Convention
CAS	Chemical Abstracts Service
CBS	Columbia Broadcasting System
CDC	Centers for Disease Control and Prevention (United States)
CNS	central nervous system
CPAP	continuous positive airway pressure
CWC	Chemical Weapons Convention
DMPS	dimercaptosuccinic acid
DMSA	dimercapto-1-propanesulfonic acid
ELISA	enzyme-linked immunoabsorbent assay
FAO	Food and Agriculture Organization of the United Nations
FBI	Federal Bureau of Investigation (United States)
GC	gas capillary column chromatography
GC–MS	gas chromatography–mass spectrometry
GMP	good manufacturing practices
GP	Geneva Protocol
HACCP	Hazard Analysis and Critical Control Point
HEPA	high-efficiency particulate arresting
HPLC	high-performance liquid chromatography
ICGEB	International Centre for Genetic Engineering and Biotechnology
IHR	International Health Regulations
ILO	International Labour Organization
IPCS	International Programme on Chemical Safety

IPE	individual protective equipment
MCDU	Military and Civil Defence Unit (OCHA)
NBC	National Broadcasting Company
NMDA	*N*-methyl-D-aspartate
OCHA	Office for the Coordination of Humanitarian Affairs (United Nations)
OIE	World Organisation for Animal Health
OPCW	Organisation for the Prohibition of Chemical Weapons
OPIDN	organophosphate-induced delayed neuropathy
OSOCC	On Site Operations Coordination Centre (OCHA)
PAVA	pelargonic acid vanillylamide
PCR	polymerase chain reaction
PEEP	positive-end expiratory pressure
PFIB	Perfluoroisobutene
PVC	polyvinyl chloride
RADS	reactive airways dysfunction syndrome
SEB	staphylococcal enterotoxin B
SIPRI	Stockholm International Peace Research Institute
TEPP	tetraethyl pyrophosphate
TICs	toxic industrial chemicals
UNDAC	United Nations Disaster Assessment and Coordination (OCHA)
UNEP	United Nations Environment Programme
UNSCOM	United Nations Special Commission
USAMRIID	United States Army Research Institute for Infectious Diseases
USPS	United States Postal Service
WFP	World Food Programme (United Nations)
WHO	World Health Organization

CONTRIBUTORS

Executive Editor

*Professor J. P. Perry Robinson, SPRU — Science and Technology Policy Research, University of Sussex, United Kingdom

Secretary to the Group

Dr *Ottorino Cosivi*, Communicable Diseases, World Health Organization, Geneva, Switzerland

Major contribution to the text and conceptual development of this publication was made by the following individuals:

Dr *Brian J. Davey*, Organisation for the Prohibition of Chemical Weapons

Professor *Alastair W. M. Hay*, University of Leeds, United Kingdom

*Dr *Martin Kaplan*, former Scientific Adviser to WHO Director-General, Switzerland

Mr *Ian R. Kenyon*, former Executive Secretary, Preparatory Commission for the Organisation for the Prohibition of Chemical Weapons

Dr *Walter Krutzsch*, Chemical Weapons Convention consultant, Germany

*Professor *Matthew Meselson*, Harvard University, United States

Dr *Graham S. Pearson*, former Director-General, Chemical and Biological Defence Establishment, Porton Down, United Kingdom

Dr *Emmanuelle Tuerlings*, University of Sussex, United Kingdom

*: identifies those who contributed to the original 1970 edition.

The Executive Editor gratefully acknowledges the contribution to this publication made by the following individuals:

Dr Mahdi Balali-Mood, Islamic Republic of Iran
Dr H. V. Batra, India
Dr Hendrik Benschop, Netherlands
Dr Raffaele D'Amelio, Italy
Dr Flavio Del Ponte, Switzerland
Dr David R. Franz, United States
Professor Jeanne Guillemin, United States
Mr Jerome M. Hauer, United States
Ms Iris Hunger, Germany
Professor Le Cao Dai, Viet Nam
Dr Roque Monteleone-Neto, Brazil
Mr Claus-Peter Polster, Netherlands
Mr Michael Sharpe, Canada
Dr Nikolay A. Staritsin, Russian Federation
Professor Robert Steffen, Switzerland
Dr Katsuaki Sugiura, Japan
Dr Jan Willems, Belgium

Additionally, valuable suggestions or review inputs were made by:

Dr Anfeng Guo, China
Dr David Ashford, United States
Dr Camille Boulet, Canada
Dr Ake Bovallius, Sweden
Mr Peter Channells, Australia
Mr Nicholas Dragffy, United Kingdom
Colonel Edward Eitzen, United States
Mr Simon Evans, United Kingdom
Dr John Fountain, New Zealand
Dr Bruno Garin-Bastuji, France

Professor Christine Gosden, United Kingdom
Dr Murray Hamilton, Canada
Dr Donald A. Henderson, United States
Dr Michael Hills, Australia
Dr Martin Hugh-Jones, United States
Dr David L. Huxsoll, United States
Dr Goran A. Jamal, United Kingdom
Dr Dennis Juranek, United States
Dr Ali S. Khan, United States
Dr Robert Knouss, United States
Dr Takeshi Kurata, Japan
*Professor Joshua Lederberg, United States
Mr Li Yimin, China
Dr Jennifer McQuiston, United States
Dr Jack Melling, Austria
Dr Jane Mocellin, France
Dr Virginia Murray, United Kingdom
Dr Eric Noji, United States
Professor Phan thi Phi, Viet Nam
Dr Alexander Ryzhikov, Russian Federation
Dr Lev Sandakhchiev, Russian Federation
Professor Alexander Sergeev, Russian Federation
Sir Joseph Smith, United Kingdom
Dr H. Sohrabpour, Islamic Republic of Iran
Dr Frank Souter, Canada
Dr Ben P. Steyn, South Africa
Dr David Swerdlow, United States
Professor Ladislaus Szinicz, Germany
Dr Noriko Tsunoda, Japan
Dr Peter Turnbull, United Kingdom
Professor Scott Weaver, United States
Dr Mark Wheelis, United States
Dr Riccardo Wittek, Switzerland

Individuals from the following international organizations also provided valuable comments and suggestions, review input, or editorial assistance

International Centre for Genetic Engineering and Biotechnology (ICGEB)
Professor Arturo Falaschi, Dr Decio Ripandelli

Organisation for the Prohibition of Chemical Weapons (OPCW)
Dr Brian Davey, Mr Clou, Peter Polster, the late Dr Johan Santesson, Ms Lisa Tabassi

Food and Agriculture Organization of the United Nations (FAO)
Mr Manfred Luetzow, Professor Juhani Paakkanen, Dr David Ward

United Nations Office for the Coordination of Humanitarian Affairs (OCHA)
Dr Arjun Katoch

World Organisation for Animal Health (OIE)
Dr Yoshiyuki Oketani, Dr Jim E. Pearson

World Food Programme (WFP)
Mr Allan Jury, Ms Christine van Nieuwenhuyse

World Health Organization (WHO)
Dr James Bartram, Ms Karen Ciceri, Dr Ottorino Cosivi, Dr Pierre Formenty, Dr Kersten Gutschmidt, Dr Randall Hyer, Dr Alessandro Loretti, Dr Gerry Moy, Dr Samuel Page, Dr Jenny Pronczuk, Dr Cathy Roth, Dr Philip Rushbrook, Dr Gita Uppal, Ms Mary Vallanjon, Dr Stephane Vandam, Dr Williamina Wilson, Dr Samir Ben Yahmed

1. INTRODUCTION

1.1 Developments since the first edition

Thirty years have passed since the World Health Organization (WHO) published its 1970 report *Health aspects of chemical and biological weapons (1)*, and there have been significant changes during this period. On the negative side, there has been the large-scale use of both mustard gas and nerve gas in the the war between Iraq and the Islamic Republic of Iran; the reported use of these agents by the Iraqi Government against its own citizens, most conspicuously at Halabja in March 1988;[1] and the use of sarin on two occasions (in 1994 and 1995) by the Aum Shinrikyo religious cult in public places in Japan, including the Tokyo subway. The cult also made preparations, fortunately ineffective, to use biological weapons. The dissemination of anthrax spores through the United States postal system in 2001, killing five people, has now further increased fears of bioterrorism. On the positive side, the Biological Weapons Convention and the Chemical Weapons Convention came into force in 1975 and 1997, respectively, and the Organisation for the Prohibition of Chemical Weapons (OPCW) has started its work of supervising the destruction of chemical-weapon stocks and factories, including those of the Russian Federation and the United States, and monitoring the world's chemical industry to prevent future misuse. From large populations of Europe and Asia, therefore, have now been lifted the immense biological and chemical threats that existed during the Cold War, when there were large active stockpiles of chemical weapons and active preparations for continent-wide biological warfare. These and other developments, both technical and political, over this period, led to a need for a review. This second edition is the result.

Technically, there has been further development along already identified lines rather than totally new concepts. The most important agents of biological and chemical warfare still include some of those

---

[1] Statement by the Secretary-General of the United Nations to the General Assembly on 12 October 1998, document A/C.1/53/PV.3, 3–5.

listed in the 1970 edition. There have been rumours of nerve gases of greater power than VX or VR, but the most important development in chemical weapons has been the "binary munition", in which the final stage of synthesis of the agent from precursors is carried out in the bomb, shell or warhead immediately before or during delivery to the target. As for biological weapons, the genetic modification techniques foreshadowed in 1972 by the first laboratory-made "recombinant" DNA, as well as other developments in molecular biology, seem to offer possibilities for producing new biological-warfare agents. The accessibility of biological agents on a militarily significant scale has been substantially increased by advances in industrial microbiology and its greater use throughout the world.

The year 1970 was a watershed in international legal attempts to deal with the problem of biological and chemical weapons. Following the public renunciation of bioweapons by the United States in 1969, the multilateral conference on disarmament in Geneva, then called the Conference of the Committee on Disarmament, decided to consider biological and chemical weapons separately; these had previously been considered together, as in the 1925 Geneva Protocol prohibiting their use. The Conference thereupon started work on a convention banning the development, production and stockpiling of biological weapons, leaving consideration of a counterpart treaty on chemical weapons for later. The resultant Biological and Toxin Weapons Convention (BWC) was opened for signature in 1972 and entered into force three years later. Concerns about the continuing threat of biological warfare, accentuated by revelations during the early 1990s about bioweapons programmes in the former Soviet Union and in Iraq, led the States Parties to establish an ad hoc group mandated to negotiate a protocol that would strengthen the BWC, particularly through mechanisms intended to ensure compliance, including verification. Work on the protocol was suspended in the latter part of 2001.

The Geneva disarmament conference intensified its efforts on the problem of chemical weapons in the 1980s, and submitted the complete draft of a chemical disarmament treaty to the United Nations General Assembly in 1992. In contrast to the biological treaty, the Convention on the Prohibition of Chemical Weapons (CWC) contained elaborate provisions on verification, to be operated through a new international organization, OPCW, with its headquarters in The Hague. CWC was opened for signature in 1993 and entered into force four years later.

The threat of use of biological or chemical weapons by the armed forces of states has clearly changed since the 1970 report, and is now a particular concern in regions of the world where states have still not joined the two Conventions. In addition, the risk that non-state entities might use such weapons remains a possibility. Vigilance and preparedness to react effectively will therefore continue to be important, as will means of rapid response by the international community. This new edition is intended as a contribution to that effort.

1.2 Origin and purpose of the present report

The first edition originated in a request from the Secretary-General of the United Nations to the Director-General of the World Health Organization in January 1969 to cooperate with a group of experts then being established to prepare a report for the United Nations on biological and chemical weapons and the effects of their possible use. This report was duly completed and released in July 1969 *(2)*. It drew from a submission by WHO prepared by a group of consultants appointed by the Director-General, including consultants from two nongovernmental organizations engaged in the study of the subject, namely Pugwash[2] and the Stockholm International Peace Research Institute (SIPRI).[3] Shortly afterwards, the Twenty-second World Health Assembly, in resolution WHA22.58, requested the Director-General to continue the work *(5)*. The result, which expanded the original submission to the United Nations, became the 1970 WHO report.

---

[2] The Pugwash Conferences on Science and World Affairs is an international organization of scientists, to which the Nobel Peace Prize was awarded in 1995: its interests have included, since the 1950s, matters of biological and chemical warfare *(3)*.

[3] SIPRI, funded by the Swedish Parliament, was then working, in consultation with Pugwash, on its six-volume study of the historical, technical, military, legal and political aspects of biological and chemical warfare armament and disarmament *(4)*.

Since then, WHO has taken steps to keep itself informed of relevant developments. At the Fortieth World Health Assembly in 1987, the subject of chemical warfare was raised and referred to the Executive Board, which, at its eighty-first session in January 1988, noted a report by the Director-General entitled *Effects on health of chemical weapons*, based on a study updating parts of the 1970 report *(6)*. Information on the health effects of chemical weapons and the availability of such information was then reviewed by a Working Group on 7–9 February 1989 *(7)*.

In view of the need to be able to respond under Article 2(d) of the WHO Constitution to emergencies that might be caused by biological weapons, contacts were made by WHO towards the end of 1990 with the Swiss Federal Department of Foreign Affairs. There was also concern at that time about unpreparedness to respond to the consequences of any attack that might be made with weapons of mass destruction, and especially bioweapons, on civilians during military operations in Kuwait. This led to collaboration between WHO and Swiss Humanitarian Aid of the Federal Department of Foreign Affairs, Switzerland, and the consequent establishment of Task Force Scorpio, a team of appropriately equipped and trained specialists who could have been dispatched to an affected area by air ambulance at short notice *(8)*. More generally, as the public has become more conscious of the possibility that biological or chemical agents may be released for hostile purposes, WHO has become concerned about the information on the subject available to the public health authorities of Member States. The Swiss Federal Department of Foreign Affairs has continued to provide support for WHO's efforts in the biological/chemical field, including financial support for the present publication.

In May 2001, the Fifty-fourth World Health Assembly, in resolution WHA54.14, requested the Director-General "to provide technical support to Member States for developing or strengthening preparedness and response activities against risks posed by biological agents, as an integral part of their emergency management programmes" *(9)*. A year later, in resolution WHA55.16, the Assembly requested the Director-General "to continue to issue international guidance and technical information on recommended public health measures to deal with the deliberate use of biological and chemical agents to cause harm" *(10)*. This second edition has been published in response to these requests from the World Health Assembly.

The 1970 report considered biological and chemical weapons at the technical and policy levels. It was intended not only for public health and medical authorities but also for those concerned with emergency response to the suspected or actual use of such weapons. This second edition is intended for much the same readership: government policy-makers, public health authorities, health practitioners and related sectors, especially those concerned with risk- and consequence-management, and their specialist advisers. Not all of the material in the first edition has been included in the second, and some parts of it may still be of interest to specialists.

The present report also considers, in Chapter 5, the 1972 BWC and the 1993 CWC, to which the majority of WHO Member States are party. These two conventions and their national implementing legislation constitute a form of protection against biological and chemical weapons, and also a guide to international assistance if the weapons are nevertheless used.

1.3 Some working definitions

The definitions of biological and chemical weapons contained in the BWC and CWC are set out on pages 28–29 below. For the purposes of this report, however, *biological weapons* are taken to be those that achieve their intended target effects through the infectivity of disease-causing microorganisms and other such entities, including viruses, infectious nucleic acids and prions. Such weapons can be used to attack human beings, other animals or plants, but it is with human beings that the report is primarily concerned.

Some of these biological agents may owe their pathogenicity to toxic substances that they themselves generate. Such *toxins* can sometimes be isolated and used as weapons. Since they would then achieve their effects as a result not of infectivity but of toxicity, they fall within the definition given below of chemical weapons, even though they are also biological weapons within the meaning of the BWC. Microorganisms are not the only life forms that can generate toxins. The BWC, where it refers to toxins, means toxic substances produced by any living organism, even when such substances are actually produced by other means, including chemical synthesis. The present report gives the same meaning to toxins as does the BWC, while recognizing that toxins are also covered by the CWC.

Chemical weapons are taken to be those weapons that are effective because of the toxicity of their active principles, i.e. their chemical action on life processes being capable of causing death, temporary incapacitation or permanent harm. They too can be used against human beings, other animals or plants, but again this report is focused on their effects in human beings. Weapons in which chemicals such as propellants, explosives, incendiaries or obscurants are the active principles are not regarded as chemical weapons, even though the chemicals may also have toxic effects. Only if producing such toxic effects is an intended purpose of the weapon can it be regarded as a chemical weapon. Some toxic chemicals, such as phosgene, hydrogen cyanide and tear gas, may be used both for civil purposes and for hostile purposes. In the latter case, they, too, are chemical weapons.

1.4 Structure

The main part of the report consists of six chapters. These are supported by seven annexes that contain more detailed technical information.

Chapters 2 and 3 describe how biological and chemical agents may endanger public health. Their purpose is to identify what is essential in any planning to avert or at least mitigate the consequences of the deliberate release of such agents.

In Chapter 4, standard principles of risk management are used to outline the steps that Member States may take to prepare themselves for the possibility that biological or chemical agents may be deliberately released with the aim of harming their population. The intention here is to provide not the detailed guidance of an operational manual, but a review of the components of preparedness together with a guide to sources of more detailed information.

Chapter 5 considers the part that law, both national and international, can play in preparedness planning, including its potentially vital role in mobilizing international assistance, while Chapter 6 identifies available sources of such assistance.

REFERENCES

1. *Health aspects of chemical and biological weapons: report of a WHO group of consultants.* Geneva, World Health Organization, 1970.

2. *Chemical and bacteriological (biological) weapons and the effects of their possible use: report of the Secretary-General.* New York, United Nations, 1969.

3. Perry Robinson JP. The impact of Pugwash on the debates over chemical and biological weapons. In: De Cerreño ALC, Keynan A, eds. Scientific cooperation, state conflict: the role of scientists in mitigating international discord. *Annals of the New York Academy of Sciences,* 1998, 866:224–252.

4. Stockholm International Peace Research Institute. *The problem of chemical and biological warfare.* Vols. 1–6. Stockholm, Almqvist & Wicksell, 1971–1975.

5. Twenty-second World Health Assembly, resolution WHA22.58, 25 July 1969.

6. World Health Organization Executive Board, report EB81/27, 10 November 1987.

7. *Report of a working group meeting on information concerning health effects of chemical weapons, Geneva, 7–9 February 1989.* Geneva, World Health Organization, 1989.

8. Steffen R et al. Preparation for emergency relief after biological warfare. *Journal of Infection,* 1997, 34(2):127–132.

9. Fifty-fourth World Health Assembly, resolution WHA54.14, 21 May 2001.

10. Fifty-fifth World Health Assembly, resolution WHA55.16, 18 May 2002.

2. ASSESSING THE THREAT TO PUBLIC HEALTH

Among the many emergencies or disasters to which public health authorities may be called upon to respond is the deliberate use of biological or chemical agents to cause harm. For public health authorities, the problem this raises is one of priorities. What priority should be given to preparedness for such releases as compared with other emergencies or disasters and the regular needs of public health? This chapter provides an historical introduction to this problem and to the more detailed discussion of threat assessment in Chapter 3.

2.1 Background

Poisons and pathogenic microorganisms are among the natural health hazards with which human beings are obliged to coexist. Difficult to perceive and therefore to avoid, they present a threat that is both insidious and damaging or deadly. Humans have survived by adaptation, partly physiological, as in the development of the immune system far back in vertebrate evolution, and partly social, as in the development of both individual and public health practices that serve to limit exposure to the dangers or to alleviate the illness they cause.

Historically, the codes of professional behaviour adopted by the military that forbid the use of poison and therefore also of disease may be regarded as a part of that same social adaptation. From the Manu Laws of India to, for example, the Saracen code of warfare based on the Koran, the Lieber Code of 1863 in the United States and the 1925 Geneva Protocol (1), this taboo seems so widespread, ancient and specific as to require some such explanation (2).

International law relating to biological and chemical warfare is considered in Chapter 5, which describes how the multilateral treaties of 1972 and 1993 on the total prohibition of biological and chemical weapons have extended that law. Underlying this extension was a widespread concern that powerful new weapons were on the verge of proliferating and spreading within a global security system poorly capable of containing the destabilization that they could cause. The United Nations, almost from its inception, has distinguished between *conventional weapons* and *weapons of mass destruction*. It defined the latter in terms of their operating principles and destructiveness,[4] but the main concern was with their consequences, namely their potential for bringing devastation, death and disease to human societies on a scale incompatible with their survival. New weapons technology might, in other words, be generating threats to humanity that called for improved forms of protection: a strengthening of social adaptation to present dangers. At its summit session in January 1992, the Security Council determined that the "proliferation of all weapons of mass destruction constitutes a threat to international peace and security". Moreover, the 15 Member States of the Council also committed themselves "to working to prevent the spread of technology related to the research for or production of such weapons and to take appropriate action to that end" *(4)*.

Throughout most of the world, the public health infrastructure is stretched to its limits coping with natural health hazards. In 1998, a quarter of the world's 53.9 million deaths were due to infectious disease, and in developing countries such disease caused one in two deaths *(5)*. It poses a major threat to economic development and the alleviation of poverty. Against such a background, the additional threat to public health of disease caused in a country by biological or chemical warfare might be no more than a slight addition to the existing burden. Conceivably, however, it might also be on such a scale or of such a nature as to be beyond the capability of the health-care system to cope. For deliberate use (or threats of use) of biological or chemical agents, a spectrum of threat can therefore be envisaged that ranges between those two

---

4   In September 1947, weapons of mass destruction were defined in a Security Council document as "atomic explosive weapons, radioactive material weapons, lethal chemical and biological weapons, and any weapons developed in the future which have characteristics comparable in destructive effect to those of the atomic bomb or other weapons mentioned above" *(3)*. It was this wording, proposed by the United States, that the United Nations subsequently used to differentiate the two broad categories of weapon in order to guide its work on the "system for the regulation of armaments" required under Article 26 of the Charter of the United Nations. Note, however, that, as is described in Chapter 5, the BWC and the CWC are not limited to weapons of mass destruction.

extremes: relative insignificance at one end, mass destruction of life or mass casualties at the other. Where along this spectrum a particular biological or chemical menace is situated will be determined by the characteristics of the agent and the way it is used, and by the vulnerability of the threatened population, reflecting such factors as the health status and degree of preparedness of that population. Particularly threatening would be the possibility of a pandemic resulting from the intentional or inadvertent release of infective agents that cause contagious disease, such as smallpox, for which effective hygienic measures, prophylaxis or therapy may be unavailable. Towards the mass-destruction end of the spectrum, remedies or countermeasures may be beyond the resources of many countries and therefore available, if at all, only through international cooperation.

There is some historical guidance on the likelihood of such a catastrophe. Biological or chemical weapons have only rarely been used by military forces. Unsubstantiated accusations of use have been more common, but this may reflect the difficulty of proving that they have or have not been used because of the lack of reliable information on such unverified episodes, or the readiness with which the emotions aroused by anything to do with poison gas or germ warfare lend themselves to calumny and disinformation. Biological or chemical warfare may have recurred sporadically for at least as long as its proscription. Poison is no novelty as a weapon of murder, and the deliberate pollution, for example, of water supplies is an expedient that retreating forces must often have found attractive. Only in recent times, however, owing to advances in technology, has the position of chemical and biological weapons moved from the insignificant towards the mass-destruction end of the spectrum.

2.2 Technological developments

The event that most clearly marked the emergence of this form of warfare from its prehistory took place near Ypres in Belgium on 22 April 1915, eight months into what was becoming the First World War. Alone among the belligerents, Germany possessed the industrial capacity needed for the large-scale liquefaction of chlorine gas and, as the war progressed, it turned to this comparative advantage as a possible way out both from the trench warfare that was immobilizing its armies in the field and from the shortage of explosives brought about by enemy naval blockade. These military necessities were given precedence, in keeping with the primacy (since disavowed) given to the German legal doctrine of *Kriegsraison* over the ancient prohibition of the use of poisons in warfare that had been reaffirmed at The Hague less than a decade previously. On the late afternoon of that day, 180 tonnes of liquid chlorine contained in 5730 pressure cylinders were released into the breeze that would carry the resultant cloud of asphyxiating vapour towards enemy lines. The available records are sparse but it is said that as many as 15 000 French, Algerian and Canadian soldiers became casualties in this onslaught, one-third of them dead. The actual numbers may have been different but, whatever they were, this was the world's first experience of a weapon of mass destruction.

This new weapon polluted the air that its target population was obliged to breathe, so protection, in the form of air filters, was not impossible to arrange. The first filters contained chemicals that reacted with the poison gas, and were therefore easily circumvented as the weaponeers turned to toxicants of different chemical composition, notably phosgene, or to ways of establishing airborne dosages more than large enough to consume the reactant contained in the filter. Improved filters were then introduced in which the pollutant was physically adsorbed, as in the activated charcoal and particle-retaining paper filters of the respirators, or "gas masks", that today remain the principal and most dependable countermeasure against vapours or aerosols. By 1917, the growing efficacy of gas masks had stimulated the development of chemicals that could attack on or through the skin, the paramount example being an oily liquid known as "mustard gas". The skin is harder to protect effectively than the lungs if those protected are to remain mobile and active, but effective skin attack commonly requires much larger quantities of agent than does inhalation attack, so that the weapons are effective over a substantially smaller area. Mustard gas used in hot weather is an exception to this general rule, as even its vapour attacks the skin. This is one of several reasons why this particular chemical agent remains so menacing even now.

Another way forward for the weaponeers was to use special methods of disseminating the chosen agent, capable of surprising target populations before they could put on their masks. Such a result could be achieved with sudden heavy airborne concentrations of agent delivered by massed artillery or, later, by aerial bombardment. Alternatively, it could be achieved with the imperceptible airborne casualty-producing dosages that could, with the right agent, be established by upwind spray-systems or aerosol-generators. Yet here, too, protective countermeasures were available, some more effective than others, but, taken together, capable today of negating the mass destructiveness of the weapons, at least when used against military forces. Comparable protection of larger and less disciplined civilian populations would be much harder, but not necessarily impossible, to achieve. Countermeasures may be of the following types: (i) medical (therapy and, for some agents, prophylaxis); (ii) technical (respirators that can be worn for many hours, and automatic agent-detection equipment able to give early warning of the need to mask or to enter air-conditioned protective shelter and when to leave); and (iii) organizational (specially developed intelligence systems, standard operating procedures, and training). More recently, new instruments of international law have been included in this range of measures, notably the BWC, the CWC, and the Statute of the International Criminal Court.

Vulnerabilities remain of course, especially in countries where the economic or technological base is not capable of providing even rudimentary protection. This is why, when chemical warfare has recurred since the First World War, it has invariably taken place within the less industrialized regions of the world, e.g. Morocco (1923–1926), Tripolitania (1930), Sinkiang (1934), Abyssinia (1935–1940), Manchuria (1937–1942), Viet Nam (1961–1975), Yemen (1963–1967) and Iraq/Islamic Republic of Iran (1982–1988) (6). In other conflicts, notably the Second World War, the widespread deployment of antichemical protection served to reduce the relative attraction of chemical weapons as compared with those against which protection is less effective. There was no significant strategic or battlefield use of chemical warfare in that conflict.

Vulnerabilities are not absent even in situations where the best protective measures are available. The struggle for supremacy between offence and defence that characterized the development of chemical warfare during the First World War continued after it, and the search for novel agents was one of the forms taken by that struggle. Thus, agents were sought capable of inducing new types of physiological effect from which military advantage might be gained, e.g. casualty-producing agents of low lethality, which promised to reduce the political costs of resort to armed force, or agents causing percutaneous casualty effects more quickly so that chemical weapons could be used like landmines to deny terrain to unprotected personnel. Above all, there was a search for agents of increased potency that would enable weapon-delivery systems to be used more economically and more efficiently. Toxic chemicals having effective doses measurable in tens of milligrams per person, e.g. phosgene and hydrogen cyanide, were replaced in the 1940s and 1950s by organophosphate acetylcholinesterase inhibitors ("nerve gases") that were active in milligram or submilligram quantities, so that substantially fewer munitions might be needed to attack a given target, thereby conferring logistic advantage. The most important of these nerve gases and other new chemical-warfare agents are identified in Chapter 3 and described in Annex 1.

Beyond the nerve gases on the scale of increasing toxicity are certain toxins, such as those described in Annex 2, and beyond them, in the nanogram and smaller effective-dose range, are pathogenic bacteria and viruses. As understanding of the microbiology and airborne spread of infectious diseases rapidly increased during the 1920s and 1930s, so too did the idea of weaponizing microbial pathogens as a more powerful form of poison gas. By the time of the Second World War, biological weapons of this type were being studied as a natural development of chemical weapons, exploiting the same delivery technology and the same understanding of cloud physics, meteorology and airborne dispersion. Before the end of that war, the feasibility of such aero-biological warfare had been demonstrated on weapon-proving grounds in, at least, Europe and North America. There were reports, too, of field experiments in which invading forces had disseminated bacterial pathogens from aircraft over populated areas of China *(7–8)*.

Other concepts of biological warfare were being considered. The vulnerability of draught animals to deliberate infection with diseases such as anthrax or glanders was exploited by saboteurs during the First World War in covert attacks on war-related transportation systems. In the interwar years, as the vulnerability of municipal infrastructures to air raids became increasingly apparent, the idea of spreading contagious disease by the bombardment of public health facilities (such as water-treatment and sewage-disposal plants) attracted attention. This, in turn, gave rise to investigations of other possible ways of deliberately initiating the spread of infectious disease. One thought was to establish foci of a contagious disease that would then spread of its own accord to parts of the target population not initially exposed to the biological agent concerned. Because of the uncertainties associated with the epidemic spread of disease, such an approach could not be accommodated at all readily within military doctrine except in the context of certain types of strategic or clandestine operation. In their selection of biological agents to weaponize or to take precautions against, military staffs therefore tended to place greater emphasis on non-contagious than on contagious diseases. In the context of terrorism, however, the objective and the consequent choice of agent may be different.

During the first half of the Cold War era, arsenals of biological weapons exploiting some of these, and other, approaches were accumulated, together with nerve gases and other chemical weapons, on both sides of the superpower confrontation. After 1970, preparations to produce biological weapons appear to have continued on one side only. The principal biological agents known with reasonable certainty to have entered the process of weaponization during the Cold War are identified in Chapter 3 and described in Annex 3. The biological weapons developed ranged from devices for clandestine use by special forces to those designed for large guided missiles or heavy bomber aircraft capable of generating large clouds of aerosol inhabited by live causative agents of contagious disease intended for far-distant rear targets, or of non-contagious disease for closer targets. Here were biological weapons that could, in principle, produce mass-casualty effects greatly exceeding those of the chemical weapons that their progenitors had emulated.

Weapons capable of producing effects comparable even with the life-destroying potential of nuclear weapons seemed to be emerging. The field testing, in large-scale open-air trials at sea during 1964–1968, of aerial weapons each capable of laying down a cross-wind line source of pathogenic aerosol tens of kilometres long demonstrated the capability of infecting experimental animals at ground level up to several tens of kilometres downwind. It thus appeared that people living within areas of the order of thousands, even tens of thousands, of square kilometres in size could now be threatened with disease by a single aircraft. At the same time, some defence science advisers were anticipating a new generation of chemical weapons having a comparable area-effectiveness *(9)*.

Despite the variety of these different weapon concepts, the chief lesson here from history is that biological warfare and, to a somewhat lesser extent, chemical warfare remained a perverse enterprise of extremely rare occurrence, notwithstanding the elaborate preparations made during the Cold War.

Large-area weapons for exploiting the damage potential of chemical or biological agents made new categories of target, such as food crops and livestock, open to attack. At the time of the Second World War, chemicals had been discovered that were as toxic to plants as the new nerve gases were to people. These herbicides, notably derivatives of 2,4-dichloro- and 2,4,5-trichlorophenoxyacetic acid in formulations such as Trioxone and Agent Orange, were used as weapons in several conflict areas of Africa and South-East Asia during the period 1950–1975, sometimes targeted against food crops and sometimes against the forest vegetation that could offer concealment. Certain plant and animal pathogens were also weaponized. Indeed, some of the first wide-area biological and toxin antipersonnel weapons were based on agent delivery systems originally conceived for anti-agriculture purposes.

Since the possible impacts on public health of anti-animal and anti-plant biological agents are indirect, such agents and their chemical counterparts are not described in detail, but the ability of biological agents, in particular, to endanger food security should not be disregarded.

2.3 Advancing science

Technological change in biological and chemical warfare has been driven, not only by factors such as the competition between the weapon and the protection against it, but also by new user requirements stemming from changes in military doctrine. More profoundly, technological change has also been driven by advances in the basic sciences within which the technology is rooted. New knowledge in the life sciences is now accumulating so rapidly that major changes in the nature, accessibility or efficacy of biological and chemical weapons may already be possible. Increasing the resulting concern are certain non-military technologies that are emerging from the new science and diffusing around the world, for some of these, and notably biotechnology, are also potentially dual use, i.e. applicable also to biological and chemical warfare. In fact, as the old armament imperatives of the Cold War recede, the threat may not be decreasing, but it is unfortunately true that the duality of the new science is making the threat seem larger.

The advent of genetic engineering offers opportunities for the improvement of human health and nutrition, yet in principle it could also be used to produce novel and perhaps more aggressive biological agents and toxins as compared with those used in earlier weapons programmes. Ability to modify more or less at will the genetic properties of living organisms could allow the insertion of new heritable characteristics into microorganisms that will make them more resistant to the available defences, more virulent or pathogenic *(10)*, better able to withstand the stresses of an unnatural environment, or more difficult to detect by routine assays. In so doing, experience shows that other necessary characteristics of the microorganism are likely to be lost; but perhaps not invariably so.

Genetic engineering also offers the possibility of making accessible toxic substances that have hitherto been available in quantities far too small for hostile use. For example, the fact that recombinant technology has been used to insert genes for a number of non-microbial toxins into microorganisms, leading to toxin expression, could enable those toxins to be produced on a large scale.

Still other aggressive possibilities may exist, e.g. weapons may be developed that could be used to harm human populations by disrupting cell-signalling pathways, or by modifying the action of specific genes.

Given the great range and variety of pathogens already present in nature, it is not immediately obvious why a weapons programme might be based on a modified organism. Nor is it always true that the new biotechnologies necessarily favour offence over defence. Vulnerability to biological agents exists chiefly because of the current inability to detect their presence in time for prompt masking or sheltering. Rapid detection methods based on modern molecular techniques are now being brought into service, although the extent to which they have the necessary sensitivity and generality, and whether they can produce results quickly enough and exclude false positives, is not clear. Moreover, the need to detect certain agents at exceedingly low concentrations continues to impose an enormous air-sampling requirement, even when polymerase chain reaction (PCR) or other amplifying methods are used. Other new biotechnologies are transforming the development of vaccines and therapeutics, while still others are thought to promise nonspecific alternatives to vaccines. An example to be mentioned here is the recent emphasis on blocking pathways of pathogenesis that are common to many infective agents, such as overproduction of cytokines. Such measures may become more important against both natural and deliberately caused infections because they are generic rather than specific to a particular pathogen, and because pathogens are less likely to be able to evade such measures by natural or artificial mutation.

Yet, overall, there can be little doubt that the spread of advanced biotechnology and the new accessibility of information about it offer new tools to any country or hostile group intending to develop a biological weapon (11–19).

2.4 Preliminary threat assessment

Appraisals and priorities will certainly differ from country to country, but it seems clear from what has just been related that prudent Member States will have at least some organization and some plan in place to deal with deliberate releases of biological or chemical agents. It is true that the existence of vulnerability does not necessarily mean the existence of threat. Yet in that spectrum of menace to the public postulated earlier in this chapter, the far mass-destruction end has already been approached by some of the bacterial or viral aerosol weapons of the Cold War. Nor is catastrophe on the scale implicit in such weapons the principal threat with which public health authorities must concern themselves. One lesson from the still-unresolved "anthrax letters" episode in the United States (see pages 98–108 below), is the havoc that can be caused by very much smaller-scale and less technically elaborate releases of biological agents. There is a somewhat similar lesson in the fact that the chemical agent that has thus far figured most commonly in deliberate releases in the United States has been not some deadly nerve gas, but butyric acid, which is a malodorant. So public health authorities may not be at fault if they consider that the threat of less than full-scale attack using only simple means of agent delivery may be the most worrisome possibility of all.

A salient factor here is the demonstrable existence of increasingly severe technological constraint as that far mass-destruction end of the spectrum has been approached: the greater and more assured the area-effectiveness sought for the weapon, the greater the practical difficulties of achieving it. There are, in short, inherent technical limitations that the threat assessment should take into account.

Consider, for example, some of the problems of conveying an agent to its intended target. Toxic or infective materials can be spread through drinking-water or foodstuffs but, as explained in Annex 5, their effects would then be expected to remain localized unless the contaminated items were themselves widely distributed or unless any biological agent that had been used succeeded in initiating contagious disease. Otherwise, large-scale effects are possible if the materials can be dispersed in the form either of vapour or of an aerosol cloud of liquid droplets or solid particles that can then be inhaled. This mode of attack is subject to uncertainty. The movement of the vapourized or aerosolized agent towards and across its target would be by atmospheric transport, the agent then being moved both laterally and vertically, causing a possibly large fraction of it to miss the target. The rate of this dispersion will vary greatly depending on the stability of the atmosphere at the time, and the direction of travel will depend both on local meteorological conditions and on the local topography. If aerosol or vapour is released inside enclosed spaces rather than in the open, the outcome may be less uncertain or difficult to predict, meaning that such smaller-scale attacks are that much less subject to technological constraint. A further major consideration is that many agents may be unstable in the atmosphere and decay over time following their dissemination in airborne form, which process may itself also stress the agent to the point of substantial degradation or complete inactivation. Furthermore, for the agent to be retained after inhalation and to exert its intended pathological effects, other technical requirements must be satisfied. In the case of particulate material, for example, larger particles may not be able to penetrate far enough into the respiratory tract. The optimal size range is, moreover, a narrow one, and the production and maintenance of the optimal size distribution within an aerosol cloud is subject to a variety of difficulties, not least the processes of evaporation or condensation that will be taking place as the cloud travels and even within the respiratory tract. These considerations apply to the aerosol dissemination of agents of both contagious disease and non-contagious disease, though an attacker might hope to rely on epidemic spread to compensate for poor aerosol presentation. However, that spread, too, is subject to unpredictabilities of its own, and therefore to uncontrollabilities. In addition, such spread, if detected early, can be limited by hygienic and prophylactic measures.

These technical factors operate to render such large-scale forms of attack more demanding in terms of materials and skills than is commonly supposed. Particularly for non-transmissible agents or chemicals, large amounts of agent will need to be disseminated to be sure that a sufficient proportion will reach the target population for a period of time sufficient to cause the desired effect. Several uncertainties will affect the outcome. Micrometeorological variation in the atmosphere could result either in the agent becoming diluted to harmlessness or in the cloud missing the target due to some veering of the wind. Such attacks are bound, therefore, to be indiscriminate, the more so if agents of contagious disease are used.

Nor are these difficulties of delivery the only or even the most demanding technical problems. In the case of biological agents, there are, for example, the difficulties of selecting the appropriate strain in the first place, including testing it, and then of maintaining its virulence throughout culturing, harvesting, processing, storing, weapon-filling, release and aerosol travel.

The conclusion to be drawn is that, although the probability of a large-scale high-technology biological/chemical attack may be low, if it nevertheless happened with, improbably, all the many imponderables and uncertainties favouring the attacker, the consequences of the event could be great. In considering strategies for national preparedness against such attacks, therefore, the possibility of a low-probability catastrophic outcome must be weighed against that of public health hazards of higher probability but smaller magnitude. It would certainly be irresponsible to disregard the possible effects of deliberately released biological or chemical agents, but it would be prudent not to overestimate them *(20–21)*. Given the emotional shock of even an alleged threat of a biological or chemical release, it will therefore be wise for Member States at least to consider how to address such dangers, should they occur, as an integral part of the national response to other threats to public health and well-being.

Technical factors are not the only consideration. Throughout much of the world, the social constraints on resort to biological or chemical weapons, including the provisions of national and international law, will increase the practical problems of acquiring and gaining advantage from such weapons. These constraints will impede access to the necessary materials, and will also obstruct those less tangible forms of assistance otherwise available from international service providers, consultants or even academics, whose corporate image, reputation or trading status would stand to suffer once their involvement became apparent. Furthermore, there would be additional justification for concerted international action against any weapons programmes. The long and continuing period during which no substantial biological attack has occurred suggests that the number of competent groups or states actually intending to use biological weapons must be small. Indeed, the element of intent is central to the probability of use, and itself is susceptible to inhibitions including those of morality and the threat of apprehension and punishment.

Yet the "anthrax letters" episode in the USA provides serious warning against complacency on this score, especially if one asks what the consequences might have been had the anthrax mailer sent a thousand letters instead of just a few. History is not always a reliable guide to the future. Therefore, preparation for the eventuality of some form of deliberate agent release, with a response strategy and plan held at the ready, will surely be thought necessary.

Whether in relation to natural disasters such as earthquakes, or to large-scale accidents in industrial production, storage or transportation facilities, many countries will already have formulated a general response strategy and plan, which they will maintain and modify in the light of changing circumstances and experience. The principles of risk management for dealing with chemical or biological attacks will overlap with those for dealing with natural or man-made disasters or emergencies. Where deliberate biological or chemical releases pose additional risk-management problems, biological and chemical addenda to an existing disaster/emergency strategy and plan will suffice, in most circumstances, for civil preparedness.

Beyond that, Member States should also consider preparing themselves to treat any deliberate use, even the most local use, of biological or chemical agents to cause harm as a *global public health threat*, and to respond to such a threat in other countries by sharing expertise, supplies and resources in order rapidly to contain the event and mitigate its consequences. The fact that there is vulnerability, however, does not always mean that there is threat.

REFERENCES

1. Marin MA. The evolution and present status of the Laws of War. *Académie de Droit International: Receuil des Cours*, 1957, 92(2):633–749.

2. Mandelbaum M. *The nuclear revolution: international politics before and after Hiroshima*. Cambridge, Cambridge University Press, 1981.

3. United Nations Security Council document S/C.3/SC.3/7/Rev.1, 8 September 1947.

4. United Nations Security Council document S/23500, 31 January 1992.

5. *Removing obstacles to healthy development: WHO report on infectious diseases*. Geneva, World Health Organization, 1999 (document WHO/CDS/99.1).

6. Perry Robinson JP. Chemical-weapons proliferation in the Middle East. In: Karsh E, Navias MS, Sabin P, eds. *Non-conventional-weapons proliferation in the Middle East*. Oxford, Clarendon Press, 1993:69–98.

7. Williams P, Wallace D. *Unit 731: the Japanese Army's secret of secrets*. London, Hodder & Stoughton, 1989.

8. Harris SH. *Factories of death: Japanese biological warfare 1932–1945 and the American cover up*. London, Routledge, 1994.

9. North Atlantic Treaty Organization, Standing Group, von Kármán Committee. *Future developments in chemical warfare*, from the report of Working Group X on Chemical, Biological and Radiological Defence, March 1961, as distributed to the UK Ministry of Defence Advisory Council on Scientific Research and Technical Development, paper No. SAC 1928, 11 February 1969, in United Kingdom Public Record Office file WO195/16864.

10. Jackson RJ et al. Expression of mouse interleukin-4 by a recombinant ectromelia virus suppresses cytolytic lymphocyte responses and overcomes genetic resistance to mousepox. *Journal of Virology*, 2001, 75(3):1205–1210.

11. Dubuis B. *Recombinant DNA and biological warfare*. Zurich, Eidgenössische Technische Hochschule, Institut für Militärische Sicherheitstechnik, report IMS 94–10, 1994.

12. United Kingdom of Great Britain and Northern Ireland. *New scientific and technological developments relevant to the Biological and Toxin Weapons Convention*, in document BWC/CONF.IV/4, 30 October 1996.

13. *Biotechnology and genetic engineering: implications for the development of new warfare agents*. United States of America, Department of Defense, 1996.

14. British Medical Association. *Biotechnology, weapons and humanity.* London, Harwood Academic Publishers, 1999.

16. Dando M. Benefits and threats of developments in biotechnology and genetic engineering. In: *Stockholm International Peace Research Institute Yearbook 1999: armaments, disarmament and international security*. Stockholm, Stockholm International Peace Research Institute, 1999:596–611.

17. Kadlec RP, Zelicoff AP. Implications of the biotechnology revolution for weapons development and arms control. In: Zilinskas R, ed. *Biological warfare: modern offense and defense*. Boulder and London, Lynne Rienner, 2000:11–26.

18. Block SM. The growing threat of biological weapons. *American Scientist*, 2001, 89(1):28–37.

19. Dando M. *The new biological weapons*. Boulder and London, Lynne Rienner, 2001.

20. Fifth Review Conference of the States Parties to the Convention on the Prohibition of the Development, Production and Stockpiling of Bacteriological (Biological) and Toxin Weapons and on their Destruction, Geneva, 19 November–7 December 2001, documents dated 26 October 2001, *Background paper on new scientific and technological developments relevant to the Convention*.

21. *Measures for controlling the threat from biological weapons*. London, Royal Society, 2000 (document 4/00).

3. BIOLOGICAL AND CHEMICAL AGENTS

Careful advance planning is essential if a Member State or other country is adequately to manage the threat or the consequences of deliberate releases of biological or chemical agents. A central consideration in such preparedness planning is that it is neither possible nor necessary to prepare specifically for attack by all possible biological and chemical agents. If a country is seeking to increase its preparedness to counter the effects of biological and chemical attacks, the targeting of its preparation and training on a limited but well chosen group of agents will provide the necessary capability to deal with a far wider range of possibilities. Knowledge of the general properties of this representative group of agents will enable certain measures to be taken against virtually any other agent. In addition to being impractical from a preparedness perspective, long and exhaustive lists of agents also give a misleading impression of the extent of possible threats. In this chapter, an approach to identifying agents of concern is described, followed by a discussion of methods of dissemination, routes of exposure, and general characteristics of biological and chemical weapons, from which conclusions are drawn to complete the threat assessment initiated in Chapter 2.

3.1　The representative group of agents

Biological and chemical weapons have been described as the "poor man's atom bomb", but this conveys a misleading impression of their ease of production and their utility. It is not enough for biological and chemical agents to be highly infective or highly toxic. In order to be selected for weaponization, a candidate agent should have characteristics that are capable of countervailing the technical limitations that would otherwise render the weapon carrying the agent unattractive to users, such as the technical limitations just described in Chapter 2. So the agent will need to be stable enough to resist degradation during handling and storage, and during the energy-transfer processes that will, in most scenarios, be involved in disseminating it on its target. Once disseminated, the agent must be capable of establishing field dosages that are infective or toxic over a predictable area. It must also be relatively easy to produce from readily available precursor compounds or from naturally occurring or genetically modified microorganisms. Once produced and, depending on the agent, further processed and formulated, it must be filled into munitions or dissemination devices, or held ready for such filling, and be storable without undue risk to its possessor. If an agent is insufficiently stable in storage, certain expedients are available, such as, in the case of some chemicals, the use of "binary" munitions that are uploaded, not with toxic agent, but with separate containers of precursors, these being adapted to mix and generate the agent either just before or during weapon launch. For biological agents, a "warm" production base rather than a large stockpile has been relied upon in past offensive military programmes.

While many thousands of toxic chemicals and hundreds of pathogenic microorganisms have been investigated for their potential utility as military weapons, relatively few have been found capable of meeting military requirements of the kind just specified, and fewer still have found their way into weapons and actually been used. The task facing public health authorities of identifying a representative group of agents against which to prepare might therefore be thought relatively straightforward. However, the deliberate agent releases against which public health authorities would need to prepare might include attacks by non-state entities whose agent-selection principles could differ from the military ones. For example, accessibility, not overall aggressiveness and stability in storage, might be the dominant criterion in their choice of agent. Also, the types of impact sought could differ from those that direct military operations. In other words, the rank order in which public health authorities assess the different agent threats, e.g. reference (1), may not be the same as that of military authorities. In the present study, the representative group has been compiled by applying a progressively sharper focus to possible agents of concern: firstly, the broad treaty definitions of biological and chemical weapons; secondly, the lists of agents that have been negotiated to facilitate treaty implementation, or, in the case of the BWC, proposed therefor; thirdly, such authoritative information as is publicly available about which agents have been weaponized or stockpiled in recent times; fourthly, agents known to have been used as weapons; and finally, considerations regarding non-state entities. This selection process is now described.

3.1.1 Scope of the international treaties

The broadest catchment of agents of concern, and therefore the starting point for the selection process, is to be found in the treaties that outlaw possession of biological and chemical weapons. The intergovernmental negotiations that culminated in the BWC and then the CWC commenced while the first edition of the present report was being prepared. In 1969, in order to determine its scope, WHO relied on the concepts of toxicity and infectivity to distinguish chemical and biological weapons from other types of weapon. It defined chemical-warfare agents as including "all substances employed for their toxic effects on man, animals and plants", and biological-warfare agents as those "that depend for their effects on multiplication within the target organism, and that are intended for use in war to cause disease or death in man, animals or plants". The treaty negotiators had, however, to devise definitions that used a broader approach, since they were aiming to control technologies that were often dual-use in character, in other words that could be used both in warfare and for peaceful purposes. For example, the negotiators could not prohibit the pro-duction of the principal lethal gas of the First World War, phosgene, without at the same time denying feedstock to manufacturers of certain plastics and other useful products; nor could they outlaw the large-scale growth of pathogenic microorganisms without threatening vaccine production. There were many such examples, so the negotiators took the general purpose for which a biological or a chemical agent was intended as the criterion of whether activities involving that agent should or should not be subject to prohibition or control under the treaties. Such a general-purpose criterion is therefore to be found in those parts of both the BWC and the CWC where the scope of the treaty is defined. Thus, the prohibitions laid down in the two treaties extend to all biological agents and toxins, and to essentially all chemicals, unless they are intended for peaceful purposes, and unless their types and quantities are consistent with such purposes. In addition, the CWC uses the concept of toxicity, applying its general purpose criterion to "toxic chemicals" and "their precursors", and defining both of these categories of chemical in broad terms. In contrast, the BWC does not seek to define the biological agents and toxins to which it applies. The actual language used in the two Conventions to define the weapons to which they apply is given in Box 3.1 below.

Box 3.1　**How biological and chemical weapons are defined in the BWC and the CWC**

Article I of the Biological Weapons Convention reads as follows:
Each State Party to this Convention undertakes never in any circumstances to develop, produce, stockpile or otherwise acquire or retain:
1. Microbial or other biological agents, or toxins whatever their origin or method of production, of types and in quantities that have no justification for prophylactic, protective or other peaceful purposes.
2. Weapons, equipment or means of delivery designed to use such agents or toxins for hostile purposes or in armed conflict.

Article II of the Chemical Weapons Convention includes the following:
For the purposes of this Convention:
1. "Chemical Weapons" means the following, together or separately:
(a) Toxic chemicals and their precursors, except where intended for purposes not prohibited under this Convention, as long as the types and quantities are consistent with such purposes;
(b) Munitions and devices, specifically designed to cause death or other harm through the toxic properties of those toxic chemicals specified in subparagraph (a), which would be released as a result of the employment of such munitions and devices;
(c) Any equipment specifically designed for use directly in connection with the employment of munitions and devices specified in subparagraph (b).
2. "Toxic Chemical" means:
Any chemical which through its chemical action on life processes can cause death, temporary incapacitation or permanent harm to humans or animals. This includes all such chemicals, regardless of their origin or of their method of production, and regardless of whether they are produced in facilities, in munitions or elsewhere.

(For the purpose of implementing this Convention, toxic chemicals which have been identified for the application of verification measures are listed in Schedules contained in the Annex on Chemicals.)

[...]

9. "Purposes Not Prohibited Under this Convention" means:
(a) Industrial, agricultural, research, medical, pharmaceutical or other peaceful purposes;
(b) Protective purposes, namely those purposes directly related to protection against toxic chemicals and to protection against chemical weapons;
(c) Military purposes not connected with the use of chemical weapons and not dependent on the use of the toxic properties of chemicals as a method of warfare;
(d) Law enforcement including domestic riot control purposes.

In order to implement treaties of such wide-ranging scope effectively, lists of agents have been drawn up so as to focus the efforts of the implementers by providing transparency for the agents that all States Parties could agree had potential for use as chemical weapons. The CWC includes three such negotiated lists ("Schedules") in which selected toxic chemicals and precursors are "identified for the application of verification measures". These schedules are set out in the treaty's *Annex on Chemicals*, and list 29 specific chemicals and 14 families of chemicals. Some of the families are very large indeed, running into many millions of chemicals, most of which have, however, never actually been made or characterized. For example, the dialkyl alkylphosphonates that constitute only a small fraction of the chemicals in item 4 of Schedule 2 comprise 1 668 964 different chemicals (excluding stereoisomers), of which apparently only 118 have actually been synthesized (2). Even the family of alkyl alkylphosphonofluoridates, with which Schedule 1 opens, i.e. the sarin family of nerve gases, theoretically contains 3652 members. Large though these numbers are, the CWC makes it clear that its Schedules are not intended to be a definitive listing of all chemicals that constitute "risks to the object and purpose of this Convention", but simply to exemplify chemicals thought to pose a particular risk of being used in a manner contrary to its general-purpose criterion.

The BWC, which is a legal instrument much shorter and simpler than the CWC, contains no analogous schedules, but such lists have been developed for inclusion in the BWC Protocol were its negotiation to be completed. The purpose of these lists would again be to exemplify, but not to define, the scope of the general-purpose criterion. Several other authorities, including defence agencies, have compiled lists of biological agents judged most likely to be employed for hostile purposes. Some of these lists are shown in Table A3.1 in Annex 3, from which it may be seen just how much variation there can be in different agent assessments.

3.1.2 Historical experience

Toxic and infective agents that were available in weaponized forms in the past to the armed forces of states are identified in official state papers now open to the scrutiny of historians. This historical record is not complete, however, because former possessor states have not yet made all of the relevant papers available, and even those that have done so have still withheld the papers of the last 20 or 30 years (the declarations received by the United Nations Special Commission on Iraq – UNSCOM – are an exception in that they include reference, albeit not yet entirely verified, to weaponization during the period 1987–1991). An extensive list of antipersonnel agents can nevertheless be compiled. That given in Table 3.1 covers the period since January 1946 and is taken from an archive of collected state papers, works of historical scholarship and other documentation at the University of Sussex.[5] It is limited to agents identified in state papers of the country concerned as having been stockpiled or having otherwise entered the process of weaponization. For convenience, Table 3.1 groups the agents into categories that are explained later in this chapter.

For some of the toxic chemicals included in Table 3.1, an indication of relative importance historically in possessor state programmes can be gained by considering the quantities of the different agents that have

---

[5] The archive is the Sussex Harvard Information Bank, which is maintained at SPRU, University of Sussex, UK, by the Harvard Sussex Program on CBW Armament and Arms Limitation (see *www.sussex.ac.uk/spru/hsp*).

been declared to OPCW as part of the obligatory declarations of chemical weapons required from States Parties to the CWC. These declared quantities are given in Table 3.2, which shows that an aggregate total of 69 863 tonnes of chemicals have been declared as chemical weapons to OPCW by its Member States. These declared stockpiles are subject to the monitoring provisions of the CWC, and their destruction under agreed protocols is observed by OPCW officials. By 31 August 2003, a total of 7837 tonnes had been destroyed.

The information on the actual use of toxic and infective agents for hostile purposes may be even less complete than that on weaponization or stockpiling, not least because of the role of these agents in clandestine warfare, on which official records are often sparse. Moreover, there have been occasions when it has been reported that chemical and biological weapons have been used when in fact they were not, the reports originating either in misperception or other error, or in the intention to deceive. Table 3.3 summarizes the record of antipersonnel use, taken from the same archive as that used for Table 3.1. Its entries are restricted to those instances since 1918 in which the fact of use can be regarded as indisputable, and in which the toxic or infective agents employed have been identified. The use of anti-plant or anti-animal agents is not included. Table 3.3 includes in its last three entries the use of toxic or infective antipersonnel agents by non-state entities – acts of terrorism on which the historical record is still more sparse.

Tables 3.1, 3.2 and 3.3 list 40 different biological and chemical agents, which is a number considerably smaller than the number of agents described in the literature on biological and chemical warfare. Not all of the 40 are readily accessible only to state forces, for among them are widely used industrial chemicals. For inclusion within the representative group of agents, some may be disregarded on grounds of close similarity to one another. It seems necessary to add only four further agents. These are: variola major, i.e. smallpox virus; the fungal agent that causes coccidioidomycosis; perfluoroisobutene, a toxic agent now produced as a by-product in the chemical industry in tens of thousands of tonnes per year; and the chemical psychotomimetic agent lysergide, also known as LSD. Although none of these four additional agents is listed in Table 3.1, all four are known to have been studied for possible weaponization including, in some cases, actual field trials as well as laboratory study.

Described in Annexes 1, 2 and 3 are 26 of the 44 agents, which thus include those from among which a public health authority may reasonably select its representative group of agents.

Table 3.1 Toxic and infective antipersonnel agents stockpiled or otherwise weaponized for state forces since 1946 according to official documents of their possessor states

Tear gases, other sensory irritants, and other disabling chemicals
10-chloro-5,10-dihydrophenarsazine (adamsite, or DM)
ω-chloroacetophenone (CN)
α-bromophenylacetonitrile (larmine, BBC or CA)
2-chlorobenzalmalononitrile (CS)
dibenzoxazepine (CR)
oleoresin capsicum (OC)
3-quinuclidinyl benzilate (BZ)

Choking agents (lung irritants)
phosgene
chloropicrin

Blood gases
hydrogen cyanide

Vesicants (blister gases)
bis(2-chloroethyl) sulfide (mustard gas)
2-chlorovinyldichloroarsine (lewisite)
bis(2-chloroethylthioethyl) ether (agent T)
tris(2-chloroethyl)amine (a nitrogen mustard)

Nerve gases
ethyl *N,N*-dimethylphosphoramidocyanidate (tabun, or GA)
O-isopropyl methylphosphonofluoridate (sarin, or GB)
O-1,2,2-trimethylpropyl methylphosphonofluoridate (soman, or GD)
O-cyclohexyl methylphosphonofluoridate (cyclosarin, or GF)
O-ethyl S-2-diisopropylaminoethyl methylphosphonothiolate (VX)
O-isobutyl S-2-diethylaminoethyl methylphosphonothiolate (VR)

Toxins[a]
ricin
saxitoxin
Clostridium botulinum toxin
staphylococcal enterotoxin
aflatoxin

Bacteria and rickettsiae
Bacillus anthracis
Francisella tularensis
Brucella suis
Burkholderia mallei
Burkholderia pseudomallei
Yersinia pestis
Rickettsia prowazeki
Coxiella burnetii

Viruses
Venezuelan equine encephalitis virus

[a] In addition to those already listed, namely OC and hydrogen cyanide.

Table 3.2 **Aggregate quantities of chemical agents declared to the OPCW by its Member States, as of 31 December 2002**

Chemical agent	Total declared (tonnes)[a]
Category 1 chemical weapons[b]	
Agent VR	15 558
Agent VX	4 032
Difluor (precursor DF)[c]	444
EDMP (precursor QL)[d]	46
Isopropanol/isopropylamine (precursor OPA)[e]	731
Lewisite	6 745
Mustard gas[f]	13 839
Mustard/lewisite mixtures	345
Runcol (agent HT)[g]	3 536
Sarin (agent GB)	15 048
Soman (agent GD)	9 175
Tabun (agent GA)	2
Unknown	5
Category 2 chemical weapons[h]	
Chloroethanol	302
Phosgene	11
Thiodiglycol	51

Chemicals declared as "riot control agents"[i]			
Adamsite	Agent CN	Agent CS	Agent CR
Chloropicrin	Agent OC	OC/CS mixture	MPA [*sic*]
Ethyl bromoacetate	Pepperspray [*sic*]	Pelargonic acid vanillylamide	

[a] Based on figures from OPCW annual report for 2002 (*3*), rounded to the nearest tonne. Excludes chemicals declared in quantities of less than one tonne. One such chemical was the nerve-gas *O*-ethyl *S*-2-dimethylaminoethyl methylphosphonothiolate, also known as médémo or EA 1699.

[b] The CWC Verification Annex, in Part IV(A) para. 16, defines Category 1 as "chemical weapons on the basis of Schedule 1 chemicals and their parts and components". See Table 3.1 for their chemical identities.

[c] Methylphosphonyl difluoride (a binary nerve-gas component).

[d] Ethyl 2-diisopropylaminoethyl methylphosphonite (a binary nerve-gas component).

[e] A mixture of 72% isopropanol and 28% isopropylamine (a binary nerve-gas component).

[f] Including "mustard gas in oil product".

[g] A reaction product containing about 60% of mustard gas and 40% of agent T.

[h] "Chemical weapons on the basis of all other chemicals and their parts and components." The CWC goes on to define Category 3 chemical weapons as comprising "unfilled munitions and devices, and equipment specifically designed for use directly in connection with employment of chemical weapons".

[i] For chemicals declared as "riot control agents", the CWC requires disclosure of their chemical identity but not the quantities in which they are held.

Table 3.3   **Antipersonnel toxic and infective agents whose hostile use since 1918 has been verified**

Period	Agent	Location of use
1919	adamsite diphenylchloroarsine (a sensory irritant) mustard gas	Russia
1923–1926	bromomethyl ethyl ketone (a tear gas) chloropicrin mustard gas	Morocco
1935–1940	chlorine (a choking agent) ω-chloroacetophenone diphenylchlorarsine mustard gas phenyldichlorarsine (a vesicant) phosgene	Abyssinia
1937–1945	ω-chloroacetophenone diphenylcyanoarsine (a sensory irritant) hydrogen cyanide lewisite mustard gas phosgene *Yersinia pestis*	Manchuria
1963–1967	ω-chloroacetophenone mustard gas phosgene	Yemen
1965–1975	2-chlorobenzalmalononitrile	Viet Nam
1982–1988	2-chlorobenzalmalononitrile mustard gas sarin tabun	Iraq Islamic Republic of Iran
1984	*Salmonella enteritidis* serotype *typhimurium*	United States
1994–1995	sarin	Japan
2001	*Bacillus anthracis*	United States

Source: Documents and materials held in the Sussex Harvard Information Bank at SPRU – Science and Technology Policy Research, University of Sussex, United Kingdom.

3.2 Dissemination of biological and chemical agents

In any release of a chemical or biological agent, the nature and degree of hazard will depend on a multitude of factors, including the agent and the amount released, the method by which the agent is disseminated, factors that influence its toxicity, infectivity or virulence both during and after its release, its movement and dilution in the atmosphere, and the state of protection and susceptibility of those exposed. Two different types of general hazard are usually distinguished, namely inhalation hazard and contact hazard, with different characteristic implications for protection (see Chapter 4). A brief summary is given here of the methods of airborne dissemination of biological and chemical agents that may create an inhalation or contact hazard to unprotected persons. Considered elsewhere in this study are certain other methods of agent dissemination, including dissemination through drinking water and food. For biological agents there is also the possibility of using arthropod vectors.

The methods of airborne dissemination that may be used depend on the physical and chemical properties of the material to be dispersed, including those that might cause the decomposition or inactivation of chemicals or toxins or, for infective agents, the loss of viability or more subtle changes that primarily affect only virulence.

For chemical agents, an inhalation hazard may be created by the dissemination of the agent as a vapour, as liquid or solid particles sufficiently small to be inhalable, as a spray that evaporates to form a vapour while still airborne, or as a spill or spray that is deposited on surfaces and subsequently evaporates to form a vapour. For some agents, vapours or inhalable particles may also present a hazard to sensitive mucous membranes, especially those of the conjunctiva. For chemical agents able to act percutaneously, a contact hazard may be created by sprays or spills of less volatile agents deposited directly on people or on surfaces with which people are likely to come into contact. A chemical agent may be disseminated mechanically by spraying or rupturing a container, by using explosives, or by a thermal process in which a pyrotechnic composition is used as the source of heat. Pyrotechnic dissemination is effective only for heat-resistant and non-combustible agents, which may evaporate initially and then condense as a suspension in air of inhalable particles, creating principally a respiratory or conjunctival hazard.

For infective agents, the principal hazard to people will be from inhalation. This may be so even for agents for which this is not the natural route of infection. For many infective agents, the risk is greatest if the agent reaches the target population in the form of particles within the narrow aerodynamic size range where particles are small enough to penetrate to the alveoli in the depths of the lungs but not so small that most of them fail to be deposited and instead are mostly exhaled. Contact with an infective agent and its entry into the body via a lesion or via mucous membranes may also present a risk, although generally less than that from inhalation. Infective agents may be disseminated as inhalable particles by dispersal of presized powder, by explosives or by sprayers or other generators specially designed to produce particles in the inhalable size range.

Small particles may have such low gravitational settling velocities that the movement in the atmosphere of a cloud of such particles is like that of a vapour cloud. A particulate cloud of this type is a colloidal suspension of matter in air, and is known as an aerosol. For both vapours and aerosols, the rate of deposition depends not on gravity but rather on chemical and physical forces that might bind the molecules or particles to the specific surfaces with which they come into contact, thereby removing them from the cloud at a rate that also depends on surface roughness and on meteorological factors. It is the effective aerodynamic diameter that is the proper measure of size in regard to the settling and impaction propensities of small particles Only for solid spheres of unit density does the effective aerodynamic diameter reduce to actual diameter. This distinction may be important for lyophilized materials that are largely hollow or for chemical agents that are very dense. Wind and other mechanical disturbances may resuspend deposited particles, but the amount resuspended is likely to be small and even that may be bound to soil or other particles of larger diameter. In consequence, exposures to inhalable particles resulting from resuspension of particles deposited from an aerosol will generally be much lower than those caused by the initial cloud.

As a particulate or vapour cloud is carried down-wind, eddy currents in the atmosphere cause it to spread both horizontally and vertically (up to the top of the atmospheric mixing layer, if such a layer is present) at a rate that depends strongly on the degree of atmospheric turbulence, resulting in lower dosages at greater down-wind and cross-wind distances from the source. Nevertheless, if the atmosphere is relatively stable, and depending on the nature and amount of the agent, dosages may reach hazardous levels even many kilometres down-wind of the source.

3.3 Routes of exposure

3.3.1 Respiratory system

The principal hazard from agent vapours and aerosols is respiratory, although certain chemical agents, notably the mustards and sensory irritants, also pose a particular hazard to the conjunctiva.

The region of the respiratory system where the inhaled vapour of a chemical agent is adsorbed and the efficiency of its adsorption depend on the solubility properties of the agent. Vapours of water-soluble agents are largely adsorbed in the nasal passages and the upper regions of the respiratory system. Water-insoluble vapours are able to penetrate more deeply and may be adsorbed in the most distal part of the respiratory system – the alveolar spaces. For an aerosol of a non-volatile agent or for an agent adsorbed to a non-volatile carrier material, the site of deposition will depend on the size and density of the aerosol particles, as discussed below for biological agents.

Some agents, including mustard, phosgene and chlorine, damage lung tissues at the site of adsorption, while others, such as the nerve agents, penetrate respiratory tissues and are carried through the bloodstream to act on specific target receptors, as in the peripheral or central nervous system.

For chemical agents that are not significantly detoxified during the period of exposure, the severity of hazard depends on the total amount inhaled. For some chemicals, however, notably hydrogen cyanide, significant detoxification occurs in the body within minutes, so that inhalation of a given amount within a short time may cause severe intoxication or death while inhalation of the same amount over a longer time would not. Most of the chemical agents listed in Table 3.2, however, including mustard and the nerve agents, are essentially cumulative in their toxic effects, except perhaps for exposures extending over many hours.

The principal hazard to persons exposed to a passing cloud of a biological aerosol would also be respiratory. This is because the amount of aerosol deposited in the respiratory system would be greater than that deposited elsewhere on the body and because the respiratory system, although provided with impressive natural defence mechanisms, is nevertheless vulnerable to infection by the agents of concern. It is also the case that, for many agents of concern, infection via the inhalatory route generally leads to more severe disease than does cutaneous infection. Nevertheless, if an agent finds its way to a lesion, cutaneous infection may result from aerosol particles deposited on bodily surfaces or on surfaces with which the person comes in contact.

The region of the respiratory system where inhaled particles are deposited depends on their aerodynamic diameter. As an approximation, the particles in a biological agent aerosol are taken to have unit density and spherical shape. Such particles with diameter around 10 μm and larger are almost entirely deposited by inertial impaction on the fimbrae of the nose, in the nasal cavities and in the upper thoracic airways. After deposition, they are transported to the nose or to the back of the throat by mucociliary action, to be expelled in nasal secretions or to be swallowed or expelled by coughing, spitting or sneezing. Such clearance protects the lungs from particulates including infective agents deposited in the respiratory airways. Additional protection against infective agents results from the action of anti-microbial substances present in mucus and from the action of phagocytic cells. Some infective agents, however, including the viruses of influenza and smallpox, have special adaptations that enable them to infect the oropharyngeal and respiratory mucosa. Infection by such agents may therefore result, not only from inhalation of contaminated particles, but also by hand–mouth and hand–nostril transfer from contaminated materials and surfaces.

Smaller particles, in the range 1–5 μm in diameter, may also be trapped in the nasal passages but a substantial percentage of them will escape inertial impaction and pass beyond the respiratory airways to reach the alveoli, where they may deposit by gravitational sedimentation. It is here, in the approximately 300 million alveoli with a total surface area of some 140 m², that most biological agents of concern, if disseminated as aerosols sufficiently fine to reach the alveoli, may initiate infection. Because of their lower gravitational settling velocities, inhaled particles with diameters below 1 μm are not likely to deposit by sedimentation but, if not simply exhaled, may nevertheless deposit on alveolar surfaces, owing to Brownian motion *(4)*.

Consistent with their gas-exchanging function, the alveoli lack ciliated epithelium and therefore lie beyond the mucociliary surface of the respiratory airways. Instead, alveolar clearance of insoluble particles is mainly achieved by mobile phagocytic cells, the alveolar macrophages, or by polymorphonuclear leukocytes which are subsequently engulfed by alveolar macrophages. Macrophages that have engulfed deposited particles may remain permanently in the alveolar connective tissue or, by processes that are poorly understood, reach the respiratory airways and be removed from the lungs by mucociliary transport. Particles may also be transported by macrophages or pass as free particles to regional lymph nodes, to be retained there or to enter the lymphatic drainage, passing through the thoracic duct into the bloodstream.

Alveolar clearance has half-times ranging from hours to many days or longer, depending on the nature of the particle. Most microorganisms and viruses engulfed by macrophages are inactivated and digested. Some microorganisms, however, are endowed with features that enable them to resist phagocytosis or to survive or multiply within macrophages. Spores of *B. anthracis*, for example, are able to germinate in macrophages, which may transport bacteria to regional lymph nodes where proliferation and passage of bacteria into the bloodstream can initiate systemic infection.

3.3.2 Skin

Several chemical agents, such as the liquid agent VX, are able to penetrate the skin and cause systemic effects. Others, such as the blister agent mustard, either as a liquid or as vapour, cause more local effects, and, in addition, may render the underlying tissues vulnerable to infection. As a general rule, the thinner, more vascular, and moister the skin, the more prone it is to attack and penetration by such agents. High relative humidity promotes penetration. As penetration into and through the skin is not immediate, removal by washing, wiping or decontamination, if accomplished within minutes after exposure, can greatly reduce the toxic effects of such agents.

Although aerosol particles do not tend to settle on surfaces and may pass over the skin without depositing, except perhaps for hairy areas, the much larger particles that occur in a spray or a coarse dust are deposited more efficiently.

3.3.3 Oronasal mucus and conjunctiva

The mucosal tissues of the conjunctiva and the nasal passages are particularly sensitive to attack with irritant agents and the conjunctiva is especially sensitive to blister agents. Also, some infective agents, including variola, influenza and certain other viruses may enter through the oronasal mucus and, perhaps, the conjunctiva.

3.3.4 Digestive system

Biological and chemical agents can enter the digestive system via contaminated food or drinking-water, by hand–mouth contact after touching contaminated surfaces, or by swallowing of respiratory mucus after the accumulation of larger aerosol particles in the nose, throat and upper airways. Of all exposure routes, this is the easiest to control, provided that the contaminated sources are known (or at least suspected). Simple hygienic measures and control of supplies of food and drinking-water can significantly reduce the risk of exposure. If chemical agents are ingested, the delayed onset of symptoms (compared with respiratory exposure) and the increased prevalence of systemic rather than localized effects may lead to the conclusion that the persons affected are suffering from a disease or general malaise or even that they have been exposed to a biological agent.

The problems presented by the direct biological contamination of food, water or other ingestible material are considered in Annex 5.

3.4 Characteristics of biological agents

The chief characteristic of biological agents defined on pages 5–6 above is their ability to multiply in a host. It is this that gives them their aggressive potential. The disease that may be caused results from the multifactorial interaction between the biological agent, the host (including the latter's immunological, nutritional and general health status) and the environment (e.g. sanitation, temperature, water quality, population density). The consequences of using biological agents to cause disease will reflect these complex interactions.

Biological agents are commonly classified according to their taxonomy, the most important taxa being fungi, bacteria and viruses. Such classification is important to medical services because of its implications for detection, identification, prophylaxis and treatment. Biological agents can also be classified according to properties that may determine their utility for hostile purposes, such as ease of production or resistance to prophylactic and therapeutic measures. More generally they can be characterized by such other features as infectivity, virulence, incubation period, lethality, contagiousness and mechanisms of transmission, and stability, all of which influence their potential for use as weapons

Infectivity of an agent reflects its capability to enter, survive and multiply in a host, and may be expressed as the proportion of persons in a given population exposed to a given dose who become infected. The dose that, under given conditions, infects half the population receiving it is termed the ID_{50}. Doses higher or lower than this will infect a larger or smaller proportion of such a population. For some pathogens the ID_{50} may be many thousands or more of infective cells or virus particles while for others it may be only a few. It cannot be ruled out that even a single infective cell or virus particle can initiate infection, albeit with correspondingly low probability.

Virulence is the relative severity of the disease caused by a microorganism. Different strains of the same species may cause diseases of different severity. Some strains of *Francisella tularensis*, for example, are much more virulent than others.

The incubation period is the time elapsing between exposure to an infective agent and the first appearance of the signs of disease associated with the infection. This is affected by many variables, including the agent, the route of entry, the dose and specific characteristics of the host.

Lethality reflects the ability of an agent to cause death in an infected population. The case-fatality rate is the proportion of patients clinically recognized as having a specified disease who die as a result of that illness within a specified time (e.g. during outbreaks of acute disease).

For those infections that are contagious, a measure of their *contagiousness* is the number of secondary cases arising under specified conditions from exposure to a primary case. The *mechanisms of transmission* involved may be direct or indirect. Thus transmission may, for example, result from direct contact between an infected and an uninfected person, or it may be mediated through inanimate material that has become contaminated with the agent, such as soil, blood, bedding, clothes, surgical instruments, water, food or milk. There may also be airborne or vector-borne secondary transmission. Airborne transmission can occur through coughing or sneezing, which may disseminate microbial droplets or aerosol. Vector-borne transmission (primary or secondary) can occur via biting insects, arthropods, or other invertebrate hosts. The distinction between types of transmission is important when methods for controlling contagion are being selected. Thus, direct transmission can be interrupted by appropriate individual hygienic practices and precautions and by proper handling of infected persons, caregivers and other contacts. The interruption of indirect transmission requires other approaches, such as adequate ventilation, boiling or chlorination of water, disinfection of surfaces, laundering of clothing or vector control.

Stability may refer to the ability of the aerosolized agent to survive the influence of environmental factors such as sunlight, air pollution, surface forces and drying, while remaining infective. It may also refer to stability during production or to stability during storage.

3.5 Characteristics of chemical agents

As with biological agents, chemical agents may be classified in a variety of different ways depending on the type of characteristic that is of primary concern. This can lead to potentially confusing differences in the way that such agents are grouped and referred to in the literature. The most common characteristics are described below in order to introduce and explain frequently used terminology.

A common form of classification of chemical agents is according to the principal intended effect, e.g. harassing, incapacitating or lethal. A *harassing agent* disables exposed people for as long as they remain exposed. They are acutely aware of discomfort caused by the agent, but usually remain capable of removing themselves from exposure to it unless they are temporarily blinded or otherwise constrained. They will usually recover fully in a short time after exposure ends, and no medical treatment will be required. An *incapacitating agent* also disables, but people exposed to it may not be aware of their predicament, as with opioids and certain other psychotropic agents, or may be rendered unable to function or move away from the exposed environment. The effect may be prolonged, but recovery may be possible without specialized medical aid. A *lethal agent* causes the death of those exposed.

This is not a particularly precise way of classifying agents, as their effects will depend on the dose received and on the health and other factors determining the susceptibility to adverse effects of the individuals exposed. Tear gas (e.g. CS or CN), usually a harassing agent, can be lethal if a person is exposed to a large quantity in a small closed space. On the other hand, nerve agents, which are usually lethal, might only incapacitate if individuals were exposed to no more than a low concentration for a short time. Protective measures may be aimed at reducing the level of the effect if total protection is not possible. For example, the use of pretreatment and antidotes in a nerve gas victim is unlikely to provide a complete "cure", but may well reduce what would have been a lethal effect to an incapacitating one.

Another form of classification is according to the route of entry of the agent into the body (see pages 38–42 above). *Respiratory agents* are inhaled and either cause damage to the lungs, or are absorbed there and cause systemic effects. *Cutaneous agents* are absorbed through the skin, either damaging it (e.g. mustard gas) or gaining access to the body to cause systemic effects (e.g. nerve agents), or both. An agent may be taken up by either or both routes, depending on its physical properties or formulation.

A further classification is based on the duration of the hazard. *Persistent agents* will remain hazardous in the area where they are applied for long periods (sometimes up to a few weeks). They are generally substances of low volatility that contaminate surfaces and have the potential to damage the skin if they come into contact with it. A secondary danger is inhalation of any vapours that may be released. Persistent agents may consequently be used for creating obstacles, for contaminating strategic places or equipment, for area denial, or, finally, for causing casualties. Protective footwear and/or dermal protective clothing will often be required in contaminated areas, usually together with respiratory protection. Mustard gas and VX are persistent agents. *Non-persistent agents* are volatile substances that do not stay long in the area of application, but evaporate or disperse rapidly, and may consequently be used to cause casualties in an area that needs to be occupied soon afterwards. Surfaces are generally not contaminated, and the primary danger is from inhalation, and only secondarily from skin exposure. Respirators will be the main form of protection required. Protective clothing may not be necessary if concentrations are below skin toxicity levels. Hydrogen cyanide and phosgene are typical non-persistent agents.

Finally, chemical agents are often grouped according to their effect on the body, the classes being differentiated according to, for example, the primary organ system that is affected by exposure. Typical classes include: *nerve* agents or "gases" (e.g. sarin, VX, VR); *vesicants* or skin-blistering agents (e.g. mustard gas, lewisite); *lung* irritants, asphyxiants or choking agents (e.g. chlorine, phosgene); *blood* gases or systemic agents (e.g. hydrogen cyanide); sensory *irritants* (e.g. CN, CS, CR); and *psychotropic* or other centrally acting agents (e.g. the disabling agent BZ and the fentanyl opioids). This type of classification is used in Table 3.1 on page 33 above.

3.6　Consequences of using biological or chemical weapons

3.6.1　Short-term consequences

The most prominent short-term effect of biological or chemical weapons is the large number of casualties that they can cause, and it is this characteristic that determines most preparedness strategies. The potential for overwhelming medical resources and infrastructure is magnified by the fact that the psychological reaction, including possible terror and panic, of a civilian population to biological or chemical attack may be more serious than that caused by attack with conventional weapons. Psychological support strategies combined with risk communication are an integral part of the services needed to manage the many exposed and non-exposed casualties who may present at medical facilities (see Chapter 4). An instructive illustration of the nature of the short-term consequences of urban attack with chemical agents is provided by the 1994–1995 terrorist attacks in Japan in which the nerve gas sarin was used (see Appendix 4.2). The "anthrax letters"episode in the United States at the end of 2001, in which at the time of writing both the perpetrator and the motive remain to be discovered, provides some insight into the short-term consequences of biological agents being deliberately released (see Appendix 4.3).

Details of the short-term injuries caused by the various biological and chemical agents can be found in Annexes 1, 2 and 3.

3.6.2　Long-term consequences

The possible long-term consequences of the use of biological or chemical weapons, including delayed, prolonged and environmentally mediated health effects long after the time and place that the weapons were used, are more uncertain and less well understood.

Some biological and chemical agents have the potential to cause physical or mental illnesses that either remain, or only become evident, months or years after the weapons have been used. Such effects have long been recognized, and have been the subject of specific scientific monographs (5–6). They may extend the potential for harm of biological or chemical weapons beyond their immediate target both in time and space. For many agents too little is known about their long-term effects for reliable predictions to be made.

Such uncertainty carries over into the planning of medical counter-measures, and little more can be done than to outline the various possibilities needing further study. Non-military experience with disease-causing organisms, or with the presence of certain chemicals in the environment, may not be helpful guides to the effects of those same agents under the quite different conditions of deliberate release, in which greater quantities may be involved. However, useful pointers to what the consequences might be can sometimes be provided by the study of the effects of occupational exposure to chemicals. Organophosphate insecticides, e.g. methyl parathion, are hazardous for humans, and both the methods of treatment and the probable long-term effects of poisoning may be similar to those for nerve gases such as sarin.

The long-term health consequences of releases of biological or chemical agents may include chronic illness, delayed effects, new infectious diseases becoming endemic, and effects mediated by ecological changes.

The potential for *chronic illness* after exposure to some toxic chemicals and some infective agents is well known. The occurrence of chronic debilitating pulmonary disease in victims of exposure to mustard gas was reported after the First World War (7). This has also been described in reports on the current status of Iranian casualties from Iraqi mustard gas during the war between Iraq and the Islamic Republic of Iran in the 1980s (8–9). Follow-up of Iranian victims has revealed debilitating long-term disease of the lungs (chronic bronchitis, bronchiectasis, asthmatic bronchitis, pulmonary fibrosis, large airway obstructions), eyes (delayed mustard gas keratitis with blindness), and skin (dry and itchy skin, with multiple secondary complications, pigmentation disorders, and structural abnormalities ranging from hypertrophy to atrophy). Deaths from pulmonary complications were still occurring as late as 12 years after all exposure had ended *(10)*. Details of long-term effects caused by other toxicants are given in Annexes 1 and 2. Biological agents, including some of the agents of particular concern, may also cause long-lasting illness. *Brucella melitensis* infections, for example, which are typically more severe than brucellosis due to *B. suis* or *B. abortus*, especially affect bones, joints and heart (endocarditis). Relapses, fatigue, weight loss, general malaise and depression are common. *Francisella tularensis* infections result in prolonged malaise, and weakness may last for many months. The viral encephalitides may have permanent effects on the central and peripheral nervous system. Annex 3 provides further information.

The *delayed effects* in persons exposed to certain biological and chemical agents, depending on the dose received, may include carcinogenesis, teratogenesis and perhaps mutagenesis. Certain biological and chemical agents have been strongly implicated in the causation of cancer in humans, but it is not yet known whether infection by any of the microorganisms suited to biological weapons can be carcinogenic in humans, and only limited information is available on the ability of certain classes of chemicals to cause cancer, mainly in experimental animals. For example, some chemicals of particular concern, such as mustard gas, are alkylating agents, and many such agents have been found to be carcinogenic. While the evidence suggesting carcinogenesis after a single acute exposure to sulfur mustard is equivocal, there is good evidence of a significant increase in cancer of the respiratory tract among workers following prolonged low-dose exposure in factories producing mustard gas *(11)*. Experiments with animals and epidemiological data for human populations show that the incidence of chemical carcinogenesis by many carcinogens depends on a power of the duration of exposure. Single exposures are therefore expected to be much less carcinogenic than months or years of exposure to the same total dose. Certain chemicals and infective agents can cause severe damage to the developing human fetus, thalidomide and the rubella virus being particularly well-known examples. It is not known whether any of the specific chemical or biological agents considered here will have teratogenic effects at the doses that could be received by pregnant women in civilian populations that might be exposed to them. Little attention has been given to the possibility that known chemical and biological agents might cause detrimental heritable mutations in humans. Several chemicals are reported to cause such changes in experimental organisms and cultured human cells.

If biological agents are used to cause diseases that are not endemic in the country attacked, this may result in the *disease becoming endemic*, either in human populations, or in suitable vectors such as arthropods and other non-human hosts, such as rodents, birds, equids or cattle. *Bacillus anthracis* spores are highly resistant to environmental degradation, and can persist, particularly in soil, for long periods. By infecting and reproducing in animals, they can establish new foci. Microbes causing gastrointestinal infections in humans, such as *Salmonella* and *Shigella*, can establish persistent reservoirs. *Salmonella* strains can do likewise in domestic animals. A particular concern would be that a deliberate release of variola for hostile purposes could cause resurgence of smallpox, which was finally eradicated from natural occurrence in the 1970s, bringing special benefit to developing countries.

Finally, there is the possibility of *effects mediated by ecological change*. New foci of disease might become established as a result of ecological changes caused by the use of biological agents infective for humans and animals, or as a result of the use of anti-plant agents. These could have adverse long-term effects on human health via reductions in the quality and quantity of the food supply derived from plants or animals. They could also have major economic impact, either through direct effects on agriculture or through indirect effects on trade and tourism.

The broad conclusion to be drawn from the foregoing analysis is that there are great difficulties associated with assessing the long-term health effects of exposure to chemical and biological agents.

Confounding variables may affect the results of studies, and it may be difficult to distinguish genuine long-term effects of exposure from background occurrence of the same symptoms due to a wide spectrum of other causes. Conflicting data and inconclusive results often make it impossible to reach definitive conclusions.

Examples of the difficulties in determining the existence of long-term effects of chemical exposure have been provided by the ongoing investigations of medical problems apparently caused by the herbicide Agent Orange to people exposed in Viet Nam, where the chemical was widely used in the 1960s and early 1970s during the Viet Nam War *(12)*. Investigations have paid special attention to the contaminant 2,3,7,8-tetrachlorodibenzo-*p*-dioxin (TCDD), which is produced during manufacture and is persistent in the environment, detectable at elevated levels in sampled lipid and body fat, and highly toxic to certain experimental animals. In a more recent example, and with even less scientific evidence for a cause–effect relationship, chemical exposures of a variety of types were among the many factors suggested as potential causes of the so-called Gulf War syndrome. In both cases, a wide range of long-term symptoms and adverse health effects (including carcinogenesis, teratogenesis and a plethora of nonspecific somatic and psychological symptoms) are said to have been caused by exposure to chemical agents, among other possible causes *(13)*. Despite intensive investigation, definitive explanations have not yet been found in either case.

3.6.3   Psychological warfare aspects

Apart from their ability to cause physical injury and illness, biological and chemical agents may lend themselves to psychological warfare (which is a military term for attacks on morale including terrorization) because of the horror and dread that they can inspire. Even if the agents are not actually used, fear of them can cause disruption, even panic. Exacerbation of such effects can be expected from the exaggerated accounts of biological and chemical weapons that may arise in some circles. People may be better able to understand the harmful effects of conventional weapons than those of toxic or infective materials.

The emergence and spread of long-range missile delivery systems has increased the vulnerability to biological or chemical attack felt in cities, where the population may seem largely unprotectable, and this in turn has increased the psychological warfare potential. This was demonstrated in Teheran during the "war of the cities" in the final stage of the war between Iraq and the Islamic Republic of Iran in the 1980s when the threat – which never became a reality – that missiles might be used to deliver chemical agents reportedly caused greater alarm than the high-explosive warheads actually used ever did. There was a further example of this during the Gulf War of 1990–1991, when it was feared that Scud missiles aimed at Israeli cities might be armed with chemical warheads. In addition to military and civil defence personnel, many civilians were issued with antichemical protective equipment and trained in procedures for chemical defence. Considerable disruption was caused since all missile strikes were regarded as chemical until proven otherwise, despite the fact that no chemical warheads were actually used by Iraq.

3.7 Assessment and conclusions

This chapter has introduced the wide variety of toxic and infective agents that could be used for hostile purposes. It has proposed that a relatively small group of agents, identified through the evaluation process that it describes, should form the focus of protective preparation. Preparedness can thereby be built against essentially all agents.

Of the various methods available for the release of biological and chemical agents, the major risk results from their dissemination as aerosols or, for some chemicals, as vapour. Respiratory protective equipment and means of predicting the potential spread of the airborne agent can allow timely protective measures to be taken in the areas that may be affected.

Skin exposure is a problem relating mostly to chemical agents and would usually occur only in the immediate vicinity of a release. Here, an important element of protection will be protective clothing. Skin protection may be required against both direct liquid exposure and high vapour concentrations. If a vapour risk exists, respiratory protection using adsorptive filters will also be required and in some cases evacuation of people from the hazardous area can be effective.

By understanding the general properties and potential consequences of the use of biological and chemical agents, a balanced approach to preparedness may be achieved. A preparedness programme should make provision not only for the immediate casualty-producing potential of such agents, but also for possible long-term consequences.

REFERENCES

1. Khan AS, Morse S, Lillibridge S. Public-health preparedness for biological terrorism in the USA. *Lancet*, 2000, 356, 1179–1182.

2. Kireev AF et al. Identification of alkylphosphonic acid derivatives by IR and mass spectrometry. *Journal of Analytical Chemistry*, 2000, 55(9):837–845.

3. Organisation for the Prohibition of Chemical Weapons. *OPCW Annual Report for 2002*. The Hague, OPCW, C-8/5 dated 22 October 2003. Annexes 6 and 7.

4. Heyder J et al. Deposition of particles in the human respiratory track in the size range of 0.005–15 μm. *Journal of Aerosol Science*, 1986, 17(5):811–825.

5. Lohs K. *Delayed toxic effects of chemical warfare agents*. Stockholm International Peace Research Institute Monograph. Stockholm, Almqvist & Wiksell International, 1975.

6. Commitee on Toxicology, Board on Toxicology and Environmental Health Hazards, National Research Council. *Possible long-term health effects of short-term exposure to chemical agents. Vol. 3. Final report: current health status of test subjects*. Washington, DC, National Academy Press, 1985.

7. Papirmeister B et al. *Medical defence against mustard gas: toxic mechanisms and pharmacological implications*. Boca Raton, FL, CRC Press, 1991:26.

8. Emad A, Rezaian GR. The diversity of the effects of sulfur mustard gas inhalation on the respiratory system 10 years after a single, heavy exposure. *Chest*, 1997, 112:734–738.

9. Emad A, Rezaian GR. Immunoglobulins and cellular constituents of the BAL fluid of patients with sulfur mustard gas induced pulmonary fibrosis. *Chest*, 1999, 115:1346–1351.

10. Keshavarz S (Director, Baghiyat'ollah Hospital, Teheran), personal communication.

11. Pechura M, Rall DP, eds. *Veterans at risk: the health effects of mustard gas and lewisite*. Washington, DC, National Academy Press, 1993.

12. *Veterans and agent orange: health effects of herbicides used in Vietnam*, Washington, DC, US Institute of Medicine, National Academy Press, 1994.

13. Fulco CE, Liverman CT, Sox HC, eds. *Gulf war and health. Vol. I. Depleted uranium, sarin, pyridostigmine bromide, vaccines*. Washington, DC, National Academy Press, 2000.

4. PUBLIC HEALTH PREPAREDNESS AND RESPONSE

4.1 Background

The initial response to a deliberate release of infective or toxic agents targeted against civilian populations is largely a local responsibility in many parts of the world. Local authorities are in the best position to deal with such events, and will generally be held accountable should the incident be mishandled. While national and international resources will be important in the long term, it is the responsibility of local officials to ensure that response systems and plans are in place before an incident actually occurs.

This chapter provides a framework that local and national authorities can use in planning the response to incidents in which biological or chemical agents may have been released deliberately. It is not intended to provide an in-depth review of all the technologies and other matters involved, or a manual for use in training. The goal is rather to demonstrate that the standard principles of risk management are as applicable to biological or chemical incidents as they are to other emergencies or disasters *(1)*. These principles, which are outlined in Appendix 4.1 below, can be used to identify areas needing particular attention when biological or chemical agents are involved. They are described further in a recent WHO publication *(2)*. The chapter thus provides an outline of the matters that will need to be considered. Further sources of detailed information are given in Annex 6.

As far as chemical attacks are concerned, States Parties to the CWC, which have thereby become Member States of the OPCW, have access to international aid in their preparedness activities. Assistance in assessing needs and specific training can be obtained by contacting the International Cooperation and Assistance Division of the OPCW Technical Secretariat. For biological attacks, Article VII of the BWC makes some provision for assistance if a State Party is exposed to danger as a result of a violation of the Convention. For further information on this and other sources of international assistance, including WHO, see Chapter 6.

Preparedness also needs to cover situations in which a threat has been made that biological or chemical agents are to be released. While such a threat may be a hoax, the authorities concerned need to be able to allay public fears as well as to take appropriate action to locate and neutralize any suspect device.

There may be a close relationship between the public health preparedness that is to be discussed in this chapter and the preparedness of military forces to protect their capabilities and operations against biological or chemical warfare. While it may be possible, however, for some countries adequately to warn, encapsulate and otherwise protect the disciplined, centrally commanded, healthy adults who make up combat forces in an active theatre of war, the protection of a civilian population, especially in peacetime, is an altogether different matter. Indeed, there may be danger in holding out a prospect of adequate civil protection that is actually unrealistic, for it may detract from efforts at prevention.

The first to respond to an attack with a toxic substance having immediate effects are likely to be the police, fire departments and emergency medical personnel on or near the scene. In contrast, the first to respond to an initially undetected attack with an infective or toxic agent having only delayed effects are more likely to be regular health-care providers, including nurses, physicians and hospital accident and emergency personnel, who may be located in widely separated places.

While chemical weapons can place a great burden on public safety personnel, and biological weapons on the public health infrastructure, they can both place an extraordinary burden on the local health-care delivery system.

Because victims of a chemical attack may be affected immediately, a rapid response will be required, in which the main emphasis will be on evacuation, contamination control and early medical treatment.

Emergency personnel will have to locate and identify the contaminated area immediately (the "hot zone") and may have to act within minutes if lives are to be saved. On the other hand, a covert release of a biological agent will be more likely to become apparent over a longer period of time, e.g. days or even weeks, and will probably take the form of the appearance of cases of infectious disease. Because some victims are likely to move around in the symptom-free incubation period after exposure, cases of the disease may appear in different locations, even distant ones, and the full picture may become evident only after information, medical reports and surveillance data from many areas have been combined. Biological agents that are transmissible from person to person can also generate clusters of secondary outbreaks. Depending on the nature of the organism involved and the normal pattern of infectious disease in the locality concerned, the attack might initially appear to be a natural outbreak of disease.

These differences need to be borne in mind in planning public health preparedness for biological and chemical incidents. However, in the early phases of an incident, it may not be clear whether the causative agent is biological or chemical, or possibly a mixture of the two. As a result, first responders may find themselves needing to manage both types of incident before the relevant specialists for biological or chemical incidents become involved.

In order to prepare for biological or chemical attack, the authorities concerned should be encouraged to make maximum use of existing emergency-response resources, and to adopt an approach that is consistent with the principles on which the management of any other type of public health emergency is based. While attacks with biological and chemical agents will have some special features, they do not necessarily require the formation of completely new and independent response systems. A well designed public health and emergency-response system is quite capable of responding to a limited biological or chemical attack and can take the measures necessary to mitigate its effects. A sizeable attack with a chemical agent will be very similar to a major hazardous-materials accident. A community's existing capability to respond to such an accident is therefore an essential component of preparedness for such an attack. A biological agent attack will generally have the characteristics of a disease outbreak, so that city, state and regional public health authorities must be involved in the response, which will have much in common with the infection-control strategies used in any outbreak of disease.

Routine sensitive and near-real-time disease-surveillance systems are thus essential in both disease outbreaks and those caused by biological agents. Such systems should be in place well in advance of an attack, so that the background disease prevalence in the area concerned is known. The performance of a surveillance system in terms of the timeliness of its response to naturally occurring outbreaks of disease provides an indication of its probable contribution during deliberately caused outbreaks. A national centre can detect a national outbreak not noticed in any individual region and it can also economically provide epidemiological expertise for investigating the causes and sources of outbreaks. Further, it can contribute to both biological and chemical defence, as the epidemiological techniques used in the investigation of both types of attack are similar (although possibly more often relevant in biological attacks). Establishing mechanisms for the routine exchange of information between the public health and veterinary sectors is very important as many biological agents are zoonotic.

A greater role in disseminating information on disease outbreaks and other health events is now being played by the media and certain interest groups, notably the Program for Monitoring Emerging Diseases (ProMed)[6] now run by the International Society for Infectious Diseases in the United States. WHO collects, verifies and disseminates information on outbreaks of diseases of international public health concern, and this information is available on a restricted basis to WHO's partners in the Global Outbreak Alert and Response Network and Member States weekly; once officially notified, the information is published electronically through the World Wide Web and in printed form in the *Weekly Epidemiological Record (3)*.

Functioning and efficient poisons centres have proved to be invaluable for authorities charged with the management of accidents involving chemicals or individual cases of poisoning. The immediate availability of chemical and toxicological information and expertise will be equally valuable in managing a chemical incident.

---

6   See *http://www.promedmail.org*

Confirming that a covert release has taken place may be a particularly difficult task. Routine emergency-call monitoring systems (which continually track the frequency, nature and location of emergency calls) are a useful management tool, and may be of great value in drawing attention to an unusual pattern of symptoms, possibly indicating a deliberate release of biological or chemical agents.

The danger of making the response to biological and chemical incidents the task solely of dedicated specialized response units is that the relative infrequency of call-out could lead to the deterioration of skills. More seriously, excessive centralization may risk increasing the time taken to react. Mobilization of a specialized biological and chemical unit throughout a region can never match the 24-hour availability and general emergency-management experience of existing response and public health services. It is true, however, that certain activities will need to be carried out by specialists (e.g. sampling and analysis for the definitive identification of the agent involved). This suggests that a readiness and response strategy should aim at enabling the local public health, emergency-response and other authorities (fire and ambulance services, police force and civil defence) to respond to, and manage the incident scene in its early phases, specialized functions being performed later by a dedicated mobile biological and chemical response unit. Exceptionally, the pre-positioning of special response units may be necessary for highly visible events (e.g. the Olympic Games) that might be a target for terrorists.

The ability to respond to biological or chemical incidents depends on *preparedness* (what needs to be considered long before an incident takes place) and *response* (what needs to happen after a warning of a pending release is received, or after the release has actually occurred).

4.2 Preparedness

4.2.1 Threat analysis

Threat analysis is a multidisciplinary activity, with inputs from the country's law-enforcement, intelligence, and medical and scientific communities. It is aimed at identifying those who may wish to use biological or chemical weapons against the population, the agents that may be used, and the circumstances under which they may be used. This is an exercise that is broad in its scope, and requires active liaison between law-enforcement, security and health agencies (typically centralized state institutions) with the local authorities. It will only rarely be possible to identify the likelihood or precise nature of the threat, and general preparedness measures will therefore usually be required. Judgements may need to be made on the basis of a general appraisal of national or local circumstances.

Even if specific biological or chemical hazards cannot be identified, general improvements in public health will automatically improve a population's ability to manage biological incidents. The ability to manage industrial chemical accidents will provide resources that can be diverted, if needed, to managing a chemical incident.

If specific potential hazards can be identified, the probability of an incident occurring and its consequences must be evaluated. Justified and well-motivated decisions on resource allocation can be made only after this has been done. Chapter 3 has identified a group of agents representative of those that may be of particular concern.

The level of threat that exists is also a function of the potential vulnerability of the community concerned. Vulnerability analysis will identify potential scenarios as well as weaknesses in the system that may be exposed to biological or chemical hazards, and will determine the current ability to respond to and manage the emergency *(4)*. This, in turn, requires an assessment of needs and capability. When potential scenarios have been identified in the preceding steps, it will be possible to determine the resources required to respond to such incidents. Response requirements must be determined for each of the actions identified below in respect of biological and chemical incidents. When identified needs are measured against currently available resources, in what is called "gap analysis", certain deficiencies will be revealed. It is then that a country inexperienced in defence against biological and chemical weapons is most likely to need international assistance (see Chapter 6 for sources of such assistance).

4.2.2   Pre-emption of attack

The establishment of a biological and chemical response system is in itself a pre-emptive risk-reduction strategy. Historical precedent suggests that the risk of biological or chemical attack in war is considerably reduced by the mere existence of effective ability to respond to and manage an incident. If an aggressor knows that an attack will be quickly and effectively dealt with, the incentive to perpetrate such an attack will be considerably diminished. A balance needs to be struck between the level of visibility that such a vigilance and response system needs in order to serve as a deterrent, and the potentially negative results that the demonstration of concern about possible vulnerabilities could produce. Ill-considered publicity given to the perceived threat of biological or chemical terrorism might have the opposite effect to that desired.

Pre-emption of terrorist use of biological or chemical agents presupposes, first and foremost, accurate and up-to-date intelligence about terrorist groups and their activities. As the agents may be manufactured using dual-use equipment, and as the equipment required for manufacture need not be large or particularly distinctive (as seen from outside the facility), technical means of acquiring intelligence, such as reconnaissance satellites, are of little use. Intelligence on terrorism, therefore, relies heavily on human sources. While large-scale national development and production programmes and facilities for the manufacture of biological and chemical weapons are relatively easy to identify, terrorist activities may be much less conspicuous and therefore more difficult to detect.

An important prerequisite for pre-emption is the existence of national legislation that renders the development, production, possession, transfer or use of biological or chemical weapons a crime, and that empowers law-enforcement agencies to act where such activities are suspected before an actual event occurs. For details of how this is dealt with in the CWC and BWC, see Chapter 5.

Pre-emption of attacks will be aided by concerted national and international efforts to monitor and control dual-use technology and equipment as, in the case of chemical and toxin attacks, by full implementation of the CWC, including its general purpose criterion. The international norm that has been established by the majority of countries by their acceptance of the principles of the BWC and the CWC may be a decisive factor in deterring would-be users of biological or chemical weapons.

4.2.3   Preparing to respond

Pre-emptory efforts notwithstanding, the risk of a biological or chemical attack cannot be eliminated completely, and could have serious consequences if it occurred. Accordingly, a preparedness programme may be necessary, and this will require the acquisition of equipment and supplies, the development of appropriate procedures, and training. Communities will need to examine their existing hazardous-materials protocols, public-health plans, and the current training of the police, firefighters, emergency medical service personnel and public health personnel, including physicians, epidemiologists, veterinarians and laboratory staff. These will have to be adapted in the light of the features unique to deliberately released biological or chemical agents.

Most civilian health-care providers have little or no experience of illnesses caused by biological and chemical weapons, and may therefore not suspect, especially in the early phases of an incident, that a patient's symptoms could be due to such weapons. There is therefore a need to train health-care workers in the recognition and initial management of both biological and chemical casualties, and for a rapid communication system that allows sharing of information immediately an unusual incident is suspected. Education and training must cover the general characteristics of biological and chemical agents; the clinical presentation, diagnosis, prophylaxis and treatment of diseases that may be caused by deliberate agent-release; and sample handling, decontamination and barrier nursing. Training, planning and drills should be directed at physicians and staff for the management of mass casualties, providing respiratory support to large numbers of patients, the large-scale distribution of medication, and supporting the local authorities in vaccination programmes. Providing the necessary education and training is expensive and may also be manpower-intensive, yet may be the most cost-effective method of medical preparation for biological attack. Such training will also be the cornerstone of an approach to prevent anxiety and fear in health-care workers, something that might be expected after a bioweapons event and that could disrupt the provision of health-care services.

Because early diagnosis of both biological and chemical exposure will be important in the choice of treatment and response, preparation should include the establishment of a reference laboratory (or a network of laboratories in large areas) in which potential agents can be identified. In addition to the need for diagnosis for purposes of medical treatment, samples obtained from a delivery system or the environment, or from patients, will require forensic analysis. Earlier diagnosis will be facilitated if regional laboratories have the necessary equipment and staff for that purpose. New diagnostic technologies mean that biological agents can be identified quickly, perhaps even at the attack site. Such state-of-the-art techniques may not, however, be available everywhere.

Failure adequately to prepare the health-care system and its staff for biological attack may not only result in late detection of an outbreak, but may also facilitate the spread of an outbreak caused by an agent transmitted by person-to-person contact. Should the local health-care facilities and personnel be perceived as unable to manage the outbreak and the clinical cases, the population, including potentially infectious patients, may travel long distances to seek treatment, thus contributing to spread of the disease.

Where a particular need for equipment, antidotes, antibiotics or vaccines has been identified, pre-attack stockpiling and planning of distribution systems, or designation of sources of rapid supply, to make them available to the exposed population will be necessary. The financial cost of such stockpiles, depending on the items chosen and the quantities stockpiled, may then be very high indeed. Spending such large sums exclusively on responding to possible attack with biological or chemical weapons can be justified only when there is an extremely unusual and very specific threat. In high-risk situations, the supply to each person or family of protective equipment (e.g. respiratory protection), antidotes (e.g. syringes loaded with antidotes for self-injection) or antibiotics can be considered. The cost and logistic burden of this type of preparation may be prohibitive, however, and may not be feasible in poor countries or those in which large numbers of people will need protection. In such cases, and depending on the agent involved, selective protective measures may still be considered for high-risk groups (e.g. prophylactic antibiotics for those most likely to be, or having been, exposed).

It is vital not to make the mistake of assuming that availability of equipment is synonymous with the ability to respond, or that a community without all the latest equipment is doomed to failure. Furthermore, ensuring the availability of specialized equipment is generally a more important part of preparation for chemical attack than for biological attack. The use of biological and chemical protective equipment requires special training, and the adaptation of existing procedures for emergency management. Without careful development of the necessary procedures and intensive training, the introduction of such equipment can hamper the ability to respond, and can even be dangerous. Some of the problems associated with the use of protective equipment are described in Annex 4.

4.2.4. Preparing public information and communication packages

If it is to have any chance of success, a plan for providing information to the public and thus demystifying the subject of biological and chemical weapons needs to be drawn up well before an incident occurs. If this is to be effective, the public needs to know how they are expected to act if an attack takes place, long before any such attack occurs. The communication plan may include radio and television broadcasts, or the distribution of brochures to the public describing the potential threat in plain, unemotional language. Clear advice should be given on how the alarm will be raised, and what to do if that happens. Excellent examples of such communication packages are available, e.g. references (5–6). A well-constructed media plan is essential, both as part of the pre-incident education process, and to avoid overreaction after an incident. It must contain explicit and exhaustive instructions on channels of communication and clearance procedures for potentially sensitive information. Of course, any public preparedness or information programme needs to be evaluated in the context of the specific local circumstances, including the possibility that too much information may be counterproductive, or even dangerous.

4.2.5   Validation of response capabilities

As with preparation for any high-consequence but low-frequency incident, it is a major challenge to prove and validate response capabilities if they are not being constantly practised or used. Realistic training simulations are a useful tool *(7–8)*, and must be evaluated critically to identify areas that can be improved.

In addition, careful analysis of actual incidents, wherever they occur, should provide valuable information that could help the international community to respond, and the lessons learned should be incorporated into future planning. Since the first edition of this report was published, a serious incident of terrorist attack on civilians in which chemical weapons were used occurred in Japan. This incident warrants careful analysis, as many lessons on the nature of, and response to, civilian attacks with chemicals can be learned. For example, the fact that most of the victims went to hospitals on their own initiative, using their own transport, has important implications for the distribution of triage and decontamination facilities. Further information on this incident is given in Appendix 4.2 below.

The deliberate use of biological agents to cause harm has fortunately been rare. In 1984, and apparently with a view to influencing a local electoral process, a religious cult known as the Rajneeshees caused 751 people in a small town in Oregon, United States, to become ill by using cultures of *Salmonella enterica typhimurium* bacteria to contaminate the salad bars of 10 restaurants over a period of some two months *(9–10)*. More recently, and with far more media exposure, letters containing *Bacillus anthracis* spores were distributed in the United States postal system. This incident is described in Appendix 4.3 below.

4.3   Response

4.3.1   Response before any overt release
of a biological or chemical agent

If a warning of an impending release of biological or chemical agents is received, a number of activities can and should be carried out before the release, if any, actually happens. The sequence in which these activities are performed will depend on the particular circumstances of the incident. The first indication of an incident may be a warning, or the finding of an unusual device or unusual materials as a result of normal activities within the community such as the response to a fire or the discovery of a strange package. One or more of the following may then be required:

Analysis of the available information. All the information available needs to be assessed by an appropriate group including the police, the intelligence services and technical experts who should have been trained to work together to analyse such information by means of realistic and credible exercises. Such a small group of analysts and experts will be able to evaluate the threat or the information on the incident and advise on appropriate action and the mobilization of specialist assistance, and may also help to avoid inappropriate responses to hoaxes.

Initiation of a search procedure. If sufficient information was given in the warning and the analysis warrants such action, it may be appropriate to search for a suspect device at a particular location. It may also be appropriate to search for those responsible for the warning or for witnesses who may have seen them.

Establishment of a cordon. Again depending on the circumstances and the information available, it may be appropriate to evacuate people from the area at risk and to establish an exclusion zone.

Early identification of the nature of the hazard. If a device or unusual package is found, it will be important to decide as soon as possible whether the impending hazard is chemical or biological in character (or even a mixture of the two). The presence of explosives, either as the primary hazard or as the disseminating charge for a toxic/infective agent, must also be considered, together with the possibility of the device containing a radioactive hazard. The appropriate specialists can then be called in to help in managing the incident, and the appropriate protective equipment selected. For example, an oronasal mask may provide adequate protection against a particulate biological hazard while a respirator and full protective clothing may be required to protect against a persistent chemical agent.

Risk reduction and/or neutralization. Depending on the nature of the device, the possibility of reducing the risk, or neutralizing the potential hazard, through containment or other mitigation and neutralization approaches should be considered. Whether it should be managed on-site or moved to a specialized facility would be a decision for specialists (equipment is available that allows on-site controlled and contained detonation of devices, together with decontamination of toxic/infective contents). Wherever possible, sampling for analytical and forensic purposes should be accomplished before destructive neutralization.

4.3.2 Distinguishing features of biological and chemical incidents

In the earliest phases of a release (and particularly if it is covert), it may be difficult to distinguish between a biological and a chemical attack. As a general rule, chemical attacks are more likely to produce simultaneous and similar symptoms in a relatively restricted area near the point of release relatively soon after release. Biological attacks are more likely to result in the appearance of ill individuals at medical centres and/or doctors' surgeries over a longer period of time and a much larger area. Symptoms resulting from exposure to chemicals with delayed effects will obviously be much more difficult to distinguish from those of an infectious disease. While there are no definitive and invariable distinguishing features, the indicators shown in Table 4.1 may help in deciding whether a biological or chemical attack has taken place. The differentiation of deliberate releases from natural morbidity is discussed in Annex 3.

Table 4.1 **Differentiation of biological and chemical attack**

Indicator	Chemical attack	Biological attack
Epidemiological features	Unusual numbers of patients with very similar symptoms seeking care virtually simultaneously (especially with respiratory, ocular, cutaneous or neurological symptoms, e.g. nausea, headache, eye pain or irritation, disorientation, difficulty with breathing, convulsions and even sudden death) Clusters of patients arriving from a single locality Definite pattern of symptoms clearly evident	Rapidly increasing disease incidence (over hours or days) in a normally healthy population Unusual increase in people seeking care, especially with fever, respiratory, or gastrointestinal complaints Endemic disease rapidly emerging at an unusual time or in an unusual pattern Unusual numbers of patients with rapidly fatal illness (agent-dependent) Patients with a relatively uncommon disease that has bioterrorism potential (particularly those listed in Annex 3)
Animal indicators	Sick or dying animals	Sick or dying animals
Devices, unusual liquid spray or vapour	Suspicious devices or packages Droplets, oily film Unexplained odour Low clouds or fog unrelated to weather	Suspicious devices or packages

Source: Adapted from references 11 and 12.

4.3.3   Response to biological incidents

Table 4.2 summarizes the major activities involved in responding to biological incidents. The sequence of events is based on application of the internationally accepted principles of risk analysis (see Appendix 4.1 for more detail on risk analysis).

Table 4.2   **Major response activities for biological attack**

Assess the risks	Determine that a release has occurred or an outbreak is taking place
	Identify the nature of the agent involved (hazard identification) and develop a case definition
	Evaluate the potential outbreak spread and assess current and delayed case-management requirements, having regard to the possibility that the infection may be contagious (risk characterization)
Manage the risks (introduction of risk-reduction/control measures)	Protect responders and health-care workers
	Introduce infection-prevention and control procedures
	Conduct case triage
	Ensure medical care of infected cases
Monitor all activities	Decide whether local and national resources are adequate or whether international assistance should be sought
	Implement active surveillance to monitor the effectiveness of the prevention and control procedures, follow up the distribution of cases (time, place and person), and adjust response activities as needed
	Repeat the risk-assessment/management process as required
	Implement longer term follow-up activities
Communicate the risks	Implement a risk-communication programme for the affected population that conveys information and instructions as needed

The following discussion summarizes some of the most important considerations in the activities listed in Table 4.2. Sources of more detailed information that may be needed by response planners are given in Annex 6. Since responses to both natural and intentionally caused outbreaks will follow similar lines, the information given below focuses specifically on the problems posed by outbreaks that have been caused deliberately. Information on public health action in emergencies caused by epidemics is available in a WHO publication (13).

Determination that a release has occurred or an outbreak is taking place

All outbreaks of infectious disease should be considered natural events unless there is good reason to suppose otherwise (see Annex 3). Initiating a response to an intentional outbreak thus requires prior confirmation that a release has actually occurred or the suspicion that an outbreak has been caused deliberately. Many factors will influence the decision to initiate such a response, particularly whether the release was overt or covert. A covert release, just like any other outbreak of disease, will be detected only when patients begin to present at medical facilities. The existing surveillance system should be able to detect the outbreak and an epidemiological investigation will then be triggered. The results of the investigation, coupled with clinical, laboratory or environmental data, may indicate that the outbreak could have been the result of a deliberate release. The importance of routine surveillance and the prompt investigation of all outbreaks so that warning can be given that an unusual outbreak may be under way have been discussed in section 4.1 above. A threatened or overt release will generate response requirements more akin to those in the early stages of a chemical release, described below. While it is probable that signs and symptoms in people and animals will provide confirmation that a release has taken place, the sampling and detection of biological agents in environmental substrates may also be required.

Identification of the agent involved

Prompt identification of the agent involved is required to ensure that the appropriate preventive and medical measures are taken. Because some agents may cause a contagious infection, it may not be advisable to wait for laboratory confirmation of the identity of the agent. It may then be necessary to introduce risk-reduction strategies soon after starting the investigation of the outbreak.

The development of sensitive and rapid methods of detecting and identifying biological agents in the environment will be difficult because of the large number of potential agents. Significant advances will have to be made in technology before such methods can be made widely accessible, and they may therefore not be available for some time.

The extent to which laboratory support will be able to aid initial diagnosis and treatment will depend on both the level of pre-incident preparation, and the availability of a network of diagnostic laboratories. The nature of the biological sample required, and the specific laboratory techniques required for agent identification, will vary according to the nature of the organism suspected. Definitive identification of a biological agent used in a deliberate attack will also be forensically important. Detailed analysis of the organism and its properties may allow it to be traced to a source laboratory. This is a highly specialized activity, distinct from the basic diagnostic procedures needed in outbreak management, and is often outside the immediate interests and responsibility of the public health sector.

Biological hoaxes may be difficult to evaluate or confirm immediately because of the long incubation periods of biological agents. One proven method of increasing the likelihood of identifying a hoax accurately is to establish a small on-call committee of experts who have trained together and are able to evaluate the situation quickly and efficiently by telephone conference or computer link at very short notice (see also section 4.3.1). The committee should include a biologist and a physician who are familiar with the classification of threat agents, representatives of law-enforcement agencies and possibly the military, a forensic psychologist, a representative of the public health community, and the on-scene authorities. A group such as this, furnished with all the information available at the time, can make the best decision possible on the steps to be taken.

Once the agent is identified, it is important to develop an initial hypothesis as to the exposure that is causing disease (source of the agent and mode of transmission). This hypothesis should be tested with clinical, laboratory or environmental data, field investigations and application of analytical epidemiology tools in comparing subgroups of the population

Evaluation of potential spread

If the incident involves the release of a biological aerosol, computer modelling may help to predict the spread of the aerosol particles. The first steps must, however, be to gather information on the wind direction and speed and on possible sources of the aerosol. With an ongoing outbreak, retrospective analysis may indicate that cases originate from specific areas, and may be a valuable indicator of an up-wind site of original release. For example, investigators of the accidental release of anthrax spores in 1979 from the military biological facility in Sverdlovsk, the former Soviet Union, were able to use aerosol spread analysis to show the striking occurrence of cases of pulmonary anthrax in persons located within specific isopleths originating from the point of suspected release (14–15).

If the release involves an agent that has potential for person-to-person transmission, an epidemic is likely to spread through secondary outbreaks. Standard epidemiological methods should then be used to predict the probable spread of the disease, and medical resources mobilized and deployed accordingly.

Protection of responders and health-care workers

The protection of responders and health-care workers is obviously essential. In addition to compromising the ability to manage the incident, the occurrence of infection in health-care workers may lead to the perception among the population that health centres and hospitals themselves constitute a high-risk source of infection. This may discourage potentially infected persons from seeking treatment from the local health-care providers, and lead them to travel to other health-care facilities, thereby increasing the risk of secondary transmission if the infection is contagious.

During the spread of a biological aerosol, the primary route of exposure will be via the airways and respiratory tract. Respiratory protection will then be the most important component of physical protection. Particulate filters are generally adequate for biological agents (in contrast to the activated-charcoal or similar filters that will be needed for the filtration of air contaminated with chemical vapour).

Most of the agents of special concern do not cause contagious disease, but some do, and if these become established in the population, the spread of aerosol droplets, contact between infected body fluids and mucous membranes or broken skin, and even ingestion may all be involved in the secondary spread of the agent. Universal precautions for dealing with potentially infective materials should therefore always be taken. The protection of responders should be based on the standard principles of barrier nursing and infection control *(12, 16–17)*.

Vaccination or prophylactic antibiotic treatment of those involved in response may have to be considered. This is more likely to be useful in the management of any secondary spread of the infection than for the primary manifestations of the attack. Pre-attack vaccination of health-care providers may be considered if appropriate vaccines are widely available (e.g. for smallpox, plague and possibly anthrax).

Infection control

If agents of transmissible (contagious) diseases are released, basic hygiene and infection-control measures, e.g. washing hands after contact, avoiding direct contact with secretions from infected individuals, keeping exposed persons away from public places, and isolating suspected or symptomatic cases, may be essential in limiting secondary spread. The dissemination of such basic information on the precautions necessary, not only to health-care providers but also to the general public, will be an important step in infection control. The population should be told what signs and symptoms to watch out for and whom to call or where to go if they appear. Lack of specificity in such advice to the public may result in local health facilities becoming overwhelmed by uninfected patients.

Large-scale evacuation as a preventive measure is not likely to form part of the response to biological incidents. Where contagious disease is involved, it may aggravate the situation by increasing both the spread of infection and the number of secondary outbreaks. Movement of patients should be restricted to the minimum necessary to provide treatment and care.

Special measures may be required to limit the nosocomial spread of such diseases as the viral haemorrhagic fevers (e.g. Ebola or Marburg), plague and smallpox. The frequent suggestion that special rooms under negative pressure should be provided is impractical because of the sheer number of probable cases. Provision may be made to care for patients at sites other than health-care centres, such as gymnasia, sports arenas or at home.

Immediate decontamination for people who may be exposed to biological attack is not so critical as it is for chemical casualties, since biological agents are non-volatile, are difficult to re-aerosolize and leave little residue on skin or surfaces. Many pathogens deposited on surfaces will rapidly die, though some may survive for longer periods *(18)*. However, it would be prudent to be prepared to decontaminate both materials and persons, particularly if a site of release can be identified. Defining a "hot zone" (as in hazardous-materials incidents) may be extremely difficult or impossible, and it may not be possible to define the contaminated zone until the outbreak has been characterized. At or near the release point of a biological agent, where large particles may have been deposited, area decontamination (or whole-body decontamination of persons who were present in the area) may be appropriate. Decontamination solutions used for chemical decontamination will usually also be suitable for biological decontamination. Hypochlorite is the recommended disinfectant for use in outbreak response. An all-purpose disinfectant should have a concentration of 0.05% (i.e. 1 g/litre) of available chlorine, a stronger solution with a concentration of 0.5% (i.e. 10 g/litre) available chlorine being used, for example, in suspected outbreaks of Lassa and Ebola virus diseases. The use of the solution with 0.5% available chlorine is recommended for disinfecting excreta, cadavers, and spills of blood and body fluids, and that of the solution with 0.05% available chlorine for disinfecting gloved or bare hands and skin, floors, clothing, equipment and bedding *(19)*. Most experts now agree that water, or soap and water, may be adequate, and probably safer, for the removal of most biological agents from human skin. Buildings can be decontaminated by means of chlorine-based liquid sprays, formaldehyde vapour produced by heating paraformaldehyde, or other disinfecting fumigants. Because of the lack of other effective tools, the decontamination of a building may be psychologically beneficial. It may, however, be extremely difficult to certify that a building is clean after an agent release. In addition to the standard principles of barrier nursing referred to above for highly transmissible agents, the disposal of waste materials, safe burial practices, and cleaning or disinfection of patients' clothing should be considered *(20)*.

Where transmissible-disease agents are involved, quarantine of the affected area via the establishment of a sanitary cordon may need to be considered. The coordinated efforts of several public service groups will be required to inform the people affected, control water and food supplies, regulate the movement of people into and out of the area, and establish medical services.

In addition, where there is a danger of the international spread of human diseases, the provisions of the International Health Regulations (IHR) *(21)*, currently under revision, should be borne in mind. The IHR provide an essential global regulatory framework to prevent the international spread of diseases through permanent preventive measures for travellers and cargo, and at border crossing points.

Triage

Any suspected or actual dissemination of biological agents is likely to lead to large numbers of people seeking care. The development of scientifically sound case definition(s) suitable for the local circumstances and the definition of the population at risk of becoming ill are very important for triage (the initial reception, assessment and prioritization of casualties). Such information can generally be gathered from the epidemiological description of the outbreak, or sometimes from more specific surveys. Fear and panic can be expected in genuinely symptomatic patients, the public and the health-care providers involved. All health-care facilities will need to plan in advance for dealing with overwhelming numbers of people seeking care or advice simultaneously, and to ensure that resources are used to help those who are most likely to benefit. Both psychological support and active treatment of anxiety will play an important part in the triage process.

Medical care

The specific medical treatment of exposed individuals will depend entirely on the nature of the organism involved (see Annex 3).

Immunization or prophylactic antibiotic treatment of certain segments of the population (contacts, health-care personnel and first responders) against potential biological agents may be warranted. This treatment will depend on the availability of such treatment and its effectiveness against the agent involved, e.g. immunization will be an important means of controlling an outbreak of smallpox or plague, and all those who enter hospitals where patients are housed and treated should be immunized against these diseases.

Because immunity generally takes several weeks to develop fully after vaccination, drugs (antibiotics) and symptomatic care may be the mainstay of management. Immune serum may be used to confer passive immunity.

If stockpiles of antibiotics or vaccines have been prepared or identified, plans for their distribution must be activated. In essence, the choice is either to take the drug to the potentially exposed person or for the person to come to the drug. The latter option generally requires fewer personnel. The stocks should be larger than needed to treat only those exposed because it may be difficult to distinguish between those who have actually been exposed and those who simply believe themselves to have been exposed. Cases may be much greater in number than the total number of available hospital beds and additional care facilities may need to be established.

International assistance

The management of a large-scale outbreak, whether of natural, accidental or intentional origin, will be beyond the resources of many countries. An early decision to enlist the assistance of international aid (see Chapter 6) may save many lives. WHO is able to offer public health assistance to countries experiencing outbreaks of infectious disease, and such aid will be available regardless of the source of the outbreak.

Monitoring the outbreak

Because of the delay in the onset of symptoms, the movement of exposed individuals during the incubation period and the possibility that a transmissible disease agent has been used, outbreaks may affect a large area. Efficient and coordinated collection of national data will therefore be necessary to track the outbreak, and to direct resources to the areas most in need. Again, good public health and near-real-time surveillance programmes will be essential in monitoring, irrespective of whether the causative agent has appeared naturally or been spread deliberately.

Follow-up activities

The sequelae of a biological attack may be present for many years after the incident. Careful case identification, record keeping and monitored follow-up will be required both from the practical viewpoint of comprehensive medical care and because of the need to study such incidents and improve preventive and response measures. Outside the medical field, follow-up forensic or arms-control activities may also be appropriate.

Risk communication and distribution of information

Because of the potential for widespread fear and panic following a biological incident, the provision of clear and accurate information on the risks to the public is essential. People must be told that medical evaluation and treatment are available and how to obtain them. If preventive measures are available to minimize the chance of exposure and infection, the public must be clearly and rapidly informed.

If the incident involves the release of a potential airborne agent from a specific point, and if there is time to issue a warning, an appropriately prepared room or building may possibly provide some protection from a biological agent cloud for those living nearby. A sealed area may be improvised by moving into a single room and sealing openings with adhesive tape. Wet towels or clothing can also be pressed into gaps to make a seal. Such improvisation, however, needs to be accompanied by an understanding of its limitations, including its potential dangers. Thus, simulations have shown that improvised shelter within buildings may only be beneficial initially, and that the total dose of the substance indoors may eventually approach or even exceed that receivable outdoors. People should therefore leave the shelter as soon as the cloud has passed, but this will not be easy to determine in the absence of agent detectors. If improvised protection is to be recommended, it must be well considered, communicated, understood and practised before any release actually occurs.

It is unlikely that military or approved industrial masks will be widely available (or, indeed, appropriate) for the local population. If respiratory protection is considered appropriate, oronasal particulate or smog masks, or even improvised multilayer cloth filters, will provide some degree of protection.

Command, control and communication

The response mechanisms described for biological incidents may involve a large number of different groups. Effective coordination and training are essential if such a multidisciplinary response is to be successful. The person who will be in overall command at each level of responsibility must therefore be identified in advance and must be an individual who is able to exert the necessary authority over the various parties involved in the response. This requirement may be in conflict with other considerations, e.g. the law-enforcement officers who usually take overall responsibility for the response in criminal incidents may not have the necessary background and expertise to deal with biological or chemical incidents. A high-level, authoritative overall command, directly supported by appropriate trained technical and specialist advisers who will ensure that the specific features of the incident are given appropriate consideration, must therefore be established.

4.3.4   Response to chemical incidents

The activities required in response to a chemical attack can be identified, as described above for biological incidents, by following the steps of the risk analysis process. This process is described in more detail in Appendix 4.1.

Table 4.3	**Major response activities for chemical attack**	
Assess the risks	Use rapid chemical detection and identification techniques to determine the causative chemical agent (hazard identification)
	Recruit the aid of specialists for definitive identification, needed for forensic and legal purposes
	With initial response initiated (see below), activate more detailed assessments regarding dose–response relationships, exposure assessment and risk characterizations (see Appendix 4.1)
Manage the risks (introduction of risk-reduction/control measures)	Protect responders
	Control contamination: establish "hot-zone" scene control to limit contamination spread; conduct immediate operational decontamination onsite, and decontamination of all persons leaving the "hot-zone"
	Conduct casualty triage
	Ensure medical care and evacuation of casualties
	Conduct definitive decontamination of the site
Monitor all activities	Decide whether local and national resources are adequate, and whether international assistance should be sought
	Continuously monitor the residual hazard level on the site, and adjust response activities as needed
	Repeat the risk-assessment/management process as required
	Implement follow-up activities (e.g. of long-term injuries and rehabilitation)
Communicate the risks	Implement a risk-communication programme for the affected population that conveys information and instructions as needed

The following discussion summarizes some of the most important considerations in the activities listed in Table 4.3. Sources of more detailed information that may be needed by response planners are given in Annex 6.

Hazard identification

Detection and identification are necessary to determine the nature of the chemical hazard being confronted, if any. It begins with the reasoned and logical application of observation skills, including the analysis of all the available information, the appearance and function of delivery devices, the appearance and odour of the substance itself (if it is an overt release), and the signs and symptoms of those who have been exposed. It is instructive to note that, after the terrorist chemical attacks in Japan, the recognition of characteristic symptoms by emergency medical personnel provided the first indication that nerve gas had been released. This clinical diagnosis guided response activities for some time before analysis confirmed the nature of the chemical used (see Appendix 4.2).

Detection strategies may include the use of a variety of devices that can provide an early indication of the agent involved. This is needed to guide initial operational response activities. A large variety of devices are available, ranging from simple colour-changing paper to sophisticated electronic contamination monitors. The choice of detection equipment must be guided by the preparedness phase risk assessment, and specific local requirements. Detection strategies must be linked to warning or alert mechanisms that will be used to activate response, whether by primary responders, specialist responders or the population. Decisions are needed on the basic philosophy of response activation. The approach whereby all suspicious incidents are treated as chemical attacks until proved otherwise may be warranted in high-risk scenarios (as exemplified by the Israeli attitude towards Scud missiles during the Gulf War). Lower-risk scenarios may be more efficiently dealt with by an approach calling for further response only if chemical detection tests are positive.

Definitive identification of chemicals used will involve a longer-term forensically based analytical process, requiring the use of sophisticated laboratory facilities. Such identification will be needed both as evidence and to determine the appropriate strategic response. As with other crimes, chemical attacks require the integration of the forensic investigation with rescue and medical operations. Response personnel must operate without disturbing the integrity of the crime scene, while forensic investigators need to allow rescue efforts to proceed effectively. For example, responders must be careful to maintain chain of custody procedures with clothes and personal effects that may be removed as part of the decontamination process. This will allow later use of such objects in an international investigation or a criminal trial.

Under the provisions of the CWC, Member States of OPCW can initiate an "investigation of alleged use", whereby an international inspection team will undertake a complete investigation of an incident, including sampling followed by analysis, making use of a worldwide network of laboratories accredited specifically for this purpose. Such investigative procedures have been practised but not yet invoked.

In an overt chemical release, an important component of exposure assessment is the prediction of the spread of the agent cloud. This will be useful in deciding where to focus protective and incident-management procedures. A variety of computerized prediction models are available to assist with this process. Depending on their sophistication, they take account to a varying degree of agent characteristics, nature of release (point or line source, instantaneous or continuous), initial concentration, wind and weather conditions, and topography to produce predictions of spread. Isopleths indicate the position of expected concentrations over time, and can be used to indicate where effects are likely to be greatest and to direct the deployment of resources.

Where high-risk areas have been identified during the pre-incident preparedness phase, it is possible to use computerized models that take into account the specific local topography and population distribution. This enables more precise information to be generated on the numbers of casualties that may result as the cloud spreads, and the available resources to be deployed to appropriate sites.

While such models may be useful as planning tools, their limitations must also be appreciated. Results tend to be more accurate when wind speeds are higher, wind speed and direction are constant, and local topography is relatively flat. Wide and commonly occurring variations in these and other relevant variables, however, often reduce the accuracy of predictions to the level of generalized estimates.

Protection of responders

Individual protective equipment (IPE) must be available to responders and must allow them to carry out a wide range of activities in a contaminated area without becoming casualties themselves. Many types of IPE are available, ranging from simple aprons and half-mask respiratory protection to fully encapsulating self-contained impermeable ensembles. The types that are stockpiled, and the choice of IPE for particular incidents, will depend on the risk assessment and the nature of the chemicals involved. In areas where the threat is significant, it may be necessary to make collective protection facilities available, i.e. large protected areas supplied with filtered air where people can shelter without the need for IPE. An outstanding example of this approach can be found in Switzerland, where threat assessments during the Cold War era led to the construction of a network of public and private collective protection facilities capable of sheltering the majority of the population in times of need. A more detailed discussion of the issues surrounding protection can be found in Annex 4.

Contamination control

The most distinctive element of disaster management for chemical incidents is contamination control, which requires:

• the rapid establishment of a well demarcated "hot zone" (with clearly visible "clean" and "dirty" areas);

• the limitation of contamination spread by means of strictly controlled entry and exit procedures;

• on-site decontamination procedures, ensuring that all persons or items leaving the dirty areas are cleaned and monitored before entering the clean environment.

Patients should be decontaminated as soon as possible, and before transport to specialized facilities (to avoid the contamination of vehicles and overburdened accident and emergency departments). However, the nature of human response to mass casualty incidents is such that many patients are likely to arrive at medical centres on vehicles other than those of the emergency services, bypassing on-site decontamination facilities. For this reason, triage at casualty reception centres should also incorporate decontamination.

Triage

Triage will need to include casualty-reception procedures suitable for contamination control purposes, since conventional triage techniques will not be adequate during a chemical incident. Normally, medical personnel separate the triage and treatment phases of a response, but because of the rapidity of onset of effects with some chemical agents, responders to a chemical incident may be required to triage and administer antidotes simultaneously. As with any mass casualty situation, it will be necessary to ensure that potentially limited resources are used to help those who are most likely to benefit from them. This can lead to difficult triage decisions, requiring the attention of the most experienced clinical personnel available. Depending on the casualty load, it may be necessary to activate additional accident and emergency departments and hospital beds to handle the sudden influx. It must be expected that many more will seek treatment than were actually exposed. Psychological support teams should be available to provide assistance, thereby reducing the number of people occupying hospital beds.

Medical care and evacuation of casualties

Medical care includes prophylaxis (pre-exposure treatment measures for high-risk personnel to prevent or minimize the effects of exposure), diagnosis and treatment.

There are not many examples of true prophylaxis, but certain medications (e.g. pyridostigmine bromide) can improve the response to treatment of those affected by nerve agents. However, such medications can have adverse side-effects, and case-by-case decisions on their use will be needed. They will normally be used only by military personnel in wartime or by emergency responders who must be able to work in a high-risk area known to be contaminated with liquid nerve agent.

Specific diagnostic aids may be required for detecting exposure to chemical warfare agents, ranging from established techniques, such as the observation of typical symptoms and the measurement of acetylcholinesterase activity (after nerve agent exposure), to newer advanced techniques, such as the detection of specific DNA adducts (after mustard gas exposure).

Initial prehospital treatment will provide symptomatic and life-saving support to allow decontamination and transport to medical centres. If the nature of the substance is known, specific treatment protocols may be required for on-site emergency antidote administration (possibly using auto-injectors), and definitive treatment of the medium- and long-term effects of exposure. As for all response measures, detailed discussion of medical protocols is outside the scope of this publication, but references to the relevant literature can be found in Annex 6.

Definitive decontamination

The decontamination strategies described above are aimed at meeting immediate operational needs, and minimizing the spread of contamination during response activities. Once the immediate manifestations of the incident have been dealt with, a final decontamination of the site will be required. This is a specialized activity and will usually need to be handled by specialist response units.

International assistance

National authorities will have to decide at an early stage whether to seek international assistance, either for the management of the incident or in order to draw international attention to it. As for many other aspects of the response to a chemical incident, Member States of OPCW have access to a carefully considered package of international assistance measures (see Chapter 6). Because of the instability of some chemicals and the transient nature of their effects, this assistance must be mobilized as quickly as possible.

Monitoring of the residual hazard

There will be an ongoing need to evaluate the hazard remaining in the contaminated area, the risk it poses to response activities, and when the area can be reopened to the public without further risk. Monitoring must continue until the "all clear" has been sounded, i.e. after definitive decontamination and certification of the removal of all residual hazard. This will be the task of specialists in the management of hazardous-materials incidents.

Follow-up

While the immediate problem after a chemical attack will be the management of the acute effects of exposure, some chemical agents have long-term effects that may appear over a period of many years (see section 3.6.2). Well-organized and well-administered follow-up programmes are therefore required, not only for the benefit of the patients, but also for the advancement of medical science in this area. An outstanding example of what may be required is the extensive patient follow-up programme still being implemented by Iranian public health authorities, many years after the exposure of individuals to chemical weapons during the war between Iraq and the Islamic Republic of Iran in the 1980s *(22–23)*.

Risk communication and distribution of information

If it is suspected that the hazard may spread to affect the downwind population (as predicted in the hazard evaluation step above), a warning and public address system will need to be activated. This may provide evacuation instructions, or information on what people should do to protect themselves against the potential spread of the hazard. Even if the hazard is not expected to spread, a large-scale incident is likely to generate widespread fear and public reaction. Rapid distribution of accurate and helpful information is essential if panic is to be avoided.

Depending on circumstances, it may be considered advisable for the population to stay indoors and to close all windows and doors. A sealed area might be improvised (as described in section 4.3.3 on pages 75–76 above for sealed areas for protection from biological agents, and with the same limitations).

Command, control, and communication

The response mechanisms described above may involve a large number of different groups. Effective coordination of this multidisciplinary response is essential for successful results. As mentioned in the preceding discussion, response is likely to involve the usual primary responders (ambulance teams, firefighters, police, etc.), specialist responders (such as military chemical defence units) and the public. Overall site command must be assigned to an authority able to exercise the control required to limit the hazard and to achieve the required coordination of all the groups involved.

REFERENCES

1. United Nations International Strategy for Disaster Reduction. *Living with risk: a global review of disaster reduction initiatives*, July 2002 (available at *http://www.unisdr.org*).

2. *Community emergency preparedness: a manual for managers and policy-makers*. Geneva, World Health Organization, 1999.

3. Grein TW et al. Rumors of disease in the global village: outbreak verification. *Emerging Infectious Diseases*, 2000, 6(2):97–102.

4. *Natural disasters: protecting the public's health*. Washington, DC, Pan American Health Organization, 2000 (Scientific Publication No. 575).

5. Norlander L et al., eds. *A FOA briefing book on biological weapons*. Umeå, National Defence Research Establishment, 1995.

6. Ivarsson U, Nilsson H, Santesson J, eds. *A FOA briefing book on chemical weapons: threat, effects, and protection*. Umeå, National Defence Research Establishment, 1992.

7. Inglesby TV et al. Observations from the Top Off exercise. *Public Health Reports*, 2001, 116(Suppl. 2):64–68.

8. Henderson DA, Inglesby TV, O'Toole T. Shining light on Dark Winter. *Clinical Infectious Diseases*, 2002, 34:972–983.

9. Török TJ et al. A large community outbreak of salmonellosis caused by intentional contamination of restaurant salad bars. *Journal of the American Medical Association*, 1997, 278(5):389–395.

10. Carus WS. The Rajneeshees (1984). In: Tucker JB, ed. *Toxic terror: assessing terrorist use of chemical and biological weapons*. Cambridge, MA, MIT Press, 2000, 115–137.

11. Sidell FR, Patrick WC, Dashiell TR. *Jane's chem-bio handbook*. Alexandria, VA, Jane's Information Group, 1998.

12. APIC Bioterrorism Task Force, Centers for Disease Control Hospital Infections Program Bioterrorism Working Group. *Bioterrorism readiness plan: a template for healthcare facilities*. Atlanta, GA, Centers for Disease Control and Prevention, 1999 (available at *www.cdc.gov/ncidod/hip/Bio/13apr99APIC-CDCBioterrorism.PDF* and at *http://www.apic.org/educ/readinow.html*).

13. Brès P. *Public health action in emergencies caused by epidemics: a practical guide*. Geneva, World Health Organization, 1986.

14. Meselson M et al. The Sverdlovsk anthrax outbreak of 1979. *Science,* 1994, 266:1202–1208.

15. Guillemin J. *Anthrax: the investigation of a deadly outbreak.* Berkeley, CA, University of California Press, 1999.

16. Garner JS. *Guidelines for isolation precautions in hospitals.* Atlanta, GA, Centers for Disease Control and Prevention, Hospital Infection Control Advisory Committee, 1996.

17. *Infection control for viral haemorrhagic fevers in the African health care setting.* Geneva, World Health Organization, 1998 (document WHO/EMC/ESR/98.2).

18. Mitscherlich E, Marth EH. *Microbial survival on the environment.* Berlin, Springer-Verlag, 1984.

19. *Guidelines for the collection of clinical specimens during field investigation of outbreaks.* Geneva, World Health Organization, 2000 (document WHO/CDS/CSR/EDC/2000.4).

20. Dunsmore DJ. *Safety measures for use in outbreaks of communicable disease.* Geneva, World Health Organization, 1986.

21. *International Health Regulations (1969) adopted by the Twenty-second World Health Assembly in 1969 and amended by the Twenty-sixth World Health Assembly in 1973 and the Thirty-fourth World Health Assembly in 1981 (3rd annotated ed.).* Geneva, World Health Organization, 1969. Full text also available on WHO web site *(http://www.who.org).*

22. Sohrabpour H. The current status of mustard gas victims in Iran. *ASA Newsletter,* 1995, 47(1):14–15.

23. Khateri S. Statistical views on late complications of chemical weapons on Iranian CW victims. *ASA Newsletter,* 2001, 85:16–19.

APPENDIX 4.1: PRINCIPLES OF RISK ANALYSIS

Responding to biological or chemical attacks is a multidisciplinary and complex task. With an array of issues and questions, a means of ordering and prioritizing an approach to response is needed. The requisite response activities, and a logically ordered sequence for their implementation, can be identified using the risk analysis approach. This is an organized way in which to identify and evaluate hazardous conditions, and to take actions to eliminate, reduce or control the risk(s) posed by such conditions. These steps can be used to structure planning, and to identify areas needing attention during both the pre-attack "preparedness" phase, and the post-warning or post-attack "response" phase (and is the way in which the preceding chapter was structured). Although some detailed considerations for biological and chemical agents may differ (e.g. population vulnerability may be a more important consideration for biological than for chemical agents), the basic principles of approach remain the same.

The risk analysis approach is generally accepted to consist of risk assessment, risk management and risk communication. In this Appendix, risk assessment and risk management are further described inasmuch as they are applicable to chemical incidents. Risk communication has been detailed in the chapter itself.

Risk assessment

Risk assessment includes hazard identification, hazard characterization (dose–response), exposure and consequence assessment, and risk characterization.

The first, and perhaps most difficult step in the process is to identify all hazardous conditions. Risk cannot be controlled unless hazardous conditions are recognized before they cause injury, damage to equipment or other accident. Once a hazardous condition is recognized it must be evaluated to determine the threat or risk it presents. The level of risk is a function of the probability of exposure to the hazard and the severity of the potential harm that would be caused by that exposure. Some hazards may present very little risk to people or equipment (e.g. a toxic chemical well enclosed in a strong container). Other hazards may cause death or serious injury if not controlled (e.g. a toxic chemical that has spilled into a busy workspace). In these two examples, the former situation carries a much lower probability of exposure than the latter. Even though the hazardous chemical may be the same substance, and the harm caused by exposure would be similar, the lower probability of exposure in the first situation results in a lower risk.

Chemicals generally can be divided into two groups: (i) chemicals causing toxic effects for which it is generally considered that there is a dose, exposure or concentration below which adverse effects will not occur (e.g. a chemical causing organ-specific, neurological/behavioural, immunological, non-genotoxic carcinogenesis, reproductive or developmental effects); and (ii) chemicals causing other types of effect, for which it is assumed that there is some probability of harm at any level of exposure – this currently applies primarily for mutagenesis and carcinogenesis. Many chemicals have been evaluated and the literature offers guidance values of levels of exposure below which it is believed that there are no adverse effects (i.e. threshold substances) and risks per unit exposure for those chemicals for which it is believed that there is a risk for health at any level of exposure (i.e. non-threshold substances).

Exposure or precursors of exposure such as concentrations in air, water or food can be measured and/or modelled. Transport and fate of chemical agents depends on their physico-chemical properties and can vary dramatically. During the risk-assessment phase of an incident, it is important to measure and/or model actual or future concentration/exposure/dose, as well as the spread of the causative chemical agent.

Risk characterization aims to provide a synthesis of the intrinsic (eco)toxicological properties of the causative chemical derived from hazard identification and dose–response relationship assessment with the actual or prognostic exposure. It takes into account uncertainties and provides the major input for making risk-management decisions. The process involves comparison of the outcome of the dose–response relationship assessment with the outcome of the risk assessment in order to characterize the risk with which populations are faced so as to recognize potential adverse health outcomes (e.g. there is a high, moderate or low risk).

Risk management

Risk management encompasses all those activities required to reach and implement decisions on risk reduction or elimination. Once a risk has been characterized, an informed decision can be made as to what control measures, if any, are needed to reduce the risks or eliminate the hazard. Control measures can consist of any action for risk reduction or elimination. Usually, however, control measures involve reducing the probability of occurrence or the severity of an incident. When toxic chemicals or infectious organisms are involved, control measures usually include administrative measures, engineering controls or physical protection. There is more detailed discussion of these measures in Annex 4. Control measures must be implemented before personnel or equipment are exposed to the hazardous condition. When controls are implemented, care must be taken to ensure that new hazardous conditions are not introduced as a result of the control measures.

There is no such thing as "no risk". It may not always be possible to control all hazardous conditions completely. When some risk remains, a conscious decision must be made at the proper level as to whether the remaining risk is an "acceptable risk". The concept of "acceptable risk" should not be unfamiliar as it is part of daily life. Everyone accepts a certain degree of risk in order to accomplish something beneficial. There is risk associated with flying on a commercial aeroplane. Most people (but not all) will accept the very small chance of an aeroplane accident in exchange for being able to reach their destination quickly.

The potential benefit to be gained from accepting a risk must always be worth the potential consequences of the risk itself. In some cases, a high potential benefit may justify acceptance of a risk that would normally be unacceptable. Unnecessary risk, risk taken without a potential benefit, or risk taken without an appropriate risk assessment must not be accepted. The decision to accept risk must always be made at the proper level. If the evaluated worst-case result of an accident during a particular activity was, for example a minor injury, it might be appropriate for an on-site supervisor or area manager to accept the risk and to proceed without further hazard control measures. At the other end of the spectrum, a decision that could place the lives of many people in jeopardy should be made only at the highest level of authority. Of course, one never plans for an injury. Risk-reduction measures are always applied. What is referred to here is the consequence of an unexpected occurrence of an accident, despite taking reasonable precautions. If the residual risk is still assessed as being too high, the risk-control process needs to be repeated to lower the probability of occurrence or consequence of exposure even further.

A fundamental principle must always be observed when addressing "acceptable risk". The number of personnel exposed to a hazardous condition, the amount of time for which they are exposed, and the level/concentration of hazard to which they are exposed must always be kept to the absolute minimum required to accomplish the task.

When applying the concept of "acceptable risk" to the possibility of chemical or biological attack, the level of residual risk that can be accepted will depend on the circumstances of the region concerned. One country may need to address a significant risk of terrorist use of biological or chemical agents by devoting considerable resources to response. In a different part of the world, the assessed low risk of biological or chemical incidents will not justify major expenditure, and acceptance of a reduced ability to respond may be justified. Such decisions are clearly extremely difficult to take and will be influenced by political factors as well as by practical considerations.

When a risk management process is being implemented, it is crucial that the control measures should be evaluated and monitored continuously to ensure that they are working as planned. If it is found that the control measures are not effective, they must be changed or modified immediately. Effective control measures should be recorded for use in controlling similar hazardous conditions in the future. Lessons should be learned by studying simulation exercises, or similar hazards or incidents in other areas/countries, and adapting one's own risk-management programme accordingly.

APPENDIX 4.2: THE SARIN INCIDENTS IN JAPAN

On 20 March 1995, a terrorist group launched a coordinated attack with the nerve gas sarin on commuters on the Tokyo subway system. This highly publicized attack killed 12 people and caused more than 5000 to seek care. Without the prompt and massive emergency response by the Japanese authorities, and some fortunate mistakes by the terrorist group, the incident could have been much more devastating. While this is the most widely publicized incident of this type, it is not the first nerve-gas attack in Japan. In June 1994, 7 people were killed and more than 300 injured in an attack by the same group on a residential apartment building in Matsumoto. In December 1994, an opponent of the group was murdered by the skin application of VX.

This Appendix provides a brief summary of the background and features of these incidents and the lessons learned from them. It draws heavily on a number of excellent and comprehensive reviews that have appeared in the international literature *(1–6)*.

Background

The Aum Shinrikyo sect was the brainchild of Chizuo Matsumoto, whose childhood aspirations apparently included the leadership of Japan. In 1984, he started a small publishing house and yoga school, which gradually developed into a cult. He renamed himself Shoko Asahara ("Bright Light"), embarked on a course of cult expansion, with increasingly bizarre teachings and rituals for devotees, and ultimately subversion with the aim of achieving supremacy for his followers in Japan. The group attracted a surprisingly large international membership, numbering in the tens of thousands, and actively recruited graduate scientists and technicians to develop armament programmes that were highly ambitious in their scope. Plans included the development and use of biological and chemical weapons.

Aum Shinrikyo's chemical weapons made worldwide news after the Tokyo subway attack in 1995, but a quest for biological weapons actually pre-dated the chemical programme. Despite the expenditure of large sums of money and great efforts to acquire the means to develop and disseminate biological agents, attempted attacks (with botulinum toxin in April 1990 and anthrax in 1993) failed, fortunately causing no noticeable effects on the target population of Tokyo.

The cult had more success with its chemical programme, which was launched in 1993 and reportedly cost around US$ 30 million. After experiments with VX, tabun, soman, mustard gas, hydrogen cyanide and phosgene, the cult's final choice was the nerve gas sarin, and a plan was developed for the production of about 70 tonnes of this substance at Aum Shinrikyo's facilities in Kamikuisiki, at the foot of Mount Fuji.

The Matsumoto incident

During 1994, Aum Shinrikyo was involved in legal proceedings concerning a land purchase, and a gas attack on the overnight premises of the three judges involved was planned for 27 June of that year, apparently to pre-empt an unfavourable ruling. An improvised sarin-dissemination system was used, consisting of a heater, fan and drip system, sarin vapour being vented from the window of a disguised delivery van. After a 20-minute release period, the gas spread over an elliptical area measuring about 800 by 570 metres (most effects occurring within a smaller area of 400 by 300 metres). While the judges survived, 7 unfortunate residents died as a result of the attack, there were 54 other hospital admissions, and 253 persons sought care at outpatient facilities. In the absence of formal identification of the toxic substance, doctors could rely only on what they observed to guide treatment, namely clinical symptomatology consistent with organophosphate poisoning. On 4 July, an official report revealed that the cause of the poisoning had been the chemical warfare agent sarin, which had been identified by gas chromatography–mass spectrometry (GC–MS) in a water specimen taken from a pond in the affected area. No evidence found at that time incriminated Aum Shinrikyo.

The Tokyo incident

The Japanese authorities were collecting increasing evidence suggestive of Aum Shinrikyo's interest in chemical weapons. Ironically, they had been unable to prevent the suspected acquisition or production of chemical weapons' since such activities were not illegal at that time. The pretext for a raid on the suspected production plant was provided when evidence linked an Aum member to a suspected kidnapping, but cult members employed by the authorities warned Asahara of the imminent raid, for which the police were being trained in chemical defence. In an apparent attempt to dissuade the police from making the raid, an attack on the Tokyo subway system was hastily planned. On the morning of 20 March 1995, five two-man teams carried out the attack, each team consisting of one getaway driver and one subway rider. Four subway riders carried two double-layered plastic bags and one rider carried three, each bag containing about half a litre of sarin. The sarin was only about 30% pure because it had been hastily produced for use in the attack. Five subway lines converging on the station of Kasumigaseki (where many Japanese government buildings and the Tokyo Metropolitan Police Department are located) had been selected. At around 08:00, i.e. during peak commuting time, the five assailants placed their sarin-filled bags on the train floor, pierced them with sharpened umbrella tips,[7] and left the trains several stations away from Kasumigaseki.

The first emergency call was received by the Tokyo fire department at 08:09, and the emergency services were soon inundated with calls for aid from the numerous subway stations where affected passengers were disembarking and seeking medical help. A total of 131 ambulances and 1364 emergency medical technicians were dispatched, and 688 people were transported to hospital by the emergency medical and fire services. More than 4000 people found their own way to hospitals and doctors using taxis and private cars or on foot. The lack of emergency decontamination facilities and protective equipment resulted in the secondary exposure of medical staff (135 ambulance staff and 110 staff in the main receiving hospital reported symptoms).

Having initially been misinformed that a gas explosion had caused burns and carbon monoxide poisoning, medical centres began treating for organophosphate exposure based on the typical symptomatology encountered, supported by the results of tests indicating depressed acetylcholinesterase activity in symptomatic victims (see Annex 1). An official announcement by the police that sarin had been identified reached the hospitals, via the television news, about three hours after the release.

---

[7] Of the 11 bags, only 8 were actually ruptured: 3 were subsequently recovered intact. It is estimated that around 4.5 kg of sarin were released.

Overall, 12 heavily exposed commuters died, and around 980 were mildly to moderately affected, while about 500 required hospital admission. More than 5000 people sought medical assistance.

Observations

Much can be learned from the analysis of these attacks, at both the general level (i.e. in terms of the international threat), and at the specific level (i.e. in terms of the immediate effect and response).

• **Magnitude of the event.** While the human consequences of the attack should not be underestimated, they should also not be exaggerated. The frequently encountered casualty toll of "over 5000" must be seen in its true perspective. The attack was serious – 12 people died, 54 were severely injured, and around 980 were mildly to moderately affected. The majority of the 5000 seeking help, many of them with psychogenic symptoms, were (understandably) worried that they might have been exposed. This demonstrates the value of rapid information dissemination via the media in reassuring the public. It also shows the importance of effective triage at receiving centres in ensuring that medical resources are reserved for those who really have been exposed. Before this attack is taken as evidence of the effectiveness of toxic chemicals in the hands of terrorists, however, the figure of 12 dead should be compared with the death tolls of recent terrorist attacks using conventional explosives, such as the bombing of the United States embassies in Nairobi and Dar es Salaam (257), the Federal Building in Oklahoma City, USA (168), and the United States Marine barracks in Lebanon (241). These, in turn, must now be regarded as relatively slight in comparison with what happened on 11 September 2001, when hijacked long-haul passenger aircraft were flown into the Pentagon outside Washington, DC, and into each of the twin towers of the World Trade Center in New York City, killing, it is now believed, more than 3100 people. Equally, it should be realized that the sarin casualty figures might have been many times worse.

• **The utility of chemical weapons in achieving terrorist objectives.** While many reports (particularly in the media) have touted the sarin incidents as evidence of a frightening new era in terrorist methodology, a sober assessment of the actual results shows otherwise. It is true that, before 11 September 2001, this was one of the most highly publicized terrorist attacks in history. The result for Aum Shinrikyo, however, can hardly be judged a success. The immediate objective of the attack was the disruption of an anticipated raid on cult premises and, on a broader level, the incitement of social upheaval. In fact, the raid was delayed for only 48 hours, the Japanese Government remained firmly in power, and most of the cult's senior members are now in prison.

• **The ease of acquisition and use of biological and chemical weapons**. Despite its ample financial resources, equipment and expertise, and years in which to develop its weapons, Aum Shinrikyo attempted but failed to use biological agents effectively *(7–9)* and achieved only relatively limited success with its chemical programme. Aspirant terrorists thinking of using biological or chemical weapons may well find these results a deterrent, not an encouragement.

• **The importance of national legislation on chemical weapons**. Despite compelling evidence of the cult's growing interest in chemical agents, which started well before the Tokyo subway attack, no Japanese laws prohibited its activities at the time, and pre-emptive action could therefore not be taken. Since the entry into force of the CWC in 1997, however, all Member States (including Japan) have been able to share their experiences and planning concepts to fulfil their obligation to enact and implement legislation forbidding persons on their territory, or under their jurisdiction, from undertaking any activities that are prohibited to the State Party itself.[8] When such legislation has been introduced, pre-emptive action against terrorist groups developing or using chemical weapons can be taken. Likewise, the entry into force of the BWC in 1975 has obliged all its States Parties (including Japan) to take the measures necessary for its implementation

• **The importance of detection and identification abilities**. In both the Matsumoto and Tokyo incidents, medical staff had to rely on clinical observation to guide their initial treatment of victims. If portable detection apparatus had been available to emergency-response personnel, this would have facilitated the earlier identification of the nature of the event. The follow-up forensic and legal process was considerably aided by the laboratory identification of sarin using

---

8   See also Appendix 5.2.

sophisticated GC–MS techniques available to the police forensic toxicologists *(10)*. In an interesting development of new biomedical testing methods, scientists in the Netherlands were later able to retrieve sarin from the stored blood samples of 10 out of 11 of the victims of the Tokyo incident, and from 2 out of 7 samples from the Matsumoto incident – unequivocal evidence of exposure to sarin *(11)*.

• **The importance of decontamination abilities and protection.** About 10% of the ambulance staff who responded to the incident reported symptoms of exposure, as did 110 members of the staff at the major receiving hospital (although these symptoms were generally mild). A contributing factor was the lack of decontamination facilities on site and of protective equipment for initial responders and hospital staff. Before this is taken to mean that high-level protection is always required, it should be remembered that the figure of 10% reporting mild effects also means that at least 90% were not affected at all. A reasonable conclusion is that the availability of protective equipment would have been of considerable benefit to responders. However, an approach based on graded protection appropriate to the level of contamination is required to prevent the unnecessary immobilization of helpers as a result of the ergonomic problems of wearing protective clothing (see Annex 4). Rapidly deployable decontamination equipment is needed both on site (to avoid secondary contamination of emergency transport) and at receiving facilities. However, it is important to remember that the majority of people who sought medical help did so on their own initiative and using their own transport. This would have effectively negated much of the utility of on-site decontamination systems, even had they been available, as they would generally be used for victims being treated in the course of evacuation by the emergency services.

• **The importance of command, control and communication.** Communication channels available to emergency-response personnel were not able to cope with the flood of calls that the attack precipitated. In particular, overload prevented effective communications between the on-site and mobile emergency medical technicians and their supervising hospital-based doctors, whether to seek medical instructions or to determine which hospitals could receive patients. As a result, a number of patients did not benefit from interventions such as airway support, intubation or intravenous therapy until after they arrived at hospitals. The timely provision of accurate information to responders is crucial to their own safety and to their ability to provide appropriate assistance. Pre-planned systems for tapping the expert knowledge of experienced toxicologists, poison information centres and chemical warfare specialists would have been of major assistance to the receiving medical facilities. A single responsible local authority with the ability to communicate with, and coordinate the activities of, the various response elements would have been a considerable advantage. Complicated formalities and the need for high-level approval prevented the rapid mobilization of the specialists in chemical defence within the Japanese military.

• **The readiness of medical personnel to handle chemical casualties.** The majority of the Tokyo hospital staff, like medical personnel in most parts of the world, were untrained in the care of casualties caused by chemical weapons and had no immediate access to treatment protocols for the victims of such weapons. This is not something that can be left to military specialists, as it is the local hospitals that will be the first to receive the casualties. Inclusion of the effects of chemical weapons and treatment of the resulting casualties both in standard medical curricula and in the training of first responders and the staff of local hospital accident and emergency departments, is an essential component of medical preparedness for responding to chemical incidents.

Conclusions

The release of sarin by a terrorist group in Japan resulted in a highly publicized incident with mass casualties. In scale, however, it did not approach the human and environmental toll that has resulted from a number of recent terrorist attacks using conventional explosives, and it falls far short of what happened in the United States on 11 September 2001. Despite many difficulties, Japanese emergency units and local hospitals were able to achieve a remarkably rapid response, without which the casualty figures might have been considerably higher. While analysis of the event reveals a number of important lessons for authorities to consider when preparing for such incidents, it also reveals many of the technical difficulties associated with toxic chemicals and their limitations as weapons for use by terrorist groups.

REFERENCES

1. Smithson AE. Rethinking the lessons of Tokyo. In: Smithson AE, Levy LA, eds. *Ataxia: the chemical and biological terrorism threat and the US response.* Washington, DC, The Henry L. Stimson Center, 2000, 71–111 (Report No. 35).

2. Tu AT. Overview of sarin terrorist attacks in Japan. In: *Natural and selected synthetic toxins: biological implications.* Washington, DC, American Chemical Society, 2000:304–317 (American Society Symposium Series, No. 745).

3. Okumura T et al. Tokyo subway Sarin attack: disaster management. Part 1: community emergency response. *Academic Emergency Medicine,* 1998, 5:613–617.

4. Okumura T et al. Tokyo subway Sarin attack: disaster management. Part 2: hospital response. *Academic Emergency Medicine,* 1998, 5:618–624.

5. Okumura T et al. Tokyo subway Sarin attack: disaster management. Part 3: national and international responses. *Academic Emergency Medicine,* 1998, 5:625–628.

6. Kulling P. *The terrorist attack with sarin in Tokyo. Socialstyrelsen report.* Stockholm, Modin-Tryck, 2000.

7. Leitenberg M. Aum Shinrikyo's efforts to produce biological weapons. *Terrorism and Political Violence,* 1999, 11(4):149–158.

8. Smithson A, Levy LA. *Ataxia: the chemical and biological terrorism threat and the US response.* Washington, DC, The Henry L. Stimson Center, 1999.

9. Takahashi H et al. *The Kameido incident: documentation of a failed bioterrorist attack.* Poster presented at the 4th International Conference on Anthrax, St John's College, Annapolis, MD, USA, 10–13 June 2001.

10. Seto Y et al. Toxicological analysis of victims' blood and crime scene evidence samples in the Sarin gas attack caused by the Aum Shinrikyo cult. In: *Natural and selected synthetic toxins: biological implications.* Washington, DC, American Chemical Society, 2000, 318–332 (American Chemical Society Symposium Series, No. 745).

11. Polhuijs M, Langenberg JP, Benschop HP. New method for retrospective detection of exposure to organophosphorus anticholinesterases: application to alleged Sarin victims of Japanese terrorists. *Toxicology and Applied Pharmacology,* 1997, 146:156–161.

APPENDIX 4.3: THE DELIBERATE RELEASE OF ANTHRAX SPORES THROUGH THE UNITED STATES POSTAL SYSTEM

During the autumn of 2001, several letters containing spores of *Bacillus anthracis* were sent through the United States postal system, causing 11 cases of inhalational anthrax, five of them fatal, and 11 confirmed or suspected cases of non-fatal cutaneous anthrax. The first onset, of cutaneous anthrax, occurred in late September and the last, of inhalational anthrax, in mid-November. Of the four letters that were recovered, one was addressed to a television newscaster, another to the editor of a newspaper, both in the city of New York, and two were addressed to United States senators in Washington, DC.

Twenty of the 22 patients were exposed to work sites that were found to be contaminated with anthrax spores. Nine of these had worked in United States Postal Service (USPS) mail-processing facilities through which the anthrax letters had passed. Two patients, both with fatal inhalational anthrax, had no known exposure to contaminated mail or contaminated premises.

Polymerase chain reaction (PCR) tests and DNA sequencing indicated that all attacks involved the same strain of *B. anthracis*. A year after the attacks, two United States mail-processing facilities remained shut down pending decontamination, and accountability for the letters remains a mystery.

This appendix outlines some of the relevant background and summarizes information about the letters, the patients, the public health response, and the clean-up operations. Sources include reports and publications by the United States Centers for Disease Control and Prevention (CDC), the United States Federal Bureau of Investigation (FBI), and the USPS, as well as United States Congressional hearings, official statements to the press, the medical literature, and accounts of USPS officials and postal workers.

Background

In 1990, immediately before the Gulf War, the United States' concern about potential anthrax attacks led to the vaccination of more than 100 000 military personnel. In 1995, this concern was again aroused when the United Nations Special Commission (UNSCOM) learned that Iraq had been developing and testing anthrax weapons during the Kuwait War. In 1998, a programme was initiated to vaccinate all United States military personnel and a Presidential Decision Directive further defined the authority and responsibilities of United States government agencies for responding to possible biological or chemical terrorist attacks on United States civilian centres. This reaffirmed and refined a 1995 Directive designating the FBI, as assigned by the Department of Justice, as the lead agency in charge of investigation and overall response management, with authority to designate other government agencies as lead agencies for specific operational tasks. By 2001, with federal assistance, most American state and large-city governments had begun to develop plans to deal with bioterrorism and many had staged mock attacks to test local emergency response capacity.

Starting in 1997, the United States experienced an increasing number of anthrax threats and hoaxes that, by the end of 1998, were almost a daily occurrence. Prominent among these were envelopes containing various powders and materials sent through the postal service to abortion and reproductive health clinics, government offices, and other locations. Until the events of autumn 2001, none of these materials tested positive for pathogenic *B. anthracis* nor had there been a case of inhalational anthrax in the United States since 1976.

In Canada, after several anthrax hoax letters there, the Defence Research Establishment, Suffield conducted experiments during February–April 2001 to estimate the hazards arising from opening a letter containing spores of *B. anthracis*. The Canadian researchers used as a simulant spores of non-pathogenic *B. globigii*, donated by the United States Department of Defense, Dugway Proving Ground, Utah. It was found, contrary to the expectation of those conducting the tests, that large numbers of spores were released into the air upon opening an envelope containing even as little as a tenth of a gram of spores, and that large doses would be inhaled by an unprotected individual in the room in which the letter was opened. The ensuing report, released in September 2001, also warned that envelopes not thoroughly sealed could pose a threat to individuals in the mail-handling system. Following the United States anthrax-letter attacks, however, it was realized that anthrax spores might escape even from fully sealed envelopes, depending on the type and grade of paper.

Dose–response measurements over a range of doses of anthrax spores to cynomolgus monkeys conducted in the pre-1969 United States offensive biological weapons programme had shown that under the experimental conditions employed, the inhalational median lethal dose (LD_{50}) was about 4000 spores. Although other measurements carried out with monkeys under various experimental conditions gave a wide range of LD_{50} values and although there are no reliable dose–response data for inhalational anthrax in any human population, it was subsequently assumed for military planning purposes that the human LD_{50} was approximately 8000–10 000 spores. While it is self-evident that doses below the LD_{50} will infect less than 50% of an exposed population, it is not known whether inhalation of even a single spore can initiate infection, albeit with very low probability. Uncertainty regarding dose–response relationships for human populations continues to make hazard prediction for inhalational anthrax problematic.

In contrast to inadequate or insufficiently appreciated knowledge regarding the dispersibility of dry spore powders, the permeability of sealed envelopes and dose–response relationships, effective medical measures for prophylaxis and therapy of cutaneous and inhalational anthrax were established and published in the medical literature well before the anthrax-letter attacks. Long experience with human cutaneous anthrax had shown it to be readily curable with several antimicrobials. Although penicillins were recommended for treatment of cutaneous anthrax, recent studies of experimental inhalation anthrax in monkeys led to the designation of doxycycline and ciprofloxacin as the antimicrobials of choice, both for prophylaxis in cases of known or suspected exposure and, if given soon after the onset of clinical disease, as therapy. Because of the possible retention of infective spores in the lungs for many days before an infection starts, suggested by United States monkey studies and human data from the

1979 Sverdlovsk (former Soviet Union) epidemic, it was recommended that antimicrobial therapy be continued for as long as 60 days following inhalatory exposure.

The anthrax letters

All four of the recovered spore-containing envelopes were sealed with tape and postmarked from Trenton, New Jersey. Envelopes, postmarked 18 September 2001, were addressed to a National Broadcasting Company (NBC) television newscaster and to the editor of the *New York Post* at their New York City offices. Two other envelopes, postmarked 9 October 2001, were addressed to Senator Tom Daschle and Senator Patrick Leahy at their Washington offices. All four recovered envelopes were postmarked and sorted at a mail-processing facility in Hamilton Township, near Trenton, before being sent to other processing and distribution centres. Those addressed to the two senators were processed at the Brentwood facility in Washington. Both facilities were found to be heavily contaminated with anthrax spores.

There are indications that at least three additional anthrax letters were sent but were lost or discarded. There were confirmed cases of cutaneous anthrax at the offices of American Broadcasting Company (ABC) and of Columbia Broadcasting System (CBS) Television News in New York and of inhalational anthrax at American Media Incorporated (AMI) in Boca Raton, Florida. Positive nasal swabs were obtained and environmental contamination was found at all three sites, and contamination was found at several mail-processing facilities through which their mail passed. Individuals at all three locations fell ill before 9 October, making it possible that three unrecovered letters were posted together with the two recovered letters of 18 September.

Both of the letters postmarked 18 September contained identical hand-printed messages in block letters that included the words "TAKE PENACILIN NOW" [sic], and both letters postmarked 9 October contained identical messages with the words "WE HAVE THIS ANTHRAX". Given that penicillin has historically been a recommended antimicrobial therapy against anthrax, that the strain used was subsequently found to be sensitive to penicillin, and that identification of the pathogen would facilitate appropriate therapy, it appears that the perpetrator sought to convey information that would enable the recipients to take protective action.

All four recovered letters included the words "ALLAH IS GREAT" and the date "09–11–01", the day of the aircraft attacks on the World Trade Center in New York and the Pentagon in Virginia, apparently with the intention to portray the sender as an Islamic terrorist.

The two letters dated 18 September and the letter addressed to Senator Daschle were recovered from the offices of their addressees, but the letter to Senator Leahy, which had been misdirected by a mechanical error to the State Department, was discovered in November only after a search of unopened government mail collected from the United States Capitol. This was collected in 635 rubbish bags that were then sealed and individually sampled for anthrax spores. Sixty-two bags were found to be contaminated, one far more than the others. Individual examination of the letters it contained then led to the discovery of the Leahy letter.

The anthrax strain was identified as the variant called Ames, originally isolated from a diseased cow in Texas in 1981 and sent to the United States Army Research Institute for Infectious Diseases (USAMRIID) at that time. From there, it was distributed to laboratories in the United States, the United Kingdom, Canada, and elsewhere. The 9 October letters contained a highly pure preparation of anthrax spores, almost entirely free of debris, while the 18 September material was decidedly less pure, containing an appreciable proportion of vegetative *B. anthracis* cells. No additives have been confirmed to have been present. Carbon isotope ratio analysis of the material in the Leahy envelope indicated that it had been produced within the two years preceding its mailing.

The patients

On or about 25 September, an assistant in the office where the NBC anthrax letter had been received and taken into custody by the FBI developed a lesion diagnosed by her physician as possibly being cutaneous anthrax, but this was not confirmed by laboratory testing until 12 October. The first case to reach public notice was that of an AMI photo editor in Florida. After an illness of several days, he died of inhalational anthrax on 5 October, one day after laboratory confirmation of the diagnosis by the Florida Department of Health and CDC. Although the federal authorities at first considered naturally occurring anthrax infection to be a possibility, the discovery of environmental contamination at AMI caused the FBI on 7 October to declare the site a crime scene. On 1 October, a second AMI employee, a mailroom worker, was hospitalized with a misdiagnosis of community-acquired pneumonia, later diagnosed as anthrax by laboratory testing on 15 October. He recovered and was discharged on 23 October.

Of the 22 confirmed or suspect cases, 12 (eight inhalational and four cutaneous) were mail handlers. These included nine USPS workers, two media company mailroom workers, and an employee in the State Department mailroom through which the Leahy letter had mistakenly passed. An additional case of cutaneous anthrax was a Texas laboratory worker engaged in testing samples from the outbreak.

Recorded onsets of symptoms fall into two clusters, 22 September–1 October and 14 October–14 November, with a 12-day gap between with no recorded onsets (Table 4.4). The two clusters may reflect the two dates on which the recovered letters were posted. Most of the inhalational cases (9 of the 11) were in the second cluster, six of them being USPS workers. This concentration of inhalational cases in the second cluster and among postal workers may reflect differences in the spore preparations; greater inhalatory exposure in mail-processing facilities, where sorting and cleaning operations generate aerosols, and/or differences between work sites in the time elapsed between exposure and the start of antimicrobial prophylaxis.

In the first cluster, 22 September–1 October, seven patients developed confirmed or suspected cutaneous anthrax. None of these cases was diagnosed by laboratory testing until 12 October or later. Overall, the time between onset and laboratory diagnosis ranged from 2 to 26 days for cutaneous anthrax and from 3 to 16 days for inhalational anthrax, with laboratory diagnosis becoming more prompt as the outbreak progressed. Although cutaneous anthrax was diagnosed by laboratory testing in two workers at the Hamilton mail-processing facility on 18 and 19 October (after which the facility was closed), the risk from leaking envelopes was not understood by officials in time to prevent inhalational anthrax in two Hamilton employees and in four employees at Brentwood (which closed on 21 October), two of whom died.

The last two cases, both inhalational and both fatal, had recorded onsets of 25 October and 14 November. Unlike any of the earlier infections, there was no known link to the anthrax letters and no evidence of environmental contamination. In the first of these perplexing cases, an employee at a New York hospital died on 31 October. Although her workplace had housed a temporary mailroom, no contamination was found there. In the second case, a 94-year-old woman residing in Connecticut died on 21 November. Whatever the source of the pathogen, these two cases emphasize the possibility that, with very low probability, perhaps depending on the health status and age of the individual, even small numbers of inhaled spores may initiate infection.

No onset of any form of anthrax was recorded among personnel at any site after they were instructed to start antimicrobial prophylaxis. Six patients diagnosed with inhalational anthrax who were admitted to hospital with only prodromal symptoms and were given antimicrobials active against B. anthracis survived. These observations are consistent with pre-existing experimental and clinical evidence and indicate that antimicrobial prophylaxis prevented clinical disease in exposed people, limiting the extent and duration of the outbreak, and that antimicrobial therapy, when begun soon after onset, prevented death.

Public health response

Most cases were detected through self-reporting and from unsolicited reports from clinical laboratories and clinicians, with the assistance of active surveillance established by local public health authorities.

After laboratory confirmation of cutaneous anthrax in an NBC employee on 12 October, an Emergency Operations Center was established at CDC to organize teams of epidemiologists and laboratory and logistics staff to support local, state and federal health investigations. Investigators responded to reports of possible cases from clinicians, law enforcement officials, and the general public.

Local and federal agencies, including the Office of the Attending Physician, United States Congress, implemented the rapid distribution of antimicrobials (ciprofloxacin and doxycycline) to individuals after an inhalational anthrax risk was officially estimated at specific sites. The United States National Pharmaceutical Stockpile, mandated by the United States Congress in 1999, facilitated the emergency availability of drugs to some 32 000 people who were potentially exposed. Altogether, National Pharmaceutical Stockpile teams distributed some 3.75 million antimicrobial tablets. Those presumed to be at higher risk were advised to remain on a prolonged course of 60 days and were encouraged to participate in a follow-up study conducted by CDC through a private contractor. At that time, they were also given the option of anthrax vaccination. Public health officials were candid about the limited data supporting the efficacy of post-exposure vaccination. Fewer than 100 people, many of them Senate staff, took advantage of the offer.

During the crisis, collection and testing of environmental and clinical samples, as well as materials from suspicious incidents and hoaxes, placed an immense burden on the FBI, Defense Department, CDC, and public health laboratories throughout the United States. The magnitude of the clinical and environmental testing undertaken would have quickly overwhelmed the United States national capacity had a significant investment not already been made in expanding laboratory training and capacity through a system called the Laboratory Response Network. This links state and local public health laboratories with advanced capacity clinical, military, veterinary, agricultural, and water- and food-testing laboratories. Established in 1999, it operates as a network of laboratories with progressively more stringent levels of technical proficiency, safety, and containment necessary to perform the essential rule-out, rule-in, and referral functions required for agent identification. The network consists of 100 core and advanced capacity public health laboratories and two higher-level laboratories, at USAMRIID and at the CDC National Center for Infectious Diseases.

During the acute phase of the outbreak, Laboratory Response Network laboratories processed and tested more than 120 000 environmental and clinical specimens for *B. anthracis*. This was accomplished chiefly by state and local public health laboratories, USAMRIID, the Naval

Medical Research Center and CDC. Forensic tests and analyses of the recovered anthrax-contaminated envelopes and their contents and of control materials were conducted by the FBI, Northern Arizona University, USAMRIID, Lawrence Livermore National Laboratory, Sandia National Laboratories and several other facilities. Epidemiological investigations were performed or coordinated by CDC.

Environmental contamination and decontamination

FBI, CDC, and USPS personnel and contractors collected surface samples from diverse locations, including offices, postal facilities and private homes. Samples collected from adjacent surfaces by swipes with wet cotton or rayon gauze and by vacuum collection through high-efficiency particulate arresting (HEPA) filters gave reasonably concordant results, but dry swipes consistently gave far less agreement and were judged unacceptable. At some sites, air sampling was also conducted. Contamination was found in at least 23 postal facilities and post offices, nearly all in New Jersey, New York, Washington, and south Florida but also as distant as Kansas City. The risk of disease associated with any level of air or surface contamination remained undefined, though more valid sampling and risk estimates quickly became a high priority for United States public health officials.

USPS mail-processing facilities were the most extensively affected environments. Mechanical agitation and air turbulence produced by high-speed sorting equipment and the use (now discontinued) of compressed air to clean machines undoubtedly contributed to the creation of dangerous aerosols and high levels of surface contamination. The Hart Senate Office Building was decontaminated with gaseous chlorine dioxide and is again in operation. After a year, the Brentwood and Hamilton mail-processing facilities remained closed, pending decontamination. In order to reduce potentially contaminated dust and aerosols from the atmosphere in its facilities, the USPS has introduced some 16 000 HEPA vacuum machines and, as a precaution, routinely sterilizes mail going to federal agencies by electron-beam irradiation. For the two fiscal years 2003–2004, it has budgeted US$ 1.7 billion for additional modifications and improvements in its ability to protect the health of its workers and to prevent pathogens and other hazardous substances from being distributed through the mail.

Table 4.4. Postal anthrax attacks 2001: demographic, clinical and exposure characteristics of the 22 cases

Case number	Date of onset of symptoms	Date of anthrax diagnosis by laboratory testing	State[a] (attack sites)	Age (years)	Sex[a]	Race[a]	Occupation[a]	Case status	Anthrax presentation	Outcome
1	22 September	19 October	NY	31	F	W	New York Post employee	Suspect	Cutaneous	Alive
2	25 September	12 October	NY	38	F	W	NBC anchor assistant	Confirmed	Cutaneous	Alive
3	26 September	18 October	NJ	39	M	W	USPS machine mechanic	Suspect	Cutaneous	Alive
4	28 September	15 October	FL	73	M	W/H	AMI mailroom worker	Confirmed	Inhalational	Alive
5	28 September	18 October	NJ	45	F	W	USPS mail carrier	Confirmed	Cutaneous	Alive
6	28 September	12 October	NY	23	F	W	NBC television news intern	Suspect	Cutaneous	Alive
7	29 September	15 October	NY	0.6	M	W	Child of ABC employee	Confirmed	Cutaneous	Alive
8	30 September	04 October	FL	63	M	W	AMI photo editor	Confirmed	Inhalational	Dead (5 October)
9	01 October	18 October	NY	27	F	W	CBS anchor assistant	Confirmed	Cutaneous	Alive
10	14 October	19 October	NJ	35	M	W	USPS mail processor	Confirmed	Cutaneous	Alive
11	14 October	28 October	NJ	56	F	B	USPS mail processor	Confirmed	Inhalational	Alive

Table 4.4. (continued) Postal anthrax attacks 2001: demographic, clinical and exposure characteristics of the 22 cases

12	15 October	29 October	NJ	43	F	A	USPS mail processor	Confirmed	Inhalational	Alive
13	16 October	21 October	DC	56	M	B	USPS mail worker	Confirmed	Inhalational	Alive
14	16 October	23 October	DC	55	M	B	USPS mail worker	Confirmed	Inhalational	Dead (21 October)
15	16 October	26 October	DC	47	M	B	USPS mail worker	Confirmed	Inhalational	Dead (22 October)
16	16 October	22 October	DC	56	M	B	USPS mail worker	Confirmed	Inhalational	Alive
17	17 October	29 October	NJ	51	F	W	Bookkeeper	Confirmed	Cutaneous	Alive
18	19 October	22 October	NY	34	M	W/H	New York Post mail handler	Suspect	Cutaneous	Alive
19	22 October	25 October	DC	59	M	W	Government mail processor	Confirmed	Inhalational	Alive
20	23 October	28 October	NY	38	M	W	New York Post employee	Confirmed	Cutaneous	Alive
21	25 October	30 October	NY	61	F	A	Hospital supply worker	Confirmed	Inhalational	Dead (31 October)
22	14 November	21 November	CT	94	F	W	Retired at home	Confirmed	Inhalational	Dead (21 November)

[a] NY, New York; NJ, New Jersey; FL, Florida; DC, District of Columbia; CT, Connecticut; F, female; M, male; W, white; W/H, white with Hispanic ethnicity; B, black; A, Asian; NBC, National Broadcasting Company; USPS, United States Postal Service; AMI, American Media Inc.; CBS, Columbia Broadcasting System.

Adapted from Jernigan DB et al. Investigation of bioterrorism-related anthrax, United States, 2001: epidemiologic findings. *Emerging Infectious Diseases*, 2002, 8(10):1019–1028 (available at http://www.cdc.gov/ncidod/EID/vol8no10/02-0353.htm).

5. LEGAL ASPECTS

National and international law was identified in Chapter 2 as an essential component of the array of measures serving to protect against the hostile release of biological or chemical agents, and to help to mitigate the consequences should such a release nevertheless take place. The present chapter describes the pertinent features of that law. At the international level, the most important legal instruments are the BWC and the CWC. Both provide for international cooperation in order to prevent the use of chemical and biological weapons, and for assistance and cooperation where breaches of these treaties are suspected, especially when such weapons have been used. The chapter begins with an account of the Geneva Protocol of 1925, which for several decades was the principal international treaty in the field. The two conventions are then described in turn, information being given about the international obligations that they establish and the national measures required to fulfil those obligations. The status of individual WHO Member States under the three treaties is set out in Annex 7.

5.1   The 1925 Geneva Protocol

At least since the early 1600s, international law has condemned what would nowadays be regarded as biological or chemical warfare, instances of which have been reported since antiquity. Subsequent development of that law *(1)* can be seen in the Brussels Declaration of 1874, which outlawed, inter alia, the use of poison or poisoned weapons, and again at the Hague Peace Conference of 1899, where agreement was reached to "abstain from the use of projectiles the sole object of which is the diffusion of asphyxiating or deleterious gases". The 1899 Conference also adopted a convention that enunciated in treaty form the Brussels Declaration's prohibition of the use of poison or poisoned weapons in land warfare, a prohibition that was later included in the 1907 Hague Convention IV concerning the laws and customs of war on land. Following the extensive use of chemical weapons, such as chlorine and mustard gas, during the First World War, the international community agreed to strengthen the existing legislation on these weapons so as to prevent their future use. This led Member States of the League of Nations to sign the *Protocol for the prohibition of the use in war of asphyxiating, poisonous or other gases and of bacteriological methods of warfare (2)* on 17 June 1925, during the Conference for the Supervision of the International Trade in Arms and Ammunition and in Implements of War. This treaty, which is usually referred to as the Geneva Protocol of 1925, entered into force on 8 February 1928, and France is its depositary. At the time of writing, it has 130 States Parties, including the five permanent members of the United Nations Security Council but not including 64 WHO Member States.[9]

The Geneva Protocol prohibits "the use in war of asphyxiating, poisonous, or other gases and of all analogous liquids, materials or devices" and also "extends this prohibition to the use of bacteriological methods of warfare". The prohibitions set out in the Protocol are now considered to have entered customary international law and are therefore binding even on states that are not parties to it. However, the Geneva Protocol prohibits only the use of such weapons, not their possession. Moreover, since many States Parties at the time reserved the right to use the weapons in retaliation against an attack with such weapons, the treaty was in effect a no-first-use agreement. Some States Parties also reserved the right to use the weapons against states not party to the protocol. For this reason, a comprehensive prohibition of the weapons themselves came to be considered necessary.

5.2   The 1972 Biological Weapons Convention

When discussion of biological and chemical weapons at the Geneva disarmament conference began in the late 1960s, when the first edition of this report was being prepared, there was much debate on whether the comprehensive prohibition of the weapons covered by the Geneva Protocol should be sought or, initially, the prohibition only of biological weapons. The United States, at that time not yet party to the Geneva Protocol, declared its unilateral renunciation of biological and toxin weapons during 1969–1970. This encouraged the international community to adopt the *Convention on the prohibition of the development, production and stockpiling of bacteriological (biological)*

---

9   See Annex 7.

and toxin weapons and on their destruction (3). Opened for signature on 10 April 1972 and entering into force on 26 March 1975, the BWC now has 151 States Parties, including the five permanent members of the United Nations Security Council but not including 42 WHO Member States.[10] The United Kingdom, the United States and the Russian Federation are the depositaries of the treaty.

5.2.1 International obligations

The BWC is designed to complement the prohibition of the use of biological weapons embodied in the Geneva Protocol. In Article I, it identifies items that each State Party "undertakes never in any circumstances to develop, produce, stockpile or otherwise acquire or retain". As has already been noted in Chapter 3, these items are not defined simply as biological weapons or biological-warfare agents. They are instead defined as: "(1) Microbial or other biological agents, or toxins whatever their origin or method of production, of types and in quantities that have no justification for prophylactic, protective or other peaceful purposes; (2) Weapons, equipment or means of delivery designed to use such agents or toxins for hostile purposes or in armed conflict." The scope of the Convention is thus specified according to a criterion of general purpose. Such an approach was adopted so as not to obstruct the many biomedical and other non-hostile applications of microbial or other biological agents and toxins, while at the same time enabling the Convention to cover any as-yet-unknown products of biotechnology and of scientific research that might find use as weapons. The treaty does not define either the "biological agents" or the "toxins" to which it refers. It is clear from the proceedings both of its negotiation and of its subsequent Review Conferences that the term "toxins" is not limited to microbial products but includes all toxic substances produced by living organisms even when they are actually produced synthetically. There is a description of toxins in Annex 2.

Another important obligation is set forth in Article II, which requires States Parties to destroy or divert to peaceful purposes all agents, toxins, weapons, equipment and means of delivery. This disarmament provision must be fulfilled no later than nine months after the entry into force of the Convention for the State Party concerned. The BWC also

---

10 See Annex 7.

requires States Parties to facilitate the exchange of equipment, material and scientific and technological information for the use for peaceful purposes of bacteriological (biological) agents and toxins (Article X), keeping in mind that the treaty prohibits the transfer of agents, toxins, weapons, equipment or means of delivery specified in Article I to any recipient whatsoever (Article III).

The operation of the BWC has been reviewed at intervals of five or six years. States Parties reaffirmed during their Review Conferences that the Convention was sufficiently comprehensive to encompass all new scientific and technological developments. They also instituted confidence-building data exchanges in order to strengthen the BWC by enhancing transparency. The Third Review Conference, in 1991, extended these data exchanges to include information on "past activities in offensive ... biological research and development programmes [since 1 January 1946]", and in the first year thereafter five States Parties affirmed that they had had such programmes, disclosing particulars. The five states were Canada, France, the Russian Federation, the United Kingdom and the United States. The periods of activity declared for the offensive programmes all terminated before the entry of the BWC into force except for the declaration by the Russian Federation, which specified "1946 to March 1992" as the period of activity.

The Third Review Conference also established an Ad Hoc Group of Government Experts (VEREX) to identify and examine potential verification measures from a scientific and technical standpoint. The VEREX Report was considered by a special conference convened in 1994 for this purpose. The conference established an Ad Hoc Group "to consider appropriate measures, including possible verification measures, and draft proposals to strengthen the convention, to be included, as appropriate, in a legally binding instrument, to be submitted for the consideration of the States Parties". The Ad Hoc Group worked from 1995 to 2001 without reaching consensus on such an instrument.

5.2.2   National implementation

The BWC stipulates that each State Party is obliged to take any necessary measures to implement the provisions of the Convention within its territory or any territory under its control anywhere (Article IV). Besides the basic obligations mentioned above, there are other areas where national measures are necessary if there is to be full implementation of the BWC. States have long taken measures to implement the obligation under Article III not to transfer to anyone agents, toxins or other items specified in Article I. In contrast, the implementation of Article X on measures for promoting technical cooperation in the field of biological activities has received relatively little direct attention.

Among their national measures under Article IV, some States Parties have enacted implementing legislation. For example, the United Kingdom introduced the *Biological Weapons Act* in 1974, Australia the *Crimes (Biological Weapons) Act* in 1976, New Zealand the *New Zealand Nuclear Free Zone, Disarmament, and Arms Control Act* in 1987, and the United States the *Biological Weapons Anti-Terrorism Act* in 1989, while already in 1972, long before the BWC had entered into force in France, that country had enacted Law No. 72–467 prohibiting the development, production, possession, stockpiling, acquisition and transfer of biological or toxin weapons.

Information on national measures is the subject of one of the confidence-building data-exchanges that BWC States Parties have agreed during Review Conferences, and the declarations made in accordance with it constitute the only readily available synoptic reference on the topic. Adopted by the Third Review Conference in 1991, it asks States Parties to provide annual returns of information about "legislation, regulations or other measures" on three different topics, namely, activities prohibited under Article I of the BWC, exports of pathogenic microbial agents and toxins, and imports of the same. Between 1992 and 1997, 46 (one-third) of the States Parties provided such information, 37 of them declaring the existence of specific measures in at least one of the three areas, and 26 declaring that they had enacted legal measures in all three areas. Examples of such legislative measures are given in Appendix 5.1.

5.3 The 1993 Chemical Weapons Convention

The CWC was negotiated over a period of more than 20 years, during which time related agreements were also concluded, notably the restrictions on warfare conducted with chemicals toxic to plant life set out in the 1977 *Convention on the prohibition of military or any other hostile use of environmental modification techniques*, and the reaffirmation of the Geneva Protocol by the 149 states represented at the Paris Conference of 1989 on the Prohibition of Chemical Weapons. The *Convention on the prohibition of the development, production, stockpiling and use of chemical weapons and on their destruction (4)* was opened for signature on 13 January 1993, entered into force on 29 April 1997 and, as of June 2004, had 164 States Parties,[11] including the five permanent members of the United Nations Security Council but not including 30 WHO Member States.[12] The CWC creates an elaborate regime to ensure compliance, and specifies in detail how its obligations are to be implemented; it also establishes an international organization (OPCW) to oversee its operation.

5.3.1 International obligations

The CWC prohibits the development, production, acquisition, stockpiling, retention, transfer and use of chemical weapons. It also forbids States Parties to assist, encourage or induce anyone to be involved in such outlawed activities. Like the BWC, the CWC uses a general purpose criterion to define its scope,[13] so that States Parties have the right to conduct activities involving toxic chemicals for purposes not prohibited under the CWC. Similarly, the provisions of the CWC must also be implemented in such a way as to avoid hampering the economic and technological development of the States Parties.

The CWC stipulates that the States Parties must totally destroy their existing stockpiles of chemical weapons and the related production facilities located on their territory or under their jurisdiction or control within 10 or, under certain conditions, 15 years after the CWC's entry into

---

11 This means that 164 states had deposited their instruments either of ratification of the CWC or of accession to it. An additional 18 states, all of which are members of WHO, had signed the treaty, but not yet ratified their signature.

12 See Annex 7.

13 The language that the CWC uses to specify the weapons that it covers is quoted and discussed further in section 3.1.1 above on pages 28–29.

force. This destruction process must be completed in such a way as to ensure the safety of the population and the protection of the environment.

Finally, the CWC establishes an international system for verifying compliance. This relies on several types of verification techniques and methods that allow for the protection of national security. This verification machinery, which includes declarations by the States Parties, routine inspections as well as means (such as challenge inspections) to investigate allegations of violations of the treaty, is operated by OPCW. The main element of the system is factual information obtained through verification procedures in accordance with the Convention that are independently conducted by the OPCW Technical Secretariat, sufficiency of such information being essential for successful operation *(5)*.

While fewer than 40% of the States Parties are directly affected by the routine verification regime, all States Parties participate in the security benefits conferred by the Convention. Accordingly, arrangements are in place for the delivery to OPCW Member States of assistance against the use and threat of use of chemical weapons (see Chapter 6). Such international cooperation is agreed between OPCW and the United Nations and will be extended to other international organizations. Cooperative measures in accordance with the CWC also extend to advice on the implementation of the Convention and in those areas in which the Technical Secretariat of OPCW has considerable expertise *(6)*.

5.3.2   National implementation

The CWC requires its States Parties to promulgate implementing legislation. Under Article VII, paragraph 4, States Parties are required to establish a National Authority. The twin pillars of the Convention's verification regime are thus (1) the OPCW Technical Secretariat (through which compliance is verified) and (2) the National Authority (through which compliance is demonstrated, including compliance with those obligations not overseen by the Technical Secretariat). The National Authority is essential to the success of the verification regime. As the national focal point for liaison with OPCW and with other States Parties, the national collection point of data and the facilitator of national implementation, effective National Authorities are essential to the effectiveness of the Convention itself. To meet its basic obligations, a State Party must be in a position to carry out the following eight fundamental functions, all of which involve its National Authority to a greater or lesser extent: (1) submit all the required declarations; (2) communicate with OPCW; (3) cooperate with other States Parties; (4) facilitate OPCW inspections; (5) respond to OPCW requests for assistance; (6) protect the confidentiality of classified information; (7) monitor and enforce national compliance; and (8) cooperate in the field of chemical activities for purposes not prohibited under the Convention, including the international exchange of scientific and technical information, and chemicals and equipment for the production, processing or use of chemicals for purposes not prohibited under the Convention.

Implementing legislation is normally necessary in order to enforce the prohibitions imposed on states by Article I of the CWC, to compel the submission of the information needed for an accurate national declaration, and for export/import controls. The requirements are described further in Appendix 5.2. Experience in the first five years of implementation has shown that comprehensive implementing legislation is essential to the reporting of reliable, complete information by States Parties. A survey of national implementing legislation showed that, in addition to the areas specified in Article VII, paragraph 1 (prohibitions, penal measures, extraterritorial application to nationals), several States Parties have found it necessary to enact legislation in 15 other areas (legal assistance; definition of chemical weapons; declaration obligations; the regime for scheduled chemicals – regulation of Schedule 1 production/use; criteria for Schedule 2 and 3 declarations; import/export controls; mixtures – licensing of industry; access to facilities; inspection equipment; application of inspectors' privileges and immunities; confidentiality; liability; mandate of the National Authority; enforcement powers of the National Authority; samples; environmental measures; and primacy of the Convention) *(7–8)*.

Five years after the entry into force of the CWC, 43% of States Parties had met their obligation to inform OPCW of the legislative and administrative measures taken to implement the Convention. At its fifth session (May 2000), the Conference of the States Parties encouraged States Parties that are in a position to do so to offer assistance to other

States Parties in their efforts to fulfil their obligations under Article VII (9). In December 2001, the OPCW Executive Council identified full implementation of the legislative measures required by Article VII as one of the five priority areas to be focused upon in OPCW's contribution to global antiterrorist efforts.

5.4 Conclusions

Through its contribution both to preventing the release of biological or chemical agents for hostile purposes and to mitigating the consequences should such release nevertheless occur, the legal regime just described stands alongside the measures of protective preparation described in Chapter 4. A complementarity is evident. Civilian populations are vulnerable to deliberate releases of biological and chemical agents to such a degree that this complementarity needs to be strengthened. Clearly, prevention and protection can be no substitute for one another but can, instead, be mutually reinforcing. The conclusion must be, then, that an emphasis on the one should not become a detraction from the other, for a danger is bound to exist that confidence in protective preparation may seem to diminish the value of preventive preparation. Full and complete implementation of the 1972 and 1993 Conventions is therefore an objective that needs continual affirmation and national support.

REFERENCES

1. Roberts A, Guelff R. *Documents on the laws of war*, 3rd ed. Oxford, Oxford University Press, 2000.

2. The text of the Geneva Protocol is available in reference 1 and also at *www.disarmament.un.org*.

3. The text of the Biological Weapons Convention is available in reference 1 and also at *www.opbw.org*.

4. *Convention on the prohibition of the development, production, stockpiling, and use of chemical weapons and on their destruction, corrected version in accordance with Depositary Notification C.N.246.1994.TREATIES-5 issued on 31 August 1994 and the change made under Article XV (new paragraph 5bis of Section B of Part VI of the Verification Annex), in accordance with Depositary Notification C.N.916.1999.TREATIES-7 issued on 8 October 1999; together with Depositary Notification C.N.157.2000. TREATIES-1 issued on 13 March 2000*. The text of the Convention is available at *http://www.opcw.org*.

5. Krutzsch W, Trapp R. *Verification practice under the Chemical Weapons Convention*. The Hague, Kluwer Law International, 1999.

6. *Opening Statement by the Director-General to the Organisation for the Prohibition of Chemical Weapons conference of the States Parties at its fifth session*, OPCW document C-V/DG.11 dated 12 May 2000.

7. *Survey of national implementing legislation*. Organisation for the Prohibition of Chemical Weapons document S/259/98, dated 16 May 2001.

8. Checklist for the legislator and model national implementing legislation and addendum. In: Tabassi L, ed. *OPCW: the legal texts*. The Hague, TMC Asser Press, 1999, 310–315.

9. *Decision on national implementation measures taken by the Organisation for the Prohibition of Chemical Weapons Conference of the States Parties at its fifth session*. OPCW document C-V/DEC.20, 19 May 2000.

APPENDIX 5.1: BWC IMPLEMENTING LEGISLATION

Legislation to enforce the prohibitions of Article I

Article IV of the BWC provides that each State Party shall take any necessary measures to prohibit and prevent the development, production, stockpiling, acquisition or retention of the agents, toxins, weapons, equipment and means of delivery specified within Article I of the Convention. It further requires that these measures apply within the territory of the State or any territory under its jurisdiction or under its control anywhere. At subsequent Review Conferences, States Parties have been invited to consider the application of such measures also to actions taken anywhere by natural persons possessing its nationality. For consistency with the Convention, the national legislation or measures should incorporate the definition of biological weapons as contained in the Convention. The fulfilment of these obligations will contribute significantly to the achievement of the object and purpose of the Convention, namely to prevent the use of biological and toxin weapons as a means of warfare or as a terrorist threat.

Examples are provided below of the relevant language in the legislation enacted by three of the States Parties.

Australia: Crimes (Biological Weapons) Act 1976

The Act makes it unlawful for Australians to develop, produce, stockpile or otherwise acquire or retain microbial or other biological agents or toxins whatever their origin or method of production, of types and in quantities that have no justification for prophylactic, protective or other peaceful purposes; or weapons, equipment or means of delivery designed to use such agents or toxins for hostile purposes or in armed conflict.

The Act extends to the acts of Australian citizens outside Australia.

Contravention of the Act is an indictable offence.

New Zealand: *New Zealand Nuclear Free Zone, Disarmament and Arms Control Act 1987*

Section 8 of the Act states:

"Prohibition of biological weapons – No person shall manufacture, station, acquire or possess, or have control over any biological weapons in the New Zealand Nuclear Free Zone."

"Biological weapon" is defined as "any agent, toxin, weapon, equipment or means of delivery referred to in Article I of the Convention".

United States of America: *Biological Weapons Anti-Terrorism Act 1989*

Paragraph 175. Prohibitions with respect to biological weapons:

"(a) IN GENERAL. – Whoever knowingly develops, produces, stockpiles, transfers, acquires, retains, or possesses any biological agents, toxin, or delivery system for use as a weapon, or knowingly assists a foreign state or any organization to do so, shall be fined under this title or imprisoned for life or any term of years, or both. There is extraterritorial Federal jurisdiction over an offense under this section committed by or against a national of the United States.

(b) DEFINITION. – For purposes of this section, the term "for use as a weapon" does not include the development, production, transfer, acquisition, retention, or possession of any biological agent, toxin, or delivery system for prophylactic, protective, or other peaceful purposes."

Legislation regulating exports of agents and toxins

Article III of the BWC provides that each State Party undertakes not to transfer to any recipient whatsoever, directly or indirectly, and not in any way to assist, encourage or induce any State, group of States or international organizations to manufacture or otherwise acquire any of the agents, toxins, weapons, equipment and means of delivery specified within Article I of the Convention. At subsequent Review Conferences, it has been stated that States Parties should also consider ways and means to ensure that individuals or subnational groups are effectively prevented from acquiring, through transfers, biological agents and toxins for other than peaceful purposes.

Examples are provided below of the relevant language in the legislation adopted by two States Parties.

Australia: *The Quarantine Act (1908) and Regulations, the Biological Control Act (1984) and Regulations, and the Therapeutic Goods Act (1989) and Regulations*

The Quarantine Act 1908 and Regulations require prior permission before a biological agent may be imported. Under the provisions of Section 13 of the Act, goods of biological origin, including human pathogenic microorganisms and toxins, may only be imported into Australia if approval has been given by the Director of Human Quarantine. Import conditions vary, depending on the nature of the organisms and the risks involved. High-risk organisms, such as serious pathogens of humans, animals and plants which might be considered as potential biological weapons, will only be permitted under the most stringent high security conditions. Very few imports are approved and these will generally be needed for diagnostic research in preparation for emergency responses to specific serious exotic disease incursions. Penalties for the importation of controlled goods without a permit, and for breaches of permit requirements, are severe and may include a fine or imprisonment or both.

Biological Control Act (1984) and Regulations

"This Act ... provides powers additional to those of the Quarantine Act in order to regulate the release of biological agents for the control of pests, diseases and weeds."

Therapeutic Goods Act (1989) and Regulations

The Act covers the import and export of therapeutic goods and will include pathogenic microorganisms where these are included in vaccines for human use.

Brazil: *Law no. 9.112 (1995) (unofficial translation)*

Article 1 – This Law regulates transactions related to the export of sensitive goods and services directly related to such goods.

...

Article 2 – The goods covered by the previous Article will be included in the Lists of Sensitive Goods that will be periodically updated and published in the Federal Government Gazette (*Diário Oficial da União*).

Article 3 – The export of the following items will depend on prior formal authorization issued by the competent federal entities in compliance with the regulations established and published in the Federal Government Gazette (*Diário Oficial da União*):

I – goods included in the Lists of Sensitive Goods; and

II – services directly linked to goods included in the Lists of Sensitive Goods.

...

Article 4 – Under the aegis of the Office of the President of Brazil, the Interministerial Commission for Controlling Exports of Sensitive Goods is established, consisting of representatives of the federal entities involved in the process of exporting the goods covered by this Law.

...

Article 6 – The export of sensitive goods and services directly linked thereto, if in violation of the provisions of this Law and its Regulations, will subject the violator to the following penalties:

I – warning;

II – fine of up to twice the value equivalent to that of the transaction;

III – loss of the goods covered by the transaction;

IV – suspension of the right to export for a period of six months to five years;

V – cancellation of qualification to work with foreign trade, in case of repeat offences.

...

Article 7 – Individuals who fail to comply with this Law either directly or indirectly, through either action or omission, will be committing a crime.

Penalty – imprisonment of one to four years.

APPENDIX 5.2: CWC IMPLEMENTING LEGISLATION

Legislation to enforce the prohibitions of Article I, including penal provisions

Article VII of the CWC provides that specific legislation must be in place prohibiting actions that would contravene a State Party's obligations under Article I. Any natural and legal person on the territory of a State Party shall be prohibited under penal law, for instance, to develop, produce or otherwise acquire chemical weapons, to transfer such weapons to anyone, to use them or to assist others in committing such crimes. Penalties will include both criminal and administrative sanctions. For consistency with the Convention, the national legislation should incorporate the definition of chemical weapons as contained in the Convention. The Convention requires States Parties to extend the application of these penal provisions to actions undertaken anywhere by natural persons possessing their nationality. Furthermore, States Parties shall assist each other and cooperate to prosecute those who contravene the prohibition of chemical weapons worldwide. The fulfilment of these obligations will contribute significantly to the achievement of the object and purpose of the Convention, namely to prevent the use of toxic chemicals as a means of warfare or as a terrorist threat. As these are the most basic violations of the very purpose of the Convention, penalties should be severe enough to deter possible violators. Legislation already promulgated by States Parties specifies that the most serious violations shall be punished by life imprisonment.

States may find it difficult to comply with their obligation under Article VII, paragraph 2, to respond to requests from other States Parties for cooperation and legal assistance. The modalities of such cooperation and legal assistance may include: (1) extradition; (2) mutual legal assistance in penal matters; (3) transfer of prisoners; (4) seizure and forfeiture of illicit proceeds of crime; (5) recognition of foreign penal judgements; or (6) transfer of penal proceedings. There is no customary practice in international cooperation and legal assistance in criminal matters; the modalities and procedures are normally prescribed in bilateral treaties or partially in a few multilateral instruments. Thus States Parties to the CWC need to check whether their municipal law and their various treaties concerning different forms of mutual legal assistance concluded with other states will allow for cooperation in this regard. If a State Party seeks mutual legal assistance and encounters obstacles, certain other non-judicial coercive techniques may be available based on comity or cooperation through organizations such as Interpol *(1)*.

Regulating and monitoring the relevant chemical industry and exports of specific chemicals

States Parties shall by law require public and private entities or persons to report if they are producing, or in some cases consuming or processing, chemicals specified in the Convention when threshold limits are exceeded. On the basis of this information, States Parties will be able to fulfil their obligation under the Convention to submit full and accurate declarations to OPCW on national activities related to chemicals listed in the schedules of the CWC. To maintain a nationwide overview of activities regulated by the CWC and ensure complete declarations, some States Parties have promulgated legislation subjecting producers of chemicals to licensing.

From the entry into force of the Convention, States Parties were required to notify OPCW 30 days in advance of any transfer of a Schedule 1 chemical to or from another State Party, and were prohibited from transferring Schedule 1 chemicals to or from states not party. From 29 April 2000, the transfer of Schedule 2 chemicals to states not party to the Convention was also prohibited. Appropriate measures of States Parties must also ensure that Schedule 3 chemicals transferred to states not party to the Convention shall only be used for purposes that are not prohibited. Each State Party's National Authority must negotiate and conclude facility agreements with OPCW governing the procedures for the implementation of verification activities by the Technical Secretariat in certain declared facilities. In order to perform these tasks, the National Authority must identify the sites, both public and private, that have to be declared and for which data for inclusion in the state's initial and annual declarations must be provided. Contacts with chemical industry associations and searches of commercial databases, and those of universities and hospitals, will usually be necessary to obtain the necessary information on the national activities that may be relevant to the Convention.

The OPCW Technical Secretariat and the Secretariat of the Organisation of Eastern Caribbean States have developed a pesticide regulation model act in which the provisions required to implement the CWC are incorporated. The result, a draft Pesticides and Toxic Chemicals Control Act and Regulations, (i) allows the parliaments concerned to consider the regulations for pesticides and toxic chemicals in a single step; (ii) facilitates ratification of, and accession to, the CWC; (iii) makes a single interministerial agency in each country responsible for pesticides and toxic chemicals and serve as the National Authority under the Convention; and (iv) enables the CWC to be enforceable in the subregion (2).

REFERENCES

1.   Yepes-Enríquez R, Tabassi L, eds. *Treaty enforcement and international cooperation in criminal matters with special reference to the Chemical Weapons Convention.* The Hague, TMC Asser Press, 2002.

2.   *An integrated approach to national implementing legislation/model act developed by the secretariat of the Organisation of Eastern Caribbean States.* OPCW document S/190/2000 dated 23 May 2000.

6. INTERNATIONAL SOURCES OF ASSISTANCE

The international community has made preparations through several organizations to support governments of states against which chemical or biological weapons might be used. These preparations may also be of assistance to governments of states subject to terrorist attack. The assistance available can be categorized as:

(a)   the application of international law;

(b)   practical protection against the weapons themselves (provision of equipment, material and scientific and technical information; and

(c)   medical and other assistance in order to prevent potentially massive harm to the population attacked by such weapons.

The principal organization providing political support is the **United Nations** (see pages 128–131 below). In the case of chemical attack, the **Organisation for the Prohibition of Chemical Weapons** (OPCW) (see pages 132–134 below) will also be important for its members. If in the future an organization is established under the BWC, this will play a role in the case of biological attack.

Practical assistance in providing protection against chemical weapons can be provided by OPCW (see pages 132–134 below). The BWC also requires its States Parties to come to each other's assistance in certain circumstances (see pages 134–135 below).

General medical assistance can be provided in either case by the **World Health Organization** (WHO) (see pages 135–137 below). The **Food and Agriculture Organization** of the United Nations (FAO) (see pages 137–138 below) and the **World Organisation for Animal Health** (OIE) (see pages 138–139 below) could be asked to provide assistance if an attack were made on plants (FAO) or animals (FAO and/or OIE), rather than on human targets. Where local resources are insufficient to cope with the humanitarian aspects of the situation, it may be appropriate to call on the **United Nations Office for the Coordination of Humanitarian Affairs** (see pages 130–131 below) or the major **nongovernmental organizations.**

Each of the above-mentioned agencies is considered briefly below.

A chemical or biological attack may overwhelm the available medical resources and pose serious logistic and organizational problems. It may then be appropriate to turn to the armed forces for help, including those of other countries. In humanitarian emergencies (e.g. refugee crises or natural disasters), such forces have supported relief efforts when invited to do so under the aegis of the United Nations (see pages 130–131 below).

6.1   United Nations

The use or threat of use of chemical or biological weapons by one state against another will clearly constitute a threat to international peace and security, and will therefore fall within the responsibility of the **United Nations Security Council**, to which the facts should promptly be reported. Both the BWC and the CWC make provision for the involvement of the Security Council when there are allegations that biological or chemical weapons have been used, and arrangements have been made for these allegations to be investigated (see below).

6.1.1   Investigation of alleged use

The United Nations General Assembly, under its resolution 42/37C of November 1987, mandated the Secretary-General to investigate "reports that may be brought to his attention by any Member State concerning the possible use of chemical and bacteriological (biological) or toxin weapons [...] in order to ascertain the facts of the matter...". Under the terms of the resolution, the Secretary-General has established a panel of experts available to carry out on-site investigations. A group of qualified experts, appointed pursuant to the resolution, has provided a report setting out guidance as to how such investigations might be carried out *(1)*.

The CWC, which entered into force on 29 April 1997, obliges OPCW to investigate any alleged use of chemical weapons against a State Party. For investigations relating to allegations of the use of chemical weapons brought to the Secretary-General by a state not party to the CWC, OPCW is obliged to cooperate with the Secretary-General in accordance with Part XI, paragraph 27, of the CWC Verification Annex and with Article II.2(c) of the Relationship Agreement between the United Nations and OPCW that entered into force on 11 October 2001.

Investigations of the alleged use of chemical weapons conducted by the United Nations up to the end of 2002 can be summarized as follows:

1981–1982: **Asia**. Investigations took place long after the alleged attacks had occurred so that on-site visits were not possible; the results were inconclusive *(2)*.

1984–1988: **Islamic Republic of Iran**. Investigations took place within days of the alleged attacks, on-site visits were made and samples taken; Iraq was identified as the perpetrator *(3–10)*.

1987–1988: **Iraq**. Chemical injuries to Iraqi soldiers were verified by the investigators *(6–7, 9)*, who reported finding no conclusive evidence of how the injuries had been caused *(11)*.

1992: **Mozambique**. Investigations were made more than a month after the alleged attack; no proof was found of the use of chemical weapons *(12)*.

1992: **Azerbaijan**. The investigation was requested by the state accused of resorting to chemical warfare in order to demonstrate its innocence; a timely on-site visit did not reveal any proof of use of chemical weapons *(13)*.

1993: **Iraq**. Investigation of the alleged internal use of chemical weapons did not reveal any proof of such use *(14)*.

In the period covered, the Secretary-General was not asked to conduct any investigations of the alleged use of biological weapons other than toxins. (However, one consultation concerning an alleged use was carried out under the BWC: see page 135 below.)

It is highly desirable for the request for an investigation to be made to the Secretary-General immediately after the incident concerned has taken place to minimize the likelihood of degradation of the evidence.

6.1.2 Humanitarian assistance

If an attack is made on a large scale with serious consequences for the population, humanitarian assistance can be sought from the United Nations. The **Emergency Relief Coordinator** of the United Nations has been mandated by General Assembly resolution A/RES/46/182 of 14 April 1992 to serve as the central focal point and coordinating official for United Nations emergency relief operations. The Coordinator is also the Under-Secretary-General for Humanitarian Affairs and is supported by the United Nations **Office for the Coordination of Humanitarian Affairs** (OCHA).

OCHA Geneva has established an emergency-response system for coordinating actions taken by the international community to deal with natural disasters and environmental emergencies, including technological accidents. It is responsible for mobilizing and coordinating international disaster response and can be contacted on a 24-hour basis in case of emergency.

In humanitarian emergencies, OCHA can:

* process requests for assistance from Member States;
* organize, in consultation with the government of the affected country, a joint interagency assessment mission;
* serve as the central coordinating body with governments, inter-governmental organizations, nongovernmental organizations and the United Nations specialized agencies concerned for all emergency relief operations;
* provide consolidated information on all humanitarian emergencies;
* actively promote, in close collaboration with the concerned organizations, the smooth transition from relief to rehabilitation.

OCHA has a Military and Civil Defence Unit (MCDU), which is the focal point in the United Nations humanitarian system for the mobilization and coordination of military and civil-defence assistance whenever these are needed in response to humanitarian emergencies.

OCHA is also in a position to provide a United Nations Disaster Assessment and Coordination (UNDAC) team and set up an On Site Operations Coordination Centre (OSOCC) in collaboration with OPCW to facilitate the coordination of all international emergency humanitarian assistance.

Member States can send requests for information and/or international assistance in natural disasters or environmental emergencies directly to the OCHA office in Geneva, or through the United Nations Resident Coordinator in the country concerned.

The **World Food Programme (WFP)** was established in 1963 as the food aid arm of the United Nations to provide, upon request, food aid and related services to meet emergency, protracted relief and recovery, and development needs.

WFP could provide, consistent with its policies and when given resources by donors, emergency food and associated logistic services in response to humanitarian disasters arising from the use of biological or chemical weapons. These include situations where: crops or food supplies are destroyed or rendered unsafe; large-scale environmental damage affects people's livelihoods; outbreaks of debilitating diseases threaten longer-term food security; or populations are displaced. WFP could provide assistance to countries whose food security is threatened by these conditions and where the government concerned does not have the capacity to respond. This is facilitated by the presence of WFP field offices and food stocks in over 80 countries.

In the event of longer-term impacts on food security, WFP could incorporate activities to address the needs of victims of biological or chemical weapons in its recovery and development programmes. When potential threats to food security arise from the use of biological or chemical weapons, these could be factored into ongoing early warning and contingency planning exercises.

6.2 Organisation for the Prohibition of Chemical Weapons

Article X, paragraph 8, of the Chemical Weapons Convention reads as follows:

Each State Party has the right to request and, subject to the procedures set forth in paragraphs 9, 10 and 11, to receive assistance and protection against the use or threat of use of chemical weapons if it considers that:

a)   chemical weapons have been used against it;[14]

b)   riot control agents have been used against it as a method of warfare; or

c)   it is threatened by actions or activities of any State that are prohibited for States Parties by Article I.

Article X, paragraphs 9, 10 and 11, require the Director-General of OPCW to take immediate action on receipt of a request. He shall, within 24 hours, initiate an investigation and submit a first report within 72 hours to the Executive Council. If required, the time for the investigation can be extended repeatedly by additional 72-hour periods. A new report must be submitted after each such period. The Executive Council is required to meet within 24 hours after receiving an investigation report to consider further action, including supplementary assistance. At the first Conference of the States Parties to the CWC in May 1997, the Organisation established a voluntary fund for action under Article X and invited States Parties to inform the Technical Secretariat of the assistance that they may elect to provide in accordance with Article X, paragraph 7. As of 31 May 2002, the voluntary fund had received about one million Euros in contributions, and 33 States Parties had made more or less specific offers of assistance in kind, ranging from protective equipment to putting assistance teams of battalion strength at the disposal of OPCW.

The assistance pledged to be delivered through OPCW, on request, can be divided into two main categories: hardware (mainly protective equipment) and a variety of assistance teams.

---

14   This provision does not specify the source of the attack, which could either be another state or a non-state entity such as a terrorist group.

Hardware offered by Member States consists largely of personal protective equipment, especially for use by civilians. The delivery of such equipment to a requesting State Party will, at best, take several days, possibly more than a week, after which the State Party concerned will have to distribute the equipment within the country.

The use of personal protective equipment requires training. To facilitate such training, a series of courses has been arranged for chief instructors by the Swiss Government in collaboration with OPCW. Such chief instructors should then be able to train local instructors who, in turn, can train the exposed population in the appropriate use of personal protective equipment.

Other assistance-related training courses are also being arranged by the Technical Secretariat of OPCW, in cooperation with various Member States. These include, for example, courses for medical personnel, courses in the use of analytical equipment, and courses on the conduct of emergency assistance and rescue operations. Information on such courses, and how to apply to attend them, is available on the OPCW web site.

Assistance teams that can be made available by Member States to assist in case of need include, inter alia, medical teams, detection teams, decontamination teams and teams for providing the necessary infrastructure support for assistance operations. Some air transport has also been offered; however, it is expected that the costs of transporting the teams may have to be covered to some extent by the Voluntary Fund for Assistance.

Article X, paragraph 5, requires the OPCW Technical Secretariat to establish and maintain a databank for the use of any requesting State Party, containing freely available information on protection against chemical weapons as well as such other information as may be provided by States Parties. This databank has now been established, and is indexed by a database using the CDS-ISIS database software developed by UNESCO. At present, requests for information from the databank have to be addressed directly to the OPCW Technical Secretariat, but it is planned to make the database available through the Internet.

Article X, paragraph 5, further requires the Technical Secretariat to provide expert advice on how a State Party can improve its protection against chemical weapons. This provision affords an opportunity to ask for assistance without having to accuse any state of using chemical weapons. To implement this provision, a protection network has been established, currently consisting of approximately 40 specialists on various aspects of chemical protection who are nationals of some 20 Member States. A State Party can request help from the protection network free of charge: specialists will be paid by the Member States putting them at the disposal of OPCW, which will cover the travel costs.

Within the framework of Article X, paragraph 5, the Secretariat can also, on request, arrange national or regional courses on protection, workshops, etc.

6.3   Biological Weapons Convention

Article VI of the Biological Weapons Convention reads as follows:

(1) Any State Party to this Convention which finds that any other State Party is acting in breach of obligations deriving from the provisions of the Convention may lodge a complaint with the Security Council of the United Nations. Such a complaint should include all possible evidence confirming its validity, as well as a request for its consideration by the Security Council.

(2) Each State Party to this Convention undertakes to cooperate in carrying out any investigation which the Security Council may initiate, in accordance with the provisions of the Charter of the United Nations, on the basis of the complaint received by the Council. The Security Council shall inform the States Parties to the Convention of the results of the investigation.

The provision of assistance is provided for under Article VII of the Convention, which reads:

Each State Party to this Convention undertakes to provide or support assistance, in accordance with the United Nations Charter, to any Party to the Convention which so requests, if the Security Council decides that such Party has been exposed to danger as a result of violation of the Convention.

Although this provision has so far not been invoked, the States Parties at their Review Conferences have reaffirmed their undertaking to provide or support assistance. They have also said that, should this Article be invoked, they consider that the United Nations, with the help of appropriate international organizations such as WHO, could play a coordinating role.

Provision for consultation is made in Article V, which reads:

> The States Parties to this Convention undertake to consult one another and to cooperate in solving any problems which may arise in relation to the objective of, or in the applications of the provisions of, the Convention. Consultation and cooperation pursuant to this Article may also be undertaken through appropriate international procedures within the framework of the United Nations and in accordance with its Charter.

At their second Review Conference in 1986, the States Parties established a procedure for convening a formal consultative meeting to facilitate any such cooperation and thus improve the implementation of this article. At their third Review Conference, in 1991, they expanded the procedure. A consultative meeting of this type was convened in 1997 to address a problem in which Cuba had alleged that, in October 1996, phytophagous insects had been released over Cuba by the United States (15).

6.4   World Health Organization

WHO is a specialized agency of the United Nations with 192 Member States. Its Secretariat includes a headquarters in Geneva, six regional offices and 141 country offices. According to its Constitution, the functions of the Organization are, inter alia, to:

- act as the directing and coordinating authority on international health work;
- furnish appropriate technical assistance and, in emergencies, necessary aid upon the request or acceptance of governments;

- provide information, counsel and assistance in the field of health;
- develop, establish and promote international standards with respect to food, biological, pharmaceutical and similar products.

The use of chemical or biological weapons may result in extremely serious public health and medical emergencies, including a sudden and significant increase in numbers of cases, and deaths from a variety of diseases. In view of its mandate outlined above, WHO would play a critical role in dealing with any such emergency.

WHO became officially engaged with the subject of biological and chemical weapons in 1969, in response to a request from the Secretary-General of the United Nations to cooperate with the United Nations Group of Consultant Experts on Chemical and Bacteriological (Biological) Weapons in the preparation of a report on this subject.[15]

A number of WHO programmes provide technical assistance on various relevant aspects of public health, such as: preparedness for, and response to, natural and man-made disasters, earthquakes being an example of the former; chemical or radiological accidents; complex humanitarian emergencies; surveillance of communicable diseases, including global outbreak alert and response; chemical safety; food safety; and mental health. These programmes rely heavily on the technical and scientific support of WHO's network of collaborating centres.

WHO contributes to global health security in the specific field of outbreak alert and response by: (i) strengthening national surveillance programmes, particularly in the field of epidemiology and laboratory techniques, preparedness for deliberate epidemics and laboratory biosafety; (ii) disseminating verified information on outbreaks of diseases and, whenever needed, following up by providing technical support for response; and (iii) collecting, analysing and disseminating information on diseases likely to cause epidemics of global importance. Several epidemic diseases coming within the scope of WHO's surveillance and response programme have been associated with biological warfare. Guidelines on specific epidemic diseases, as well as on the management of surveillance programmes, are available in printed and electronic forms; an updated listing of these documents is accessible

---

15   See section 1.2.

through the World Wide Web. WHO is responsible for the administration of the International Health Regulations (IHR), a global framework (politically neutral and technically competent) within which national and global surveillance and response networks can operate in a timely and coordinated way. A revised version of the IHR is in preparation that will take account of global developments during the last 30 years of the twentieth century.

The International Programme on Chemical Safety (IPCS), a joint venture of the United Nations Environment Programme (UNEP), the International Labour Organization (ILO) and WHO, which was established to carry out and disseminate evaluations of the effects of chemicals on human health and the quality of the environment, produces guidelines and training material on preparedness for, and response to chemical incidents of technological origin, that would also be applicable if chemical agents were released deliberately. IPCS provides technical support for national chemical safety programmes, including the establishment or strengthening of chemical information centres able to provide advice on chemicals and toxic exposure on a 24-hour basis. The INTOX programme of IPCS, which includes an electronically linked network of about 120 centres in 70 countries, allows rapid access to toxicological, analytical and clinical expertise. Such a mechanism will also be useful in the identification of, and response to incidents involving chemical agents used in warfare.

6.5   Food and Agriculture Organization of the United Nations

FAO is an autonomous agency of the United Nations system with 175 Member States, and of which the European Union is also a member organization. Its Constitution requires, inter alia, that FAO shall furnish such technical assistance as governments may request, and organize, in collaboration with the governments concerned, such missions as may be needed to assist them to fulfil the obligations arising from their acceptance of the recommendations of the United Nations Conference on Food and Agriculture and the Constitution of FAO.

FAO has not formally been involved in the control of biological and chemical weapons, but is, however, prepared to play an active part within its broad mandate in providing technical and humanitarian assistance. In recent years, FAO has contributed significantly in emergency relief and rehabilitation when droughts, floods, earthquakes, hurricanes, locust swarms, livestock plagues, war, civil strife, and natural and man-made disasters have caused immense suffering to the populations affected.

6.6 World Organisation for Animal Health (OIE)

The World Organisation for Animal Health is composed of the official veterinary services of 157 countries. Its three main goals, established since its foundation in 1924, are: (i) to inform governments of the occurrence and course of animal diseases worldwide, and of ways to control these diseases; (ii) to provide international coordination of research on, and control of, important animal diseases; and (iii) to work towards the harmonization of trade regulations for animals and animal products.

Although OIE has no programmes or activities with the specific objective of preventing or reacting to biological warfare, the ongoing sharing of information on the occurrence, prevention and control of animal diseases, including zoonoses, is relevant to this objective. Senior animal health officials from all countries meet annually to discuss recent scientific developments and to agree on matters of international importance affecting public veterinary services.

OIE has established an information system to collect and disseminate information on outbreaks of animal diseases that are the most serious from the animal and public health viewpoints. The urgency of dispatching information varies according to an internationally agreed classification of disease as List A and List B diseases.[16]

OIE has an emergency fund that is available for sending missions to developing countries in need of urgent technical assistance to investigate and control outbreaks of animal diseases. Such assistance

---

[16] *List A diseases* are transmissible diseases that have the potential for very serious and rapid spread, irrespective of national borders, which are of serious socioeconomic or public health consequence and of major importance in the international trade of animals and animal products. *List B diseases* are transmissible diseases that are considered to be of socioeconomic and/or public health importance within countries and that are significant in the international trade of animals and animal products.

is usually provided in cooperation with other international organizations such as FAO and WHO.

6.7 Nongovernmental organizations

Nongovernmental organizations are non-profit-making, voluntary citizens' groups at the local, national or international level, including scientific bodies and professional associations. Task-orientated and driven by people with a common interest, they perform a variety of services and humanitarian functions, bring citizens' concerns to the attention of governments, monitor policies, and encourage political participation at the community level. They provide analysis and expertise, serve as early warning mechanisms and help to monitor and implement international agreements. Some are organized around specific issues, such as human rights, the environment or health. Their possible involvement in the prevention and control of the health consequences of chemical and biological weapons will depend on their goals, their location, their mandate and their resources. If an accident or incident involving chemical/biological agents occurs, it is very likely that, in addition to the local administrations, they will be actively involved in providing care to the affected populations.

6.8 Contact information

Food and Agriculture Organization of the United Nations
Viale delle Terme di Caracalla – I-00100 Rome, Italy
Telephone: +(39) 06 57051
Facsimile: +(39) 06 5705 3152
Internet: *http://www.fao.org*

OCHA New York
United Nations Office for the Coordination of Humanitarian Affairs
United Nations, New York – NY 10017, USA
Telephone: +(1) 212 963 1234
Facsimile: +(1) 212 963 1312
E-mail: *ochany@un.org*
Internet: *http://www.reliefweb.int/ocha_ol/index.html*

OCHA Geneva

United Nations Office for the Coordination of Humanitarian Affairs
United Nations, Palais des Nations – CH-1211 Geneva 10, Switzerland
Telephone: +(41) 22 917 1234
Facsimile: +(41) 22 917 0023
E-mail: *ochagva@un.org*
[Outside official working hours, the Duty Officer of the OCHA office
in Geneva can be reached at any time through the emergency
telephone number +(41) 22 917 2010]

World Organisation for Animal Health (OIE)

12, rue de Prony – F-75017 Paris, France
Telephone: +(33) 1 44 15 18 88
Facsimile: +(33) 1 42 67 09 87
E-mail: *oie@oie.int*
Internet : *http://www.oie.int*

Organisation for the Prohibition of Chemical Weapons

Johan de Wittlaan 32 – NL-2517 JR The Hague, Netherlands
Telephone: +(31) 70 416 3300
Facsimile: +(31) 70 306 3535
Internet: *www.opcw.org*

World Food Programme

Via C.G. Viola 68, Parco dei Medici – I-00148 Rome, Italy
Telephone: +(39) 06 65131
Facsimile: +(39) 06 6513 2840
E-mail: *wfpinfo@wfp.org*
Internet: *http://www.wfp.org*

World Health Organization

Avenue Appia 20 – CH-1211 Geneva 27, Switzerland
Telephone: +(41) 22 791 2111
Facsimile: +(41) 22 791 3111
Internet: *http://www.who.int*

REFERENCES

1. United Nations General Assembly document. A/44/561, 4 October 1989.

2. United Nations General Assembly document A/37/259, 1 December 1982.

3. United Nations Security Council document S/16433, 26 March 1984.

4. United Nations Security Council document S/17127, 24 April 1985, plus Add.1, 30 April 1985.

5. United Nations Security Council document S/17911, 12 March 1986, plus Add.1 and Corr.1, dated 14 March 1986, and Add.2, 16 April 1986.

6. United Nations Security Council document S/18852, 8 May 1987, plus Add.1, 18 May 1987, and Corr.1, 26 May 1987.

7. United Nations Security Council document S/19823, 25 April 1988, plus Add.1, 10 May 1988, and Corr.1, 17 May 1988.

8. United Nations Security Council document S/20060, 20 July 1988, plus Add.1, 2 August 1988.

9. United Nations Security Council document S/20063, 25 July 1988, plus Add.1, 2 August 1988.

10. United Nations Security Council document S/20134, 19 August 1988.

11. McCormack TLH. International law and the use of chemical weapons in the Gulf War. *California Western International Law Journal*, 1990–1991, 21(1):1–30.

12. United Nations Security Council document S/24065, 12 June 1992.

13. United Nations Security Council document S/24344, 24 July 1992.

14. United Nations Special Commission for the destruction of Iraqi weapons of mass destruction, *Executive Summary of UNSCOM 65: Chemical Weapons Inspection No. 12, 10–22 November 1993,* transmitted to the UN Secretary-General on 7 December 1993.

15. *Report of the formal consultative meeting of States Parties to the convention on the prohibition of the development, production and stockpiling of bacteriological (biological) and toxin weapons and on their destruction.* Formal Consultative Meeting of States Parties to the Convention on the Prohibition of the Development, Production and Stockpiling of Bacteriological (Biological) and Toxin Weapons and on their Destruction. BWC/CONS/1, 29 August 1997.

ANNEX 1. CHEMICAL AGENTS

1. Introduction

The large-scale use of toxic chemicals as weapons first became possible during the First World War (1914–1918) thanks to the growth of the chemical industry. More than 110 000 tonnes were disseminated over the battlefields, the greater part on the western front. Initially, the chemicals were used, not to cause casualties in the sense of putting enemy combatants out of action, but rather to harass. Though the sensory irritants used were powerful enough to disable those who were exposed to them, they served mainly to drive enemy combatants out of the trenches or other cover that protected them from conventional fire, or to disrupt enemy artillery or supplies. About 10% of the total tonnage of chemical warfare agents used during the war were chemicals of this type, namely lacrimators (tear gases), sternutators and vomiting agents. However, use of more lethal chemicals soon followed the introduction of disabling chemicals. In all, chemical agents caused some 1.3 million casualties, including 90 000 deaths.

During the First World War, almost every known noxious chemical was screened for its potential as a weapon, and this process was repeated during the Second World War (1939–1945), when substantial stocks of chemical weapons were accumulated, although rarely used in military operations. Between the two world wars, a high proportion of all the new compounds that had been synthesized, or isolated from natural materials, were examined to determine their utility as lethal or disabling chemical weapons. After 1945, these systematic surveys continued, together with a search for novel agents based on advances in biochemistry, toxicology and pharmacology. The chemical industry, not surprisingly, was a major source of possible agents, since most of the new chemical warfare agents had initially been identified in research on pesticides and pharmaceuticals.

Few candidate chemical warfare agents satisfy the special requirements of their potential users, including acceptable production costs as well as appropriate physical, chemical and toxicological properties. Of the many hundreds of thousands of chemicals screened, only about 60 have either been used in chemical warfare or stockpiled for possible use as weapons. Two-thirds of them were used during the First World War, when battlefields also served as testing grounds. Fewer than a dozen chemicals were then found to be effective, but have since been supplemented or replaced by a similar number of more recently developed chemicals.

The properties of some of these chemicals are described below. They are grouped according to one of the classifications set out in Chapter 3: (i) *lethal chemicals*, intended either to kill or to injure the enemy so severely as to necessitate evacuation and medical treatment; and (ii) *disabling chemicals*, used to incapacitate the enemy by causing a disability from which recovery may be possible without medical aid. Their properties are summarized in Table A1.1.

The chemicals included in Table A1.1 are not the only toxicants that can kill or injure on a large scale. Before the Chemical Weapons Convention was adopted, chemicals were selected as chemical warfare agents primarily because they had characteristics that made them so aggressive that munitions disseminating them would be competitive with conventional weapons. Nowadays, less aggressive toxicants might be used, especially where accessibility or terrorizing potential rather than casualty cost-effectiveness dominates weapons choice. There are many commercial chemicals that, although less toxic than those described here, could cause great harm, as the release of methyl isocyanate in Bhopal, India, in 1984 bears witness. Information about the properties of such toxic industrial chemicals (TICs) is widely available, e.g. on pesticides. Some high-hazard TICs are shown in Table A1.2. When considering the threat from the deliberate release of chemicals, it is therefore appropriate to take account, not only of the chemical warfare agents set out in the Schedules of the Chemical Weapons Convention, but also of such TICs as may be present in hazardous quantities, their location and their transportation between industrial facilities.

Unless otherwise indicated, the information given in this Annex on each agent has been taken either from the First Edition of the present study or from the Hazardous Substances Data Bank, which is a toxicology file of the Toxicology Data Network (TOXNET®) of the United States National Library of Medicine.

Table A1.1. Some properties of selected lethal and disabling chemicals

CAS[a] Registry Number, class and properties	Common name							
	Sarin	VX	Hydrogen cyanide	Phosgene	Chloropicrin	PFIB[b]	Mustard gas	Lewisite
CAS Registry Number	107-44-8	50782-69-9	74-90-8	75-44-5	76-06-2	382-21-8	505-60-2	541-25-3
Class	Nerve gas	Nerve gas	Blood gas	Asphyxiant	Asphyxiant	Asphyxiant	Vesicant	Vesicant
Melting/freezing point (°C)	-56	-51	-14	-118	-64	-156	14	-17
Boiling point (°C)	147	298	26	8	112	-29	228	190
Volatility at 20 °C (mg/m³)	16 100	12	873 000	6 370 000	165 000	Gas	625	3000
Relative vapour density	4.86	9.2	0.93	3.5	5.7	5.5	5.4	7.2
Solubility in water at 20 °C (%)	100	1-5	100	Reacts	0.2	Insoluble	0.1	Slightly
Airborne concentration perceptible to human beings (mg/m³)	-	-	30000	6	2	-	1.3	-
Airborne concentration intolerable to human beings (mg/m³)	-	-	-	-	25	-	-	-
Lethality in rats: reported sc LD$_{50}$ (mg per kg) [or reported inhal LCt$_{50}$ (mg.min/m³)]	0.12 [220]	0.015	(cat) [1550]	-[1880]	10 (cat)	-[1235]	1.5-5.0 [420]	1.0 [1500]
Estimated median effective airborne dosage for incapacitation of human beings (mg.min/m³)	5	0.5	2000	1600	-	-	100	300
Estimated median lethal airborne dosage for human beings (mg.min/m³)	70-100	50	1000-2000	5000	20000	-	1000-1500	1200
Estimated median lethal percutaneous dosage for human beings (mg)	1700	6	7000	-	-	-	7000	2500

[a] CAS: Chemical Abstracts Service. [b] Perfluoroisobutene.

Sources: Vojvodiç V, Toksikologija bojnih otrova. [Toxicology of war gases.] Belgrade, Vojnoizdavaçki Zavod, 1981; Marrs TC, Maynard RL, Sidell FR, Chemical warfare agents: toxicology and treatment. Chichester, Wiley, 1996; Hazardous Substances Data Base, available on CD ROM from Canadian Centre for Occupational Health and Safety, 250 Main Street East, Hamilton, Ontario, Canada L8N 1H6; Aaron HS, Chemical warfare agents: a historical update from an American perspective. US Army Biological and Defense Agency, report ERDEC-SP-004, April 1993; Klimmek R, Szinicz L, Weger N, Chemische Gifte und Kampfstoffe: Wirkung und Therapie. [Chemical poisons and war agents: effect and therapy.] Stuttgart, Hippokrates Verlag, 1983; Franke S, Lehrbuch der Militärchemie [Textbook of military chemistry], Vol. 1. Berlin, Militärverlag der Deutschen Demokratischen Republik, 1977.

Table A1.1 (continued). Some properties of selected lethal and disabling chemicals

CAS[a] Registry Number, class and properties	Common name					
	Lysergide	BZ	Adamsite	CN	CS	CR
CAS Registry Number	50-37-3	6581-06-2	578-94-9	532-27-4	2698-41-1	257-07-8
Class	Psychotropic	Psychotropic	Irritant	Irritant	Irritant	Irritant
Melting/freezing point (C)	83	164	195	54–55	94–95	72
Boiling Point (C)	Decomposes	320	410	245	310	335
Volatility at 20 °C (mg/m³)	Negligible	0.5	0.02	105	0.35	0.63
Relative vapour density		11.7	9.6	5.3	6.5	6.7
Solubility in water at 20 °C (%)	Insoluble	Soluble	0.6	Insoluble	0.05	0.01
Airborne concentration perceptible to humans (mg/m³)	–	–	0.1	0.3	0.05–0.1	0.003
Airborne concentration intolerable to humans (mg/m³)	–	–	2–5	4.5	1–5	0.7
Lethality in rats: reported sc LD_{50} (mg per kg) [or reported inhal LCt_{50} (mg.min/m³)]	16 (iv)	–	–[3700]	50 [3700]	>100 [32500]	–
Estimated median effective airborne dosage for incapacitation of human beings (mg.min/m³)	10–100	100–200	20–25	50	5–10	0.15
Estimated median lethal airborne dosage for human beings (mg.min/m³)	–	200 000	15 000–30 000	8500–25 000	25 000–100 000	>100 000
Estimated median lethal percutaneous dosage for human beings (mg)	–	–	–	–	–	–

[a] CAS: Chemical Abstracts Service.

Table A1.2. **Some high-hazard toxic industrial chemicals**

Ammonia	Arsine	Boron trichloride
Boron trifluoride	Carbon disulfide	Chlorine
Diborane	Ethylene oxide	Fluorine
Formaldehyde	Hydrogen bromide	Hydrogen chloride
Hydrogen cyanide	Hydrogen fluoride	Hydrogen sulfide
Fuming nitric acid	Phosgene	Phosphorus trichloride
Sulfur dioxide	Sulfuric acid	Tungsten hexafluoride

Source: NATO International Task Force 25 (ITF-25), *Reconnaissance of industrial hazards*, as quoted in *Chemical and biological defense primer*, Washington, DC, Deputy Assistant to the US Secretary of Defense for Chemical and Biological Defense, October 2001, p. 11.

Note: ITF-25 did not rank industrial chemicals according to toxicity alone, but according to a hazard index reflecting such factors as the volume in which a chemical might be present in an area of concern, the inhalation toxicity of the chemical, and whether it existed in a state that could give rise to an inhalation hazard. Those listed here are from the high-hazard end of the ranking. Two (hydrogen cyanide and phosgene) are listed in part A of Schedule 3 of the Chemical Weapons Convention, signifying their past use as chemical-warfare agents. Another (phosphorus trichloride) is listed in part B of Schedule 3, indicating its past use as an agent precursor. Because the hazard index for a given chemical will vary from country to country, the ranking is not universal. For example, in countries where tungsten hexafluoride is present only in laboratories and in small quantities, its hazard index will be low.

2. Lethal chemicals

The lethal chemicals known to have been developed into chemical-warfare agents, and TICs too, may be divided into two groups: (i) tissue irritants; and (ii) systemic poisons. The first group contains the choking gases (lung irritants or asphyxiants) and the blister gases (vesicants); the second the blood and nerve gases.

Chlorine, an asphyxiant, was the first lethal chemical to be used in the First World War. In the spring of 1915, massive surprise attacks with the gas caused thousands of casualties, none of whom had any protection against such an airborne poison. Respirators used to protect troops were crude at first, but rapidly became more sophisticated. In parallel with these developments in the technology of defence were efforts to find agents more aggressive than chlorine. Widespread use of phosgene and diphosgene followed. Hydrogen cyanide was produced, but its physical properties (it is lighter than air) proved poorly suited to the munitions of relatively small payload capacity that were characteristic of most of the available delivery systems at that time. Another trend was the development of substances such as chloropicrin, the physical and chemical properties of which enabled them to penetrate the respirators then available. The third and most significant development was that of agents such as mustard gas and the arsenical vesicants, e.g. lewisite, which damaged the skin and poisoned through skin penetration.

Among the many new chemicals reviewed for their chemical-warfare potential during the 1920s and 1930s were *bis* (trichloromethyl) oxalate, a congener of phosgene, and the tetrachlorodinitroethanes, congeners of chloropicrin. Other chemicals examined included disulfur deca-fluoride; various arsenical vesicants; nitrogen mustards and higher sulfur mustards; metallic carbonyls; cadmium, selenium and tellurium compounds; fluoroacetates; and carbamates. A few were found to offer some advantages over existing chemical warfare agents for particular purposes and were put into production. None, however, was thought superior to phosgene or mustard gas in general utility, and it was these two agents that formed the bulk of the chemical weapons stockpiled at the start of the Second World War, just as they had at the end of the First.

The most significant development in the lethal agents occurred at the time of the Second World War, when Germany manufactured tabun, the first of what became known as the G-agent series of nerve gases. A pilot plant for producing tabun was operating when war broke out in September 1939. At the war's end in 1945, some 12 000 tonnes of tabun had been produced, much of it filled into munitions. Tabun is both more toxic and faster acting than phosgene. Inhalation is a primary route of exposure, but casualties can also be caused if nerve agents penetrate the eye or skin, albeit at higher dosages.

Work continued on the G agents in several countries after the war. Sarin, first characterized in Germany in 1938, emerged as one of the more attractive nerve gases for military purposes. It went into production when methods were developed that overcame the difficulties that had precluded its large-scale manufacture during the war. In the early 1950s, the first of what became known as the V agents was discovered in an agrochemical laboratory. Members of the series, such as VX and VR, are considerably more toxic than the G-agent nerve gases, especially if absorbed through bare skin.

During the Gulf War of 1981–1988, United Nations investigators collected evidence of the use of mustard gas and nerve agents. During the war, more than 100 000 Iranian military and civilian personnel received treatment for the acute effects of Iraqi chemical weapons *(1)*, and 25 000 people were killed by them *(2)*, a number that continues to increase. In addition, 13 years after the end of the war, 34 000 of those who had been acutely affected were still receiving treatment for long-term effects of the weapons *(1)*. Evidence also exists of the widespread use of chemical-warfare agents against centres of population in Kurdish areas of Iraq in 1988. In particular, soil and other samples collected from the vicinity of exploded munitions were later analysed and found to contain traces of mustard gas and sarin. Iranian military personnel and Kurdish civilians have been treated in hospitals in Europe and the United States for mustard gas injuries. Health surveys within the Kurdish regions affected have, however, been limited, and the present health status of the population remains to be determined *(3)*.

2.1 Lung irritants

2.1.1 Phosgene

Also known as carbonyl dichloride (CAS Registry Number 75-44-5), phosgene is a colourless gas at most ambient temperatures, but a fuming liquid below 8.2 °C. It is easily liquefied under pressure.

Sources

Phosgene does not occur naturally. First prepared in 1812, it is widely available in the chemical industry, where it is used as an intermediate in the manufacture of dyestuffs, pesticides, pharmaceuticals, polymers, resins and hardeners, among other products. Annual production in the United States is about 1 million tonnes, in Europe about 1.2 million.

Phosgene is also produced during the thermal decomposition or photo-oxidation of chlorinated solvents, and when polyvinyl chloride (PVC) is burned.

Exposure

Inhalation is the principal route. At high concentrations, skin and eye irritation occur. The lung is the main target organ, and damage to it following acute exposure to phosgene obeys Haber's Law, i.e. degree of injury is proportional to the product of the concentration and duration of exposure. Haber's Law does not apply in chronic exposures.

Phosgene is variously described as smelling like decaying fruit, fresh-cut grass or mouldy hay. Trained workers can detect it at concentrations of 0.4 ppm. The odour threshold is generally about 1.5 ppm. Eyes, nose and throat become irritated at 3–4 ppm. Dosages damaging to the lung are 30 ppm.min or greater. Pulmonary oedema occurs at dosages exceeding 150 ppm.min (600 mg.min/m³) *(4)*.

Latency period and recovery time

Irritation of the eyes, nose and throat, together with chest tightness, occur rapidly at concentrations exceeding 3 ppm, followed by shortness of breath and a cough. If these are the only symptoms, they abate rapidly after exposure ceases. At dosages exceeding 30 ppm.min, the initial irritation and respiratory symptoms are followed by a second (possibly asymptomatic) phase, the duration of which is inversely proportional to the inhaled dose. After large doses, it may be 1–4 hours; after small doses, 24–48 hours. Pulmonary oedema, sometimes fatal, occurs in the third phase. If the patient survives, clinical and radiological oedema resolve within a few days. Antibiotics can be used if signs of infection develop. Residual bronchitis can last for several days. Blood gases and carbon monoxide diffusion normalize within a week. However, exertional dyspnoea and increased bronchial resistance may persist for several months *(5)*.

Main clinical symptoms

Burning and watering of the eyes, a sore or scratchy throat, dry cough and chest tightness usually indicate exposure to concentrations exceeding 3 ppm. These symptoms are only a rough guide to the possibility of more severe lung injury. Exposures to 2 ppm for 80 minutes will not cause any irritation but result in pulmonary oedema some 12–16 hours later *(6)*.

Sense of smell is a poor guide to possible concentrations. At high concentrations, olfactory fatigue sets in, and subjects lose their sense of smell and their ability to assess the danger.

Erythema of the oral and pharyngeal mucous membranes is seen at higher concentrations.

Moist rales may be evident in lung fields and indicate the presence of pulmonary oedema. Lengthening of respiration occurs, indicating bronchiole luminal narrowing. Dyspnoea develops, and patients produce increasing amounts of sputum, which becomes frothy. Blood is viscous, and coagulates readily. Methaemoglobin concentrations increase and cyanosis and reduced arterial blood pressure follow, causing a marked increase in heart rate. The terminal clinical phase of lethal poisoning causes extreme distress with intolerable dyspnoea until respiration ceases. Phosgene intoxication always produces a metabolic acidosis and a compensatory hyperventilation. Arterial blood gases usually indicate hypoxaemia *(5)*.

At very high concentrations (> 200 ppm), phosgene passes the blood–air barrier, causing haemolysis in the pulmonary capillaries, congestion by red cell fragments and stoppage of capillary circulation. Death occurs within a few minutes from acute cor pulmonale (acute enlargement of the right ventricle). Contact with liquid phosgene may cause skin damage or blistering.

Most survivors of acute exposure have a good prognosis, but shortness of breath and reduced physical activity may persist in some for the remainder of their lives. Smoking appears to worsen the chances of recovery, and pre-existing lung disease, e.g. emphysema, will exacerbate the effects of phosgene exposure *(7)*.

Long-term health implications
Evidence suggests that phosgene is unlikely to be mutagenic. Data on carcinogenicity are insufficient for an assessment.

Detection
A number of techniques are available to determine air concentrations, including passive dosimetry, manual and automated colorimetry, infrared spectroscopy and ultraviolet spectrophotometry. Paper tape

monitors capable of detecting 5 μg/m^3 have been described. Other methods employ an absorbent and solvent *(4)*.

Principles of medical management

Rapid triage in the following order should be carried out:

1. Severe respiratory distress.
2. Dyspnoea – at first with exertion, later at rest.
3. Cough, irritation of eyes and throat.
4. Irritation only.

Victims should be removed from the source of exposure and their clothing loosened. If they are in contact with liquid phosgene, contaminated clothing and footwear should be removed and the affected area gently warmed with lukewarm water.

Patients should be observed for up to 48 hours. If oedema develops, it will be apparent by this time. Warmth, rest and quiet are vital for all patients *(4, 5)*.

Prophylaxis/treatment

Affected skin and eyes should be flushed with running water for 15–20 minutes.

It is important to differentiate between early irritant symptoms and pulmonary oedema evident on chest X-ray. Irritation will precede oedema. However, oedema may sometimes develop in the absence of lung irritation.

Early oedema may be detected by chest X-ray before evident clinical signs appear by using 50–80 kV; at 100–120 kV, this may not be seen *(6)*.

Early intubation is essential at the first sign of oedema or pulmonary failure. Adequate oxygenation is essential, and the mode of ventilation will need to be assessed for each individual *(6, 8, 9)*.

Pulmonary function tests and chest X-rays should be conducted on patients at follow-up after 2–3 months.

Stability/neutralization

Phosgene is very persistent in the atmosphere. As it does not absorb UV light, it does not undergo photolysis by sunlight in the troposphere but should photolyse at higher altitudes. The half-life in the atmosphere is estimated to be 113 years at sea level.

Phosgene reacts with hydrogen in water, and with primary and secondary amines.

The water solubility and vapour pressure of phosgene are such that it will volatilize rapidly from water.

Protection
This can be provided by a military-type respirator.

2.1.2   Chloropicrin

Also known as trichloronitromethane or nitrochloroform (CAS Registry Number 76-06-2), chloropicrin is both a lacrimator and a lung irritant. It is an oily liquid, colourless or yellowish green, at all ambient temperatures, with a highly irritating vapour. It will not burn but can decompose at high temperatures forming toxic gases such as phosgene, hydrogen chloride, nitrogen oxides and carbon monoxide. For chemical-warfare purposes, chloropicrin has been used as a casualty agent, a harassing agent and a training agent.

Sources
Chloropicrin was first prepared in 1848 from picric acid and bleach. Nowadays it is made by chlorinating nitromethane. Its peaceful applications include use as an insecticide, rodenticide and fumigant. Its former application as a riot-control agent is now rare.

Exposure
Exposure to chloropicrin is primarily through inhalation and direct contact. Concentrations of 0.3–1.35 ppm will result in painful eye irritation in 3–30 seconds, depending on the susceptibility of the individual. A 30-minute exposure to a concentration of 119 ppm and a 10-minute exposure to 297.6 ppm both resulted in the death of the individual exposed. Higher concentrations will be lethal following shorter exposure periods.

The odour threshold of chloropicrin is 1.1 ppm, above the level at which it will irritate the eye. Concentrations of 1–3 ppm will cause lacrimation.

Severe lung damage leading to pulmonary oedema and airways injury may occur. Oedema may be delayed and is exacerbated by physical activity. Complications of lung injury include secondary infections and bronchiolitis obliterans. Skin irritation is likely following direct contact, and may result in permanent scarring. Ingestion of small amounts will cause pain and is likely to result in nausea, gastroenteritis, and even death. The estimated lethal dose is 5–50 mg/kg body weight.

Chloropicrin is intermediate in toxicity between chlorine and phosgene. Chlorine in fatal concentrations produces injury primarily of the upper respiratory tract, trachea, and larger bronchi, whereas phosgene acts primarily on the alveoli. Chloropicrin causes greater injury to the medium and small bronchi than to the trachea and large bronchi. Alveolar injury is less than with phosgene, but pulmonary oedema occurs and is the most frequent cause of early deaths. Renal and hepatic damage following exposure has also been reported.

The permissible occupational exposure limit in the United States is 0.1 ppm as a time-weighted average over 8 hours.

Latency period and recovery time

Irritation of the eyes occurs rapidly and within 30 seconds following exposure to 0.3–1.35 ppm (2–9 mg/m^3). Concentrations of 1–3 ppm cause lacrimation, and a 1-minute exposure to 15 ppm will cause injury to the lung *(10)*.

The effects of exposure may be delayed, but if oedema is not present after 48 hours, it is unlikely to occur.

If exposure is substantial, symptoms such as nausea, vomiting and diarrhoea may persist for weeks *(11)*.

Individuals injured by inhalation of chloropicrin are reportedly more susceptible to the gas, and experience symptoms at concentrations lower than those that affect naive individuals.

Main clinical symptoms

Irritation of the eyes, nose and throat occur, resulting in lacrimation and coughing. Other symptoms reported in exposed individuals include vertigo, fatigue, headache and an exacerbation of orthostatic hypotension.

A concentration of 4 ppm for a few seconds renders an individual unfit for activity and 15 ppm for the same period has caused respiratory tract injury. Concentrations of 15 ppm cannot be tolerated for longer than 1 minute, even by individuals accustomed to chloropicrin.

Ingestion results in nausea, vomiting, colic and diarrhoea.

Inhalation is reported to cause anaemia in some individuals, and the haematopoietic system is also affected in animals exposed to chloropicrin, with reduced erythrocyte, haemoglobin and haematocrit (erythrocyte volume fraction) counts *(12)*.

Asthmatics exposed to chloropicrin will experience asthma attacks because of its irritant properties.

Auscultation of the lungs may reveal moist diffuse rales, but these will be present only in the most severe cases. X-ray examination of the chest may show diffuse infiltration of lung fields.

Toxic pulmonary oedema will be more severe, and appear earlier if patients undertake physical activity after exposure.

Long-term health implications
Data are inadequate to assess whether chloropicrin causes developmental, reproductive or mutagenic effects. In a carcinogenicity study in rodents, animals were exposed for too short a period to enable an assessment of carcinogenic risk to be made. Data on mutagenicity are equivocal: chloropicrin is mutagenic to bacteria but not to mammalian cells.

Detection
A range of analytical methods is available for detection purposes, including chemical assays and combinations of gas chromatography, ion-selective electrode, electron capture, spectrometry and polarography *(13, 14)*.

Principles of medical management
Patients should be removed from the source of the exposure and clothing loosened. The airway should be checked to ensure that it is clear. Patients should be observed for 48 hours, checking for hypoxia or hypercarbia; if oedema develops, it will be apparent by this time. Warmth, rest and quiet are vital for all patients.

Prophylaxis/treatment
If skin contamination occurs, the affected areas should be washed with soap and tepid water. Washing may need to be done for 20–30 minutes, and any contaminated clothing removed.

If there is contact with the eyes, they should be washed with copious amounts of tepid water for up to 20 minutes. If irritation persists, the irrigation should be repeated.

If chloropicrin is ingested, vomiting should not be induced. The patient should be encouraged to drink water or fluids.

Oedema may be delayed following inhalation but should be detectable by 48 hours. Positive airway pressure will assist breathing. Oxygen should be administered if the patient is hypoxic or cyanosed. Bacterial infection is common with oedema, and careful surveillance cultures are required. Prophylactic antibiotics are not recommended. Fluids should be administered if the patient is hypotensive.

Stability/neutralization

Chloropicrin decomposes to give phosgene, nitrosyl chloride, chlorine and nitrogen oxides on exposure to light. Heating above 150 °C causes decomposition to phosgene and nitrosyl chloride. Chloropicrin reacts violently with alkali or alkaline earths. It is sparingly soluble in water (2.2 g/litre).

If fire breaks out in the vicinity of chloropicrin, the area concerned should be approached from upwind. Water (in flooding conditions or as fog or foam), dry chemicals or carbon dioxide should be used to extinguish fires.

If spills occur, these should be contained with sand/soil or absorbent material, which should then be shovelled into a suitable container. Care must be taken in flooding an area with water as this may react with the acid chloropicrin. Large quantities of water can be added safely to small quantities of chloropicrin.

Protection

Any air-purifying, air-supplying, or chemical-cartridge full-face mask will provide adequate protection.

2.1.3   Perfluoroisobutene

Also known as 1,1,3,3,3-pentafluoro-2-(trifluoromethyl)-1-propene (CAS Registry Number 382-21-8) or PFIB, perfluoroisobutene is a rapid-acting lung irritant that damages the air–blood barrier of the lungs and causes oedema. Microscopic oedema is evident in pulmonary tissues within 5 minutes. It is a colourless, odourless gas at most ambient temperatures and is easily liquefied.

Sources

PFIB does not occur naturally. It is a by-product of the manufacture of polytetrafluoroethylene (Teflon) and is also formed when this type of polymer or the related perfluoroethylpropylenes are heated to temperatures that cause thermal decomposition. The fumes generated in decomposition contain PFIB. Teflon generates PFIB-containing fumes at temperatures in excess of 360 °C *(15)*.

The properties of organofluoride polymers, which include lubricity, high dielectric constant and chemical inertness, are such that these materials are used extensively in military vehicles such as tanks and aircraft.

Exposure

Inhalation is the principal route of exposure. High concentrations may produce irritation of the eyes, nose and throat. The lung is the main target organ and the only one reported in human studies. Systemic effects seen in animal studies occur only where there is substantial injury to the lung, and hypoxia is considered to be a major contributing factor.

Data on dosages causing symptoms in humans are sparse and, where effects have been reported, individuals have been exposed to a range of other gases as well as PFIB.

In rodents, dosages of 150–180 ppm.min (1250–1500 mg.min/m^3) will kill 50% of the test population. Comparable dosages for phosgene are 750 ppm.min *(16, 17)*.

Latency period and recovery time

A syndrome known as "polymer fume fever" has been described following inhalation of the pyrolysis products of organofluorides. Exposure to fumes has occurred when Teflon has been heated directly in welding processes and indirectly when cigarettes contaminated with micronized Teflon have been smoked *(15, 18, 19)*. Symptoms may appear 1–4 hours post-exposure and are often mistaken for influenza. Subsequent symptoms are those of pulmonary oedema with, initially, dyspnoea on exertion, followed by difficulty in breathing unless seated or standing and, later, dyspnoea at rest. Oedema, as shown by clinical and radiological evidence, becomes more marked for up to 12 hours, before it clears, with recovery usually complete by 72 hours.

Main clinical symptoms

High concentrations in animals have caused sudden death, but this has not been recorded in humans.

Irritation of the eyes, nose and throat may occur if the concentration is high enough. At lower concentrations, a sense of discomfort in the chest, especially on taking a deep breath, may be the first symptom. There may be a feeling of irritation or oppression retrosternally, but usually not severe enough to be described as pain. A dry irritating cough may or may not develop and worsen as the chest becomes increasingly sore. However, these preliminary symptoms may be absent, and the first warning of illness may only be a general malaise.

A few hours after exposure, there is a gradual increase in temperature, pulse rate and (possibly) respiration rate. Shivering and sweating usually follow. Temperatures are reported not to exceed 104 °F (40 °C) and pulse-rate is generally below 120.

Physical signs are fleeting. Auscultation of the lungs may reveal diffuse, moist rales, but these are usually present only in the most severe cases. X-ray examination of the chest may show diffuse infiltration of lung fields.

Toxic pulmonary oedema may be more severe and appear earlier if the patient exercises post-exposure.

Two human deaths from pyrolysis products of polymerized organofluorides have been reported *(16)*.

Long-term health implications

Several reports of decreased pulmonary function, including reduced carbon monoxide perfusion rate, have been documented in humans up to 6 months after exposure to polymer fume.

In one reported case, a 50 year-old woman experienced some 40 episodes of polymer-fume fever mainly related to smoking organofluoride-contaminated cigarettes, and 18 months after her last bout she was found to have progressive exercise dyspnoea. Pulmonary function tests supported a provisional diagnosis of alveolar capillary block syndrome, with decreased carbon monoxide perfusion, increased difference with exercise between the alveolar and the arterial partial pressure, and minimal airway disease. Cardiopulmonary physical examination, chest radiograph and arterial blood gases were normal, but the woman died 6 months later from a ruptured berry aneurysm and a subarachnoid haemorrhage. Histological examination of the lungs revealed moderate interstitial fibrosis. Alveolar septae were thickened by dense collagen with only focal, minimal chronic inflammatory cell infiltration. The bronchi were normal *(20)*.

No data are available on the genotoxicity, mutagenicity or carcinogenicity of PFIB.

Detection
Gas samples can be collected by using an adsorbent filter either passively or with the aid of a pump. Laboratory analysis can be effected by gas chromatography.

Principles of medical management
Victims should be removed from the source of exposure and clothing loosened. Airways should be checked to ensure adequate clearance. Patients should be observed for 48 hours, checking for hypoxia and hypercarbia; if oedema develops, it will be apparent by this time. Warmth, rest and quiet are vital for all patients.

Prophylaxis/treatment
There is no recognized prophylaxis for human PFIB exposure. Protection against the lethal effects of inhaled PFIB has been demonstrated in rats when N-acetylcysteine was administered orally 4–8 hours before gas exposure. The duration of protection was related to the plasma concentrations of thiol compounds (cysteine, glutathione and N-acetylcysteine) derived from the N-acetylcysteine administered *(21)*. No post-exposure medical or chemical therapy that impedes or reverses injury from PFIB inhalation is known *(16)*.

Early oedema may be detected by chest X-ray (and before clinical signs appear) using 50–80 kV. Pulmonary oedema responds clinically to the application of positive airway pressure. PEEP (positive-end expiratory pressure)/CPAP (continuous positive airway pressure) masks are of value initially. Intubation may be necessary. Oxygen should be administered if the patient is hypoxic or cyanosed. Fluid replacement is mandatory when the patient is hypotensive. Combined hypotension and hypoxia may damage other organs. Bacterial infection is common, and careful surveillance cultures are required. However, routine prophylactic antibiotics are not recommended. Steroid therapy has been used in two instances of PFIB exposure of the same worker. Since recovery is often spontaneous, assessing the value of steroid use is difficult *(16)*.

Stability/neutralization

When dissolved in water, PFIB decomposes rapidly to form various reactive intermediates and fluorophosgene, which, in turn, decomposes to give carbon dioxide, a radical anion and hydrogen fluoride *(22)*.

Protection

A military-type respirator can be used but some types may not be effective, since the advantage of PFIB as a chemical warfare agent is that it is poorly adsorbed by charcoal.

2.2 Blood gases

Lethal chemical agents that interfere with cell respiration have come to be known as blood gases. This is a reference to the mode of action of cyanides, which were believed to interfere with oxygen uptake from the blood (or carbon dioxide exchange between blood and tissues and between blood and the air in the lungs). The key agent is hydrogen cyanide, a toxic industrial chemical that has also been used as a chemical-warfare agent. Another such chemical, not described here, is cyanogen chloride.

2.2.1 Hydrogen cyanide

Also known as hydrocyanic acid (CAS Registry Number 74-90-8) or HCN, hydrogen cyanide is a rapid-acting lethal agent that inhibits aerobic respiration at the cellular level, preventing cells from utilizing oxygen *(23)*. Liquid HCN, which at atmospheric pressure occurs over the temperature range $-14\,°C - +26\,°C$, is colourless to yellowish brown in appearance. On standing, it polymerizes and may explode, though it can be stabilized. Some people can smell HCN at low concentrations, describing an aroma of bitter almonds or marzipan; others cannot detect it.

Sources

Hydrogen cyanide is widely available in the chemical industry as an intermediate. It is used as a pesticide, rodenticide, fumigant and, in certain countries where capital punishment is still practised, as an instrument of state killing. More general exposure to cyanide occurs through tobacco smoke, smoke inhalation from fires and, in sub-Saharan Africa, from cyanide-glycosides in the cassava tuber *(24)*.

Exposure

Inhalation is the most likely route of entry, causing hyperventilation initially. HCN vapour does not cross skin. Liquid HCN will penetrate skin, as may aerosols.

Although cyanides are rapidly detoxified by sulfur transferase enzymes, these are unlikely to play a significant role in acute poisoning, as occurs on the battlefield. Detoxification is important at lower concentrations, and exposure to 60 mg/m^3 may not cause any serious symptoms. At 200 mg/m^3, death occurs after 10 minutes. Above 2500 mg/m^3, and certainly above 5000 mg/m^3, death is likely within 1 minute *(25)*.

Latency period and recovery time

Symptoms of poisoning are rapid in onset since the gas is quickly absorbed from the lungs. Hyperventilation occurs first and increases with the dose inhaled. This is followed by rapid loss of consciousness at high concentrations.

Main clinical symptoms

The toxicity of HCN is largely attributable to the inhibition of cytochrome oxidase, which results in interference with aerobic respiration in the cell by preventing oxygen from being utilized. Lactic acid accumulates, and cells die from histotoxic anoxia. Intracellular calcium concentrations increase before cell death, a mechanism not specific to cyanide, as the phenomenon is seen in most cells before they die.

Hyperventilation is the principal initial symptom at very high concentrations, followed by loss of consciousness, convulsions and loss of corneal reflex, death being caused by cardiac and/or respiratory arrest.

At high concentrations, victims notice a sensation of throat constriction, giddiness, confusion and poorer vision. Temples on the head feel as though gripped in a vice, and pain may occur in the back of the neck and chest. Unconsciousness follows and the individual falls. Failure to remove the victim from the HCN atmosphere will result in death in 2–3 minutes, preceded by brief convulsions and failure of respiration *(26)*.

At lower but still lethal concentrations, symptoms may increase in severity over an hour or longer. Victims notice an immediate and progressive sense of warmth (due to vasodilation) with visible flushing. Prostration follows, with nausea, vomiting, probable headache, difficulty in breathing and a feeling of tight bands around the chest. Unconsciousness and asphyxia are inevitable unless exposure ceases.

At low concentrations (or doses), individuals may feel apprehensive, experience dyspnoea, headaches and vertigo, and notice a metallic taste in the mouth.

Long-term health implications

There are no long-term health implications at low concentrations. Tropical ataxic neuropathy, seen in victims of chronic cyanide poisoning caused by the consumption of poorly processed cassava, is not relevant to HCN exposure in warfare.

At near lethal concentrations, the effects of HCN on cellular respiration are likely to affect brain function. Deterioration in intellect, confusion, loss of concentration and Parkinsonian symptoms are possible.

Detection

A number of analytical methods are available for use in detection. Laboratory detection (and detection in mobile field vehicles) is by gas chromatography–mass spectrometry (GC–MS).

Cyanide is rapidly removed from blood and converted by the enzyme rhodanase into the less toxic thiocyanate, which can be measured in urine.

Principles of medical management

The patient should be removed from the source of exposure. The rapidity of action of HCN may mean that those arriving on the scene will find casualties who are asymptomatic; showing acute symptoms; recovering from them; or dead. Triage should be performed.

Victims who are asymptomatic several minutes after exposure do not require oxygen or antidotes.

Where exposure has caused acute effects (convulsions, apnoea), oxygen and antidotes should be administered immediately.

Patients recovering from acute exposures (and unconscious, but breathing) will make a faster recovery with antidotes and oxygen (27).

Resources permitting, resuscitation should be attempted on subjects with no pulse in case heart stoppage is recent.

Decontamination of clothing or equipment is unnecessary in view of the high volatility of HCN.

Prophylaxis/treatment
This is likely to be complicated on the battlefield. Exposed troops cannot be expected to self-administer antidotes *(25)*.

Treatment must be prompt. After oxygen has been administered, subsequent treatment is aimed partly at dissociating the cyanide ion from cytochrome oxidase. Therapies include sodium thiosulfate (to increase rhodanase activity), sodium nitrite or 4-dimethylaminophenol (4-DMAP) (to form methaemoglobin, which in turn combines with cyanide to form cyanmethaemoglobin) or cobalt (which also combines with cyanide ions) *(27–29)*.

Stability/neutralization
HCN is unstable and non-persistent, and degrades slowly in the atmosphere. It can travel long distances, and its concentrations will fall as the distance travelled increases. It mixes with water and decomposes slowly.

Protection
A military-style gas mask with filters treated so as to adsorb cyanide should be used.

2.3   Vesicants

The vesicants, or blister agents, are general tissue irritants with an additional systemic action. Contact with skin tissues provokes blistering in the affected region after some delay. Contact with the eyes causes more rapid injury and leads to inflammation and possible temporary loss of sight. Injury to the respiratory tract occurs, the nature of the injury varying with the agent.

The two main groups of vesicants are the dichloroarsine derivatives and the so-called "mustards". The latter are militarily the more important as they lack the initial irritant effect of the dichloroarsines and have odours that are much less readily detected, so that they are well suited to insidious attack. The dichloroarsines will cause pulmonary oedema (toxic alveolitis), whereas this is not a typical feature of mustard gas exposure. All the mustards contain at least two 2-chloroethyl groups, attached either to thioether residues (the sulfur mustards) or to amine residues (the nitrogen mustards).

2.3.1　Mustard gas

Also known as bis(2-chloroethyl) sulfide (CAS Registry Number 505-60-2), yperite or Lost, mustard gas is a colourless to amber oily liquid of neutral reaction, freezing at 14 °C when pure and boiling at 228 °C with slow decomposition. At high concentrations, it has a pungent odour resembling that of horseradish, onions or garlic, much of which may be due to contamination with ethyl sulfide or similar by-products of its synthesis. It is only slightly soluble in water, but may dissolve in organic solvents and fats. Chemically and physically, it is a relatively stable substance. When dissolved in water, it first hydrolyses and then oxidizes to the less toxic sulfoxide and sulfone.

Sources

Sulfur mustard had been synthesized by 1860 and was developed as a chemical warfare agent during the First World War. It has practically no other application.

Exposure

Exposure to both liquid and vapour occurs, mainly via inhalation and by skin contact. Mustard gas produces militarily significant effects over a wide range of dosages. Incapacitating eye injury may be sustained at about 100 mg.min/m³. Significant skin burns may begin at 200 mg.min/m³. The estimated respiratory lethal dose is 1500 mg.min/m³. On bare skin, 4–5 g of liquid mustard gas may constitute a lethal percutaneous dosage, while droplets of a few milligrams may cause incapacitation.

Mustard gas vapour can be carried long distances by the wind. Local contamination of water exposed to sulfur mustard may occur, liquid mustard tending to sink as a heavy oily layer to the bottom of pools of water, leaving a dangerous oily film on the surface.

Toxic concentrations of mustard gas in the air smell, the odour being detectable at about 1.3 mg/m^3. Experience in the First World War and in the war between Iraq and the Islamic Republic of Iran in 1980–1988 has clearly shown the incapacitating effects of mustard gas secondary to the lesions of skin and mucosa. Only a limited number of cases – 2–3% among about 400 000 exposed during the First World War *(25)* and a similar percentage in the war between Iraq and the Islamic Republic of Iran – have a fatal outcome, mainly within the first month.

Latency period from exposure to symptoms
Under field conditions without protection, signs and symptoms develop gradually after an interval of several hours. The duration of this interval depends on the mode of exposure, the environmental temperature, and probably also on the individual.

Quite soon after exposure, however, nausea, retching, vomiting and eye smarting have occasionally been reported. Acute systemic effects, central nervous excitation leading to convulsions and rapid death occur only at supra-lethal dosages.

Main clinical symptoms
Signs and symptoms usually develop in the following order. The first definite symptoms generally occur in the eyes between 30 minutes and 3 hours after exposure, starting with a feeling of grittiness, progressive soreness and a bloodshot appearance, and proceeding to oedema and all the phenomena of acute conjunctivitis, with pain, lacrimation, blepharospasm and photophobia. There is increased nasal secretion, sneezing, sore throat, coughing and hoarseness, and dyspnoea may develop. Within 4–16 hours after exposure, these symptoms become much more marked and distressing: the eyes begin discharging and are very painful, the nasal discharge is more purulent, and the voice is husky or suppressed. Nausea, retching and vomiting, associated with epigastric pains, occur in a large proportion of subjects and may recur at frequent intervals for several hours. In severe cases, they may become intense and prolonged. Diarrhoea may set in, but is rather unusual. The skin may begin to itch during this period and skin rashes may show as a dusky erythema of the exposed parts of the body

and the axilla and genitals, with blisters beginning to appear. At the end of 24 hours, all these symptoms may have increased in severity, but death almost never occurs during the first day.

Evolution and recovery

In mild cases, skin lesions may remain limited to an erythema, which turns black in about 10–15 days, while the superficial epidermal layers desquamate without causing an actual skin defect. This phenomenon, already known from the First *(26, 30)* and Second *(31)* World Wars, was also observed in Iranian casualties *(32)*. With moderate to severe exposure, large blisters develop, filled with a clear yellow fluid, which usually break, leading to erosions and full-thickness skin loss and ulceration. Blisters caused by mustard gas may heal in 2 or 3 weeks, and full-thickness erosions after 6–12 weeks. On and around the burned area, hyperpigmentation occurs. The site of healed mustard burns is hypersensitive to mechanical trauma.

In severe cases, inflammation of the upper and lower respiratory tract becomes conspicuous during the second day. The expectoration becomes abundant, mucopurulent, sometimes with large sloughs of tracheal mucosa. This is complicated by secondary infection of the necrotic respiratory membranes. Fever sets in, with rapid pulse and respiration. The infection may terminate in bronchopneumonia, with death at any time between the second day and the fourth week. Recovery is slow, and expectoration and cough may persist for several weeks.

Sulfur mustard is absorbed and distributed systemically. In severe cases, after a brief period of increasing white blood cell count in peripheral blood, a rapid fall takes place. In Iranian casualties from the war between Iraq and the Islamic Republic of Iran, leukopenia was observed between day 5 and day 20 after exposure. Severe leukopenia was accompanied by sepsis, cardiovascular shock and multi-organ failure.

Experience with Iranian casualties showed that, in those with severe lung complications requiring artificial ventilation, and where there was substantial systemic exposure leading to severe leukopenia, prognosis was very poor, even when sophisticated treatment was available *(32)*.

Long-term health implications

Recent experience after the war between Iraq and the Islamic Republic of Iran confirmed that long-term skin lesions – mainly scarring of the skin, and hyper- and hypopigmentation – itching, and lung diseases, such as chronic obstructive bronchitis and emphysema, could develop (Sohrabpour, Doulati & Javaadi, personal communication, 1999).

A most distressing phenomenon, known from the First World War but now also observed after the war between Iraq and the Islamic Republic of Iran, is the development of delayed keratitis of the eye after an interval of 6–10 years with late-onset blindness. The lesions recur even after corneal transplantation (Javaadi, personal communication, 1999).

Both sulfur and nitrogen mustards have been shown to be mutagenic, carcinogenic and teratogenic under both in vitro and in vivo experimental conditions. Studies undertaken on mustard gas factory workers in Japan and the United Kingdom demonstrated the carcinogenic effect in humans. Exposures to mustard gas in factories may have been both considerable and prolonged. A more difficult question concerns the likelihood of developing cancer as a result of exposure to sulfur mustard on the battlefield. Here the evidence is suggestive but not absolutely clear-cut *(25)*. Although 11–14 years have, at this writing, passed since the employment of mustard gas in the war between Iraq and the Islamic Republic of Iran, no increase in cancer incidence has so far been observed in exposed soldiers (Keshavarz, personal communication, 1999), but it is still too soon for definite conclusions.

Detection in the field and diagnosis of exposure

A number of techniques are available to detect liquid sulfur mustard, e.g. by means of detection paper, powder or chalk. Sulfur mustard vapour in air can be detected by the use of vapour-detection kits or by means of automated chemical agent detectors employing either ion-mobility spectrometry or flame photometry.

In the diagnosis of exposure to sulfur mustard in humans, alkylation products of sulfur mustard with haemoglobin, albumin and DNA in blood, as well as metabolites of sulfur mustard in urine, have proved to be useful targets.

Based on a monoclonal antibody that was raised against the major adduct of sulfur mustard in human DNA, namely the adduct at the 7-

position of guanine, enzyme-linked immunosorbent (ELISA) and immunoslotblot assays have been developed. With haemoglobin, the adducts with the amino function in terminal valine of the α- and ß-chains have proved to be most convenient for diagnosis. In principle, the immunoassay approach has been developed for use under field conditions, whereas the mass-spectrometric methods can be used to confirm the immunochemical result under more sophisticated conditions. In view of the long biological half-life of the protein adducts, the mass-spectrometric methods are highly useful for retrospective detection of exposure. Both the mass-spectrometric and the immuno-assay methods have been successfully applied to blood samples taken from Iranian soldiers during the war between Iraq and the Islamic Republic of Iran more than 3 weeks after alleged mild exposure to sulfur mustard *(33)*.

Metabolism of sulfur mustard leads to a complicated mixture of products excreted into the urine. Contrary to the widely held belief, the hydrolysis product of sulfur mustard, namely thiodiglycol, is only a minor metabolite in urine. However, the sulfoxide derivative of thiodiglycol is abundantly present. This is reduced to thiodiglycol for GC–MS analysis.

Unfortunately, both thiodiglycol and its sulfoxide are often present in the urine of unexposed persons. ß-Lyase activity on bis-cysteinyl conjugates of sulfur mustard (presumably derived from glutathione adducts) leads to the excretion of two sulfoxide/sulfone metabolites that can be reduced to thioether derivatives for subsequent GC–MS analysis. These products are not present in the urine of unexposed persons and were found in that of two male subjects who had suffered from extensive blistering due to accidental exposure to sulfur mustard *(34)*.

Principles of medical management

Adequate first-aid measures are very important. Attendants should wear protective clothing and respirators when dealing with contaminated casualties. Patients should be removed from the source of contamination, and areas of liquid contamination should be decontaminated. Liquid contamination of the eyes should be immediately rinsed out, using copious amounts of normal saline or water from any source.

Prophylaxis/treatment

No prophylactic treatment against mustard gas is available, prophylaxis depending entirely on the protection of skin and airways by adequate protective garments. Treatment is symptomatic.

As far as skin lesions are concerned, different patterns of management have been used, ranging from treating exposed persons at burns units to treating by bathing and the use of wet dressings. Calamine lotions have been used for erythema and minor blistering, chloramine 0.2% or 0.3% solutions or silver sulfadiazine (Flamazine) 1% cream for preventing secondary infections of the skin lesions, and local corticosteroid solutions to reduce itching and irritation. Systemic analgesics, from paracetamol to morphine, and systemic antihistamines or corticosteroids have also been used. In one patient with large full-thickness burns, skin grafts were applied and were found to take well *(25)*. Several days after exposure, removal of the surface of the skin in the affected area until capillary bleeding occurs (dermal abrasion) may hasten recovery from the lesions *(35)*.

Eye lesions should be treated by saline irrigation, petroleum jelly on follicular margins to prevent sticking, local anaesthetic drops to relieve severe pain (though these may damage the cornea) or, better still, systemic narcotic analgesics. To prevent infection, chloramphenicol eye drops or another local antibiotic should be used. In cases of severe eye damage, an ophthalmological opinion must be sought.

Inhalation of moist air was used in the treatment of Iranian casualties in the war between Iraq and the Islamic Republic of Iran, and acetylcysteine was used as a mucolytic. Bronchodilators have also been used. Antibiotic cover is recommended in view of the risk of secondary infection.

Bone-marrow depression leading to severe leukopenia and aplastic anaemia should be treated with granulocyte, platelet and red cell transfusions. Whether drugs that stimulate normal marrow are of any use is not known. Granulocyte colony-stimulating factor and related factors should be considered in severe leukopenia, but it is not known whether they would be useful *(25)*.

In order to eliminate sulfur mustard from the circulation and from the body in general, administration of thiosulfate and other thiols, as well as haemodialysis and haemoperfusion, have been used in some Iranian mustard gas casualties. There is, however, no established place for them in the treatment of mustard gas intoxication. Moreover, since there is no sound theoretical basis for haemodialysis and haemoperfusion, as no active mustard has been identified in blood taken from victims, and since, with both procedures, there may be a risk of bleeding and of secondary infection in these immunocompromised patients, these procedures should not be applied *(32)*.

In severely ill patients, appropriate intensive care measures are necessary.

Stability/neutralization

Sulfur mustard can be quite persistent in the environment, depending on the temperature. It represents a serious persistent hazard, particularly at temperatures below 0 °C. Substances such as metal, glass and glazed tiles are generally impervious to mustard, although painted surfaces may take it up for a time and then release it later. Decontamination procedures for skin, equipment and materiel have been developed by most armies, using neutralizing, active chemicals, such as chloramine solutions, or neutral adsorbing powders, e.g. fuller's earth. The use of plain water for decontamination, e.g. by showering, is of dubious value since it can disperse the agent over the body.

Protection

Military-type active-carbon-containing protective clothing and a full-face gas mask with an appropriate filter should be used.

2.3.2   Lewisite

Also known as 2-chlorovinyldichloroarsine (CAS Registry Number 541-25-3), lewisite is an odourless, colourless oily liquid, freezing at –18 °C and boiling at 190 °C. Technical preparations are often blue-black in colour and smell like geraniums. They will usually also contain lewisite-2 (bis(2-chlorovinyl)chloroarsine) and lewisite-3 (tris(2-chlorovinyl)arsine). Lewisite is practically insoluble in water but freely soluble in organic solvents. It hydrolyses rapidly when mixed with water or dissolved in alkaline aqueous solutions such as sodium hypochlorite solution.

Sources

Lewisite was studied as a potential chemical-warfare agent before 1918, but there has been no verified use on a battlefield except where it has served as a freezing-point depressant for mustard gas. It has essentially no applications for peaceful purposes.

Exposure

Exposure may occur to liquid and vapour, via inhalation and by skin contact. Lewisite is about 7 times less persistent than mustard gas. Acute toxicity figures for humans are not well known, but 0.05–0.1 mg/cm^2 produces erythema, 0.2 mg/cm^2 produces vesication and a 15-minute exposure to a vapour concentration of 10 mg/m^3 produces conjunctivitis. About 2.5 g, if applied to the skin and not washed off or otherwise decontaminated, would be expected to be fatal to an average 70-kg person because of systemic toxicity. On inhalation, the LCt$_{50}$ [inhalational toxicity of the vapour form, where C is concentration measured in mg/m^3 and t is the time of exposure measured in minutes] in humans is estimated to be about 1500 mg.min/m^3.

Latency period, and main clinical symptoms

The latency period from exposure to symptoms appears to be shorter with lewisite than with mustard gas. Otherwise, as seen in accidental exposures, lewisite produces a similar clinical picture. There is immediate eye irritation and blepharospasm, rapidly followed by coughing, sneezing, lacrimation and vomiting. On skin contact, a burning sensation is felt, and the erythema and vesication, following after a few hours, are painful. Maximal blister size, covering the whole erythematous area, develops over 4 days. Abnormal pigmentation does not occur. Breathing may be difficult, followed in severe cases by pseudomembrane formation and pulmonary oedema. Liver toxicity and systemic arsenic toxicity – diarrhoea, neuropathy, nephritis, haemolysis, shock and encephalopathy – may follow after extensive skin contamination. Eye lesions may be particularly serious with blindness following unless decontamination is very prompt.

Evolution and recovery

Healing of skin lesions proceeds in a few weeks and more readily than in the case of mustard lesions, unless there has been secondary infection. Secondary bronchopulmonary infections may occur, whereas recovery from systemic toxicity will depend on the severity of the initial lesions. Lewisite seems not to be mutagenic, teratogenic or carcinogenic.

Detection in the field and diagnosis of exposure

The detection and identification of lewisite in the environment are much more difficult than for sulfur mustard. It cannot be detected by automated chemical agent detectors, although laboratory identification by gas chromatography, after derivatization, is possible. As with sulfur mustard, techniques based on protein adducts might become available, more especially the quantification of the metabolite 2-chlorovinylarsonous acid bound to haemoglobin and detectable in blood 10 days after subcutaneous administration to experimental animals. Unbound 2-chlorovinylarsonous acid may be measured in urine for up to 12 hours after exposure *(36)*.

Principles of medical management

Adequate first-aid measures are very important. Attendants should wear protective clothing and respirators when dealing with contaminated casualties. Patients should be removed from the source of contamination, and areas of liquid contamination should be decontaminated. Liquid contamination of the eyes should be immediately rinsed out using copious amounts of normal saline or water from any source.

Prophylaxis/treatment

No prophylactic treatment against lewisite is available, so prophylaxis depends entirely on protection of the skin and airways by adequate protective clothing and by early decontamination with fuller's earth or dilute solutions of bleach.

Treatment with dimercaprol (British anti-lewisite, BAL, 2,3-dimercaptopropanol) is the standard treatment for poisoning by arsenic compounds. It acts as a chelator by binding arsenic, and is available for deep, intramuscular injection, as a skin and eye ointment, and as eye drops (5–10% in vegetable oil). Local instillation in the eyes and intramuscular injections may be painful. Intramuscular doses are limited because of systemic toxicity. Several dosing regimens have been proposed, one of which prescribes 2.5 mg/kg, 4-hourly for four doses, followed by 2.5 mg/kg twice daily. Another scheme suggests 400–800 mg i.m. in divided doses on day 1, 200–400 mg i.m. in divided doses on days 2 and 3, and 100–200 mg i.m. in divided doses on days 4–12. The magnitude of the dose depends on body weight and the severity of the symptoms.

More recently, two water-soluble analogues of dimercaprol have been introduced in the clinic as arsenical antidotes, namely *meso*-2,3-dimercaptosuccinic acid (DMSA) and 2,3-dimercapto-1-propanesulfonic acid (DMPS). They are less toxic than BAL and can be given orally; DMPS can also be given intravenously.

In severely ill patients, appropriate intensive care measures should be applied.

Decontamination/neutralization

Decontamination procedures for skin, equipment and materiel have been developed by most armies, using neutralizing, active chemicals, such as chloramine solutions, or neutral adsorbing powders, such as fuller's earth. The efficacy of decontamination by plain water, e.g. by showering, is dubious since it can disperse the agent over the body.

Protection

Military-type active-carbon-containing protective clothing and a full-face gas mask with an appropriate filter should be used.

2.4 The nerve gases

The designation "nerve gas" or "nerve agent" is used for organophosphorus and other organophosphate compounds that inhibit tissue cholinesterase in humans at small dosages. It is an allusion to the mode of action of these substances, namely the disruption of nerve impulse transmission. At the present time, two families of nerve gases are important for military purposes, namely the G agents, which are alkyl esters of methylphosphonofluoridic acid or of dialkylphosphoramido-cyanidic acid, and the V agents, which are mainly alkyl esters of S-dialkylaminoethyl methylphosphonothiolic acid. G agents are primarily designed to act via inhalation, while V agents act primarily through skin penetration and the inhalation of aerosol.

Chemically and toxicologically, the nerve gases are similar to many of the commercial organophosphate pesticides and, while information on severe nerve gas poisoning in humans is rather limited, there are extensive data on human exposure to some of these pesticides.

Insecticides such as tetraethyl pyrophosphate (TEPP) and parathion have caused a number of fatalities as a result of misuse or accidental poisoning.

Among the many different G and V agents, those that have in the past been manufactured in kilotonne quantities for chemical-warfare purposes are:

O-ethyl *N*,*N*-dimethyl phosphoroamidocyanidate	Tabun: CAS 77-81-6
O-isopropyl methylphosphonofluoridate	Sarin: CAS 107-44-8
O-1,2,2-trimethylpropyl methylphosphonofluoridate	Soman: CAS 96-64-0
O-ethyl *S*-2-(diisopropylamino)ethyl methylphosphonothiolate	VX: CAS 50782-69-9
O-isobutyl *S*-2-(diisopropylamino)ethyl methylthiophosphonothiolate	VR: CAS 159939-87-4

Others have been produced, but in lesser amounts. Those produced in the largest quantities have been sarin and VR. In the account given below, however, VX is described rather than its isomer VR because the latter is still poorly characterized in the published literature. It would seem, however, that any differences in the properties of these two agents would be unlikely to invalidate the general picture presented.

Besides the G and V agents, there are several other chemical classes of organophosphate anticholinesterase agents that have been studied for chemical-warfare application. One such class, reported to have entered weaponization in the 1980s after discovery in the 1970s, is known as novichok. Published information on the novichok agents is, however, sparse. One characteristic is said to be a toxicity exceeding that of the V agents but the absence of a direct carbon–phosphorus bond in their molecular structure. The latter might mean, as some commentators have asserted publicly, that at least some novichoks do not figure in the schedules of the Chemical Weapons Convention.

2.4.1   Sarin and VX

Nerve agents are mostly odourless and colourless to yellow-brown liquids at ambient temperature, and are soluble in water. They hydrolyse quite rapidly in strongly alkaline solutions, while between pH 4 and pH 7 hydrolysis takes place very slowly. The water solubility of VX is in the range 1–5% at room temperature. It is more resistant to hydrolysis than sarin, particularly in alkaline solution.

Exposure

Nerve gases may be absorbed through any body surface. When dispersed as a vapour or aerosol, or absorbed on dust, they are readily absorbed through the respiratory tract or conjunctivae. Absorption is most rapid and complete through the respiratory tract.

The first effect observed on exposure to low air concentrations is miosis. For sarin, it appears in 50% of exposed men at about 3 mg.min/m³. At about 10 mg.min/m³, other muscarinic symptoms appear producing an incapacitating effect. Higher exposures become more and more incapacitating and are eventually lethal. Approximate figures for the concentration–time product that would be lethal to 50% of exposed men, are 150 mg.min/m³ for tabun, 70–100 mg.min/m³ for sarin, 40–60 mg.min/m³ for soman and 50 mg.min/m³ for VX *(25)*.

Latency period

Exposure to nerve agent vapour dosages that were just lethal would probably result in death within one to a few hours. An exposure to several times the lethal dose would probably be fatal within several minutes to half an hour. Photographic evidence from Halabja in Iraqi Kurdistan suggests rapid death from exposure to what was most probably a sarin attack in March 1988. VX has been used in both a murder and an attempted murder. One man died on the fourth day after admission to hospital following an injection of VX into his neck *(37)*. In an attempted murder, VX was sprayed on to the victim's back, necessitating a 15-day stay in hospital before his discharge, at which time he was suffering from amnesia and a neuropathy affecting the nerves that innervate the muscles of the shoulder girdle and upper extremities. By 6 months, the neuropathy had resolved but not the amnesia. There are significant differences in physiological responses to VX and sarin *(38)*.

Main clinical symptoms

The effects of both nerve agents and organophosphate insecticides have been related to the inhibition of tissue cholinesterases at synaptic sites, and to an accumulation of excessive amounts of acetylcholine at nicotinic and muscarinic receptors in effector organs. These phenomena are followed by other disturbances of the nervous system. Numerous studies have demonstrated that the excitatory amino acid glutamate also plays an important role in the maintenance of organophosphorus-induced seizures and in the subsequent neuropathology, especially through an over-activation of the *N*-methyl-d-aspartate (NMDA) receptor subtype *(39)*.

Muscarinic, nicotinic and central nervous system symptoms of nerve-gas poisoning, as listed by Grob *(40)*, are given in Table A1.3. The time course of their appearance varies with the degree and route of absorption. After inhalation, bronchoconstriction and respiratory distress appear before pronounced symptoms involving the gastro-intestinal tract develop. Deaths from nerve agent poisoning can be attributed to respiratory and circulatory failure.

Evolution and recovery

After a single mild to moderate exposure, full recovery may take place. Moderate to severe poisonings necessitate treatment if there is to be survival. Inhibition of acetylcholinesterase is irreversible, but adaptation of synaptic transmission occurs. Spontaneous reactivation of the inhibited enzyme is almost non-existent in acute intoxication. If a patient survives for a number of hours or days there may be some spontaneous reactivation (with sarin, cyclohexyl sarin and VX but *not* with soman), provided that the agent does not persist and cause re-inhibition. Repeated daily exposures are cumulative and may result in severe poisoning.

Long-term effects

It is possible that persistent paralysis, organophosphate-induced delayed neuropathy (OPIDN), and axonal death followed by demyelination might develop among victims surviving many times the lethal dose of sarin. However, no such delayed effects have been observed among sarin survivors in the Islamic Republic of Iran.

Table A1.3. **Signs and symptoms of nerve-gas poisoning**[a]

Site of action	Signs and symptoms
Muscarinic	*Following local exposure*
Pupils	Miosis, marked, usually maximal (pin-point), sometimes unequal
Ciliary body	Frontal headache; eye pain on focusing; slight dimness of vision; occasional nausea and vomiting
Conjunctivae	Hyperaemia
Nasal mucosa membranes	Rhinorrhoea; hyperaemia
Bronchial tree	Tightness in chest, sometimes with prolonged wheezing, expiration suggestive of bronchoconstriction or increased secretion; cough
Sweat glands	Sweating at site of exposure to liquid
Nicotinic	
Striated muscle	Fasciculations at site of exposure to liquid
Muscarinic	*Following systemic absorption*
Bronchial tree	Tightness in chest, with prolonged wheezing expiration suggestive of bronchoconstriction or increased secretion; dyspnoea, slight pain in chest; increased bronchial secretion; cough; pulmonary oedema; cyanosis
Gastrointestinal system	Anorexia; nausea; vomiting; abdominal cramps; epigastric and substernal tightness with "heartburn" and eructation; diarrhoea; tenesmus; involuntary defecation
Sweat glands	Increased sweating
Salivary glands	Increased salivation
Lacrimal glands	Increased lacrimation
Heart	Slight bradycardia
Pupils	Slight miosis, occasionally unequal; later, more marked miosis
Ciliary body	Blurring of vision
Bladder	Frequency; involuntary micturition
Nicotinic	
Striated muscle	Easy fatigue; mild weakness; muscular twitching; fasciculations; cramps; generalized weakness, including muscles of respiration, with dyspnoea and cyanosis
Sympathetic ganglia	Pallor; occasional elevation of blood pressure
Central nervous system	Giddiness; tension; anxiety; jitteriness; restlessness; emotional lability; excessive dreaming; insomnia; nightmares; headache; tremor; apathy; withdrawal and depression; bursts of slow waves of elevated voltage in EEG, especially on hyperventilation; drowsiness; difficulty in concentrating; slowness of recall; confusion; slurred speech; ataxia; generalized weakness; coma, with absence of reflexes; Cheyne-Stokes respiration; convulsions; depression of respiratory and circulatory centres, with dyspnoea, cyanosis, and fall in blood pressure

[a] After Grob, 1963 *(40)*.

Detection

Detection may be needed for the three basic purposes – alarming, monitoring and identification – and for some additional special purposes, e.g. miosis-level warning and food and water monitoring. There are now many examples of commercially available military equipment that is capable of performing the various detection tasks. The types of equipment range from manually operated wet chemical detection kits to advanced automatic equipment for specific CW agents. Military equipment is usually robust, of limited weight and size, and usually and increasingly designed for quick and easy operation.

Diagnosis of exposure

Apart from symptomatology, the measurement of decreased cholinesterase activity in blood is the only method currently available for the rapid diagnosis of exposure to nerve agents. However, this approach has several disadvantages, since it is nonspecific for nerve agents or even for organophosphate exposure. Moreover, it is useful only when > 20% of inhibition has occurred, since blank values from the patient are usually not available.

Newer tests, which in the present state of development can be performed only in the laboratory, include: (i) analysis of intact or hydrolysed nerve agent in blood and/or urine; (ii) regeneration of nerve agent bound to proteins with fluoride ions and subsequent analysis of the phosphofluoridate; and (iii) hydrolysis of the phosphorylated protein and subsequent analysis of hydrolysed nerve agent and enzymatically formed metabolites thereof *(41–43)*.

Principles of medical management

In severe cases of nerve agent poisoning, antidotal treatment *per se* may not be sufficient for survival. Assisted ventilation and general supportive measures will be required, sometimes for several days.

Prophylaxis/treatment

Prophylaxis and treatment will depend on the biochemical mechanism that has been identified.

Prophylaxis is based on the administration of a reversible anticholinesterase agent. Pyridostigmine, which is a carbamate used in myasthenia gravis, is proposed at doses of 30 mg, 3 times daily, aimed at producing a blood cholinesterase inhibition of about 30%.

In cases of severe poisoning, these 30% protected cholinesterases will spontaneously reactivate and, assuming that the same phenomenon happens at the cholinergic synapses, the casualty will recuperate. (Reinhibition of the enzyme could occur if poison persists in the body and is available to bind to cholinesterases when pyridostigmine is removed). Further developments include a combination of the centrally acting carbamate physostigmine and the central-anticholinergic scopolamine to improve the protection of acetylcholinesterases in the central nervous system. They also include the administration of catalytic scavengers to capture the nerve agent in blood before it can be distributed into the organism.

Anticholinergic and anticonvulsant agents constitute a symptomatic drug therapy. Atropine sulfate blocks the muscarinic effects in the periphery, and partially counteracts the convulsive effects and respiratory depression in the central nervous system. Loading doses range between 1 and 5 mg i.v. every 30 minutes until full atropinization, and maintenance doses of between 0.5 and 2 mg/hour. Titration of atropine in the individual patient must be carried out on the basis of the most relevant effects for a favourable clinical outcome, i.e. a decrease in bronchial constriction and secretions as judged by auscultation and blood gas analysis. Changes in heart rate are less important but easier to follow, and a mild tachycardia of 80 beats or more per minute should be maintained. Besides atropine, a centrally acting anticonvulsant should be administered, diazepam being the drug of choice. It is used to both prevent and treat convulsions. In addition to diazepam, lorazepam, midazolam and pentobarbital have been used to treat soman-induced seizures. Seizure control declines markedly if there is any delay in treatment; 40 minutes after exposure, control is minimal. Most clinically effective antiepileptic drugs may be incapable of terminating nerve agent-induced seizures *(44)*. Because of the involvement of the glutaminergic system, the clinical utility of concomitant administration of an NMDA receptor blocker is currently under study.

Oximes, which are acetylcholinesterase reactivators, constitute a causal therapy. Most clinical experience has been gained with pralidoxime chloride, pralidoxime methanesulfonate or methylsulfate, and obidoxime chloride. More recently, the oxime HI6 (1-(2'-hydroxyiminomethyl-1'-pyridinium)-3-(4"carbamoyl-1"-pyridinium)-2-oxapropane dication) has been introduced by some countries. These agents relieve the important symptom of skeletal neuromuscular blockade but penetrate only poorly into the central nervous system. They can be administered as repeated injections or as a loading dose followed by a maintenance dose *(45)*.

Stability/neutralization

Tabun, sarin and soman are quite volatile, whereas thickened soman and VX may persist in the environment, depending on temperature. VX represents a serious persistent hazard, particularly at temperatures below 0 °C. Decontamination procedures for skin, equipment and materiel have been developed by most armies, using neutralizing, active chemicals, such as chloramine solutions, or neutral adsorbing powders, e.g. fuller's earth.

Protection

Military-type active-carbon-containing protective clothing and a full-face gas mask with an appropriate filter should be used.

3. Disabling chemicals

Over most of the past century, disabling chemicals have been widely used, e.g. by police or other forces for law-enforcement purposes; by veterinarians to capture dangerous animals; by medical doctors to sedate or calm patients; by thieves and other criminals to disable victims; and by military forces to achieve tactical objectives with diminished loss of life. A particular chemical may be used for several of these purposes.

In the context of law enforcement, sensory irritants such as tear gases or sternutators have long been used by police forces to control civil disorder and are therefore often called "riot control agents" even when used for quite other purposes. The Chemical Weapons Convention, which states that "law enforcement including domestic riot control purposes" are among the "purposes not prohibited under this Convention", defines a "riot control agent" as "any chemical not listed in a Schedule, which can produce rapidly in humans sensory irritation or disabling physical effects which disappear within a short time following termination of exposure". For law-enforcement purposes other than riot control, as in certain lawful types of anti-terrorist action, many toxic chemicals have been studied and occasionally used, including opioids and irritant agents. The CWC seems to place no restrictions on what these chemicals may be other than that they should not be on Schedule 1 and that their types and quantities should be consistent with their purposes. In the case of chemicals held for use against hostage-takers, for example, or against persons threatening to detonate bombs, a key property is that the disablement should be extremely fast. However, the heterogeneity of any population that might be exposed to such a chemical is likely to mean that the dosage required for rapidly disabling all individuals will be lethal for some of them. Disabling chemicals initially studied for military purposes have sometimes found law-enforcement application, and vice versa.

Regarding military applications, defence authorities used to differentiate three classes of disabling chemical. *Class A*: agents that cause temporary physical incapacitation such as sleep, temporary paralysis, weakness, temporary blindness or serious respiratory disturbance and give no danger of death or permanent incapacitation. *Class B*: agents that in small doses cause temporary physical incapacitation, but that in large doses may cause death or permanent effects. *Class C*: agents that cause mental incapacitation. On this classification, a likely fatality rate exceeding 2% was taken as disqualifying an agent from any class of disabling chemical. The point about agents less lethal than this was that they might allow the high casualty rates or wide-area coverage effects available from more traditional chemical weapons to be exploited even when unprotected friendly forces or non-combatants were in the target area. When the classification was enunciated, in 1960, the examples cited of actual agents were the lacrimators CN and CS for Class A, the arsenical sternutator or vomiting agent adamsite for Class B, and the psychotropic agent LSD for Class C; meanwhile there was active research to identify disabling chemicals of greater military efficacy *(46)*.

Since that time several new disabling chemicals have emerged. Among these are chemicals that cause physical incapacitation by psychotropic action, meaning that the distinction between Class A and Class C has faded. Examples include orivals, fentanyls and other opioids. The distinction between Class A and Class B was always less sharp than military authorities appeared to believe, for even an agent such as CS can cause serious damage to those who are exposed to abnormally high dosages or who are abnormally susceptible. That there is no such thing as a non-lethal or otherwise harmless disabling chemical has now become generally recognized.

The key distinction is now seen to lie in the duration of disablement. On the one hand is a chemical causing incapacitation that lasts for little longer than the period of exposure – a characteristic of many irritant agents and the property that, in the civil context, makes it possible for disabling chemicals to be used by police forces to drive back rioters – and on the other is an agent causing incapacitation that lasts for a period of time substantially longer than that of exposure, thus providing a wider variety of possible actions for users of the weapon. Toxic substances in this longer-lasting category are commonly termed "incapacitants" or "incapacitating agents", although a new term, "calmatives", is starting to emerge. For the short-term category, "irritant" or "harassing agent" is a convenient label for the disabling chemicals concerned. In both categories, time to onset of disablement is also an important determinant of utility.

3.1 Incapacitants

Many chemicals can produce a non-fatal and prolonged but temporary incapacitation under controlled laboratory conditions, but few have yet been found that can be expected to do so under less controlled conditions. There are two main obstacles. First, if fatalities are to be kept close to zero even in the immediate vicinity of the functioning munition, the agent must be one for which the incapacitating dosage is very much lower than the lethal dosage. Secondly, the agent must be one that can disable groups of individuals to an extent that is both significant from the user's point of view and predictable.

One class of potential incapacitating agents include the potent psychotropic drugs. These affect the central nervous system in a variety of ways so that the behaviour of exposed individuals is altered, rendering them incapable of performing military functions.

Interpreting the behaviour of a group of soldiers exposed to a psychochemical on the basis of experimental studies on subjects under controlled conditions is fraught with difficulties. Drug-induced behavioural changes in individuals are strongly influenced both by their environment and by the behaviour of other individuals in the vicinity. A drug does not always cause a behavioural change, particularly if there are persons in the vicinity who do not receive it. With LSD, for example, it has been demonstrated that drugged soldiers may behave in an apparently normal manner if they are in a unit with other soldiers who are not drugged. It would appear that the effects of a psycho-chemical on a group can be accurately predicted only if all of its constituent members receive a dose that would produce similar behavioural changes.

There is a more fundamental uncertainty, however, which results from the motivation of specific individuals. Where the motivation is powerful, subjects may accomplish complicated tasks even though they may be obviously quite severely drugged and behaving irrationally. Even though a drug might distort perception at an individual level, predicting the physical response and motivation of a drugged individual in a motivated fighting unit is much more difficult. Thus it is conceivable that, under the influence of a psychochemical, a combat unit is as likely to excel as it is to behave in an uncoordinated manner. Effects of exposure to psychochemicals in war are unknown, since experiments have been conducted only in peacetime. Motivation may be significantly different under fire.

In addition to behavioural effects, some psychochemicals will also cause physical incapacitation. Symptoms may include blurred vision, fainting, vomiting and incoordination. Two psychochemicals considered for weaponization and tested on many volunteers are reviewed below, but there are many other chemicals that alter mental function with and without accompanying somatic symptoms.

3.1.1 Lysergide

Also known as 9,10-didehydro-N,N-diethyl-6-methyl-ergoline-8-ß-carboxamide (CAS Registry Number 50-37-3), N,N-diethyl-D-lysergamide or LSD, lysergide is a water-soluble solid, melting at around 198 °C, that is colourless, odourless and tasteless. It can be disseminated either as a contaminant of food or water or as an inhalable aerosol. It acts on the 5-hydroxytryptamine or serotonin pathway. As an agonist for the 5-HT2 receptor – a post-synaptic receptor – its effects are excitatory, resulting in release of serotonin, which in turn causes both mental and somatic symptoms *(47)*.

Sources

Lysergide is widely available as an illegal drug.

Exposure

Lysergide is active following inhalation or after oral or intravenous administration.

The first symptoms of exposure are usually somatic and include mydriasis, dizziness, weakness, drowsiness, nausea and paraesthesia. They occur within a few minutes after either oral dosing or inhalation.

Altered mental states occur at doses as low as 25 μg. Following oral doses of 0.5–2.0 μg/kg, somatic symptoms, including dizziness and weakness, are seen within a few minutes. In the dose-range 1–16 μg/kg, the intensity of the psychophysiological effects are proportional to the dose. LSD is not an addictive substance. Lethal doses are estimated to be about 0.2 mg/kg *(48)*.

Latency period and recovery time

Anxiety, restlessness, vomiting and general paraesthesias occur within 5 minutes following inhalation. Perceptual distortions begin some 30–60 minutes after oral ingestion. Peak effects occur 3–5 hours after exposure, and recovery is usually within 12 hours. Panic attacks are one of the more serious consequences of LSD exposure and usually last less than 24 hours, but can degenerate into prolonged psychotic states. LSD toxic psychosis can last from days to months. The psychosis is generally considered not to be caused by the LSD, but to be an exacerbation of an already underlying condition. LSD has a short half-life in humans of about 3 hours *(48, 49)*.

Anxiety, fatigue, movement into a dark environment, or use of marijuana can precipitate flashbacks, which may persist intermittently for several years after exposure to LSD.

Main clinical symptoms

Panic attacks are the most common adverse effect. Somatic effects are not consistent, are usually inconsequential and include: mydriasis; increased heart rate, blood pressure and reflexes; paraesthesias; twitches; incoordination; and skin flushing and sweating. Coma may occur at higher doses/exposures. Perceptual distortions occur, with altered sense of colour, shape and distance. Auditory and visual hallucinations are common. Emotional lability is frequently evident and often triggered by sensory clues.

The emotional and behavioural effects of LSD are different for each individual, and influenced by the local environment. Heightened arousal in a group situation may be seen as greater animation, talking and elation. In unusual surroundings with unfamiliar people, initial nervousness may well lead to anxiety.

Neuroleptic malignant syndrome leading to hyperpyrexia has been recorded in only one case and is therefore likely to be a rare event.

Long-term health implications
Evidence for teratogenic and embryo-lethal effects in animals is equivocal, with effects observed in some studies but not in others. LSD crosses the placenta and distribution of the chemical is similar in mother and fetus. There is no evidence that recreational use of LSD causes infertility in women.

Detection
Methods for the detection of LSD – usually developed for drug samples – include gas capillary column chromatography (GC), high-performance liquid chromatography (HPLC), and GC–MS. Radioimmunoassay techniques are available for detecting LSD in urine samples. Detection limits are as low as 5 pg/ml with GC–MS but usually higher with other techniques *(47, 50)*.

Principles of medical management
Patients should be removed from the source of exposure, assessed, stabilized and reassured.

Prophylaxis/treatment
No specific antidotes exist. Vital signs should be monitored and airway and circulation checked. Restraints should be avoided but care must be taken to ensure that patients do not injure themselves. They should be reassured and sedated with diazepam if necessary. Gastric lavage should be avoided if ingestion is the probable route of exposure as it is ineffective (LSD is absorbed rapidly) and may exacerbate psychotic reactions. For acute panic attacks, reassurance, support and reduction

of sensory stimuli are the best management approaches. Patients should be placed in quiet environments, preferably with friends or familiar individuals. Sedation with diazepam (5–10 mg i.v.) may be needed. For acute psychotic reactions, haloperidol is the safest neuroleptic agent (but should be used only if essential). Phenothiazines should not be used as they may potentiate anticholinergic effects. Chlorpromazine should be avoided as this may cause cardiovascular collapse. Flashbacks should be treated with psychotherapy, and with anti-anxiety and neuroleptic drugs *(47)*.

Stability/neutralization

LSD is soluble in water and degraded by ultraviolet light so that persistence in the environment is therefore unlikely.

Protection

A military-type gas mask provides protection against aerosols.

3.1.2   *Agent BZ*

BZ is the hydrochloride salt of 3-quinuclidinyl benzilate (CAS Registry Number 6581-06-2). It is a water-soluble solid melting at 239–241 °C. Its free base is a solid melting at 164–167 °C. Sometimes referred to as a psychochemical, BZ is an anticholinergic compound similar structurally and pharmacologically to atropine. It affects both the peripheral autonomic and the central nervous systems. It may be disseminated in aerosol form from solutions *(51)*, pyrotechnically, or as a pre-sized powder.

Sources

3-Quinuclidinyl benzilate is produced commercially as an intermediate for the drug clidinium bromide.

Exposure

Inhalation is the most likely route, but BZ is also active by the intravenous, intramuscular and oral routes. As an aerosol, particle sizes in the 0.6–0.8 μm range are more effective than a larger particle size (2–4 μm). Cumulative effects are possible following repeated exposures *(51)*.

Symptoms are both time- and dose-dependent *(52)*. Mild incapacitation with some hallucination occurs at about 90 mg.min/m³ (the i.v. equivalent dose is 4.60 μg/kg), severe incapacitation with marked hallucinations at 135 mg.min/m³ (the i.v. equivalent dose is 6.16 μg/kg).

Based on data from animal studies and comparisons with fatalities due to atropine, the human median lethal dose is estimated to be in the range 0.5–3 mg/kg or 35–225 mg for a 70-kg individual.

Latency period from exposure to symptoms, and recovery time
Onset of symptoms is fairly rapid, regardless of the route of administration. In general, at milder incapacitating doses, symptoms abate within 48 hours. At serious incapacitating doses, delirium usually subsides within 72 hours, with recovery complete by 120 hours. Recovery is invariably gradual, simpler abilities returning initially; those requiring more complex integration (including judgement, social awareness and creative ideas) are restored last *(51)*.

Main clinical symptoms
The toxicity of BZ, which is more potent than atropine and has a longer duration of action, is largely attributable to its anticholinergic properties. Signs and symptoms of exposure include increased heart rate and blood pressure; dry skin and mouth; mydriasis; blurred vision; ataxia; disorientation and confusion leading to stupor. At lower exposures, subjects may be noticeably slower in action, less alert, and sleepy. As dosages increase, symptoms intensify – motor coordination deteriorates; confusion, apprehension and restlessness increase; and subjects lose contact with reality, becoming stuporose.

Following incapacitating doses of BZ, signs and symptoms appear in phases, as follows:

- 1–4 hours: restlessness, involuntary movements, ataxia, dizziness, nausea, vomiting, dry mouth, flushed skin, blurred vision, dilated pupils, confusion and sedation progressing to stupor.

- 4–12 hours: stuporose, even semiconscious, inability to respond to environmental stimuli, hallucinations.

- 12–96 hours: random unpredictable behaviour; increasing activity as subjects return to normal; hallucinations may dominate awareness. Real objects and individuals may be generally ignored or ludicrously interpreted. The hallucinations may be benign, entertaining or terrifying.

BZ inhibits secretory activity in the glandular cells concerned with digestion. Saliva is thick, tenacious and scanty, with dry mouth and marked pharyngeal discomfort. Swallowing can be painful, with speech reduced to a whisper. Breath has a foul odour and food and fluids may be refused for more than 24 hours. Urination may be difficult or impossible for up to 16 hours following exposure and frequent attempts to urinate may result *(51)*.

In common with atropine, BZ inhibits sweating, and exposure to the chemical in hot, dry climates may induce heatstroke. Some deaths and symptoms said to be consistent with exposure to an atropine-like chemical warfare agent and with severe heat stress have been reported *(53)*, but it has also been claimed that the symptoms are more consistent with exposure to smoke from white phosphorus *(54)*.

Long-term health implications

Evidence collected and reviewed from studies on volunteers exposed to BZ, from deliberate experimentation with the chemical, and from patients receiving repeat doses of atropine suggest that long-term effects are unlikely. There are limited mortality data on subjects following exposure to BZ in test situations. Data on mutagenicity are also limited and do not enable any conclusion to be reached. No carcinogenicity data are available *(52, 55)*.

Detection

Laboratory confirmation (and in mobile field laboratories) is by GC–MS. HPLC can also be used.

Principles of medical management

Patients should be removed from the source of exposure. Rapid triage should be conducted in the following order:

1. haemorrhage and other surgical emergencies,
2. coma,
3. stupor,
4. ataxia,
5. ambulatory.

Clothing and any equipment likely to be contaminated should be removed. Powder on clothing should be prevented from becoming airborne.

Prophylaxis/treatment

Heatstroke should be avoided. Excessive clothing should be removed if the ambient temperature is above 25 °C. Bladder distension should be checked and hydration monitored. Dehydration is not likely to be a problem in the first 12 hours, but thereafter fluids should be administered *orally* only if the patient is able to drink unaided. Support should be provided and patients should be prevented from injuring themselves.

Physostigmine is the drug treatment of choice; however, in comatose, stuporose and ataxic patients it is of limited effectiveness earlier than 4 hours after BZ exposure. Physostigmine salicylate (1 mg per 20 kg, or 1 mg per 40 lb) i.v. should be given, but if the response is not satisfactory (fall in heart rate, mental clearing), a second, identical dose should be given. Thereafter, patients should be maintained on oral doses of 2–5 mg every 1–2 hours, as necessary. Solutions of the drug – which are bitter – should be added to a more palatable beverage. The frequency of treatment and the dosage should be reduced over 2–4 days.

With effective treatment, the supine heart rate will be 70–80 beats per minute and accompanied by clearer mental function. Treatment should be under the control of a physician. If no doctor is available, oral doses of physostigmine (1 mg per 10 kg) every 2 hours will provide partial control with safety. Both the frequency of treatment and the dose should be reduced 2–4 days after exposure.

Physostigmine is a toxic drug and care is needed to avoid overdosing, the signs of which are profuse sweating, clammy skin, abdominal cramps, vomiting, muscle twitching, tremors, weakness and other cholinergic symptoms. These are usually mild, and the short half-life of physostigmine (30 minutes) means that they are of short duration and rarely require additional treatment. If these symptoms do occur, the treatment should be delayed by 30 minutes and the dose of physostigmine reduced by one-third. Treatment should not be discontinued because the delirium of BZ may return rapidly *(56)*.

Large overdoses of physostigmine may cause apnoea secondary to neuromuscular block. If apnoea does occur, mouth-to-mouth resuscitation should be given.

Barbiturates should not be used. Neostigmine and pilocarpine are ineffective antagonists of the effects of BZ on the CNS and should not be used instead of physostigmine.

If the number of patients is very large, mass confinement in a safe, cool area is the most important single measure.

Ambulatory patients should be observed for 8 hours and released if no more than mildly affected.

Stability/neutralization

Hydrolysis of BZ solutions is both time- and pH-dependent. Increasing pH will increase the rate of hydrolysis. An alkaline pH > 13, achieved with 5% solutions of sodium hydroxide, will cause rapid hydrolysis.

To dispose of BZ, powder should be collected on a flammable material (e.g. paper or card) and incinerated in a well-ventilated area. Alternatively, BZ should be dissolved in a suitable solvent, such as water. If the BZ powder dissolves, 5% sodium hydroxide should be added to neutralize the solution and diluted after 2 hours with additional water and discarded. If the BZ powder fails to dissolve in water, it is likely to be the free base, and should be dissolved in an organic solvent, e.g. chloroform or methylene chloride. BZ base is less soluble in acetone or alcohols, but will dissolve slowly in them. The mixture of BZ and the organic solvent should be incinerated.

BZ is likely to persist in the environment for some time. Data are not available on its half-life in or on soil.

Protection

A military-type gas mask will provide protection.

3.2 Harassing agents and other irritants

The harassing effects of the irritant disabling chemicals arise from the body's reflex responses to sensory irritation, and include lacrimation, sternutation, vomiting and pain (57). Any sensory irritant can provoke all these responses, and it is both the concentration and the tissue with which the agent comes in contact that will determine the response. The conjunctiva of the eyes is particularly sensitive to some irritants. If the predominant response is the secretion of tears, the irritant will be classed as a lacrimator. The inner surfaces of the nose or upper respiratory tract may be particularly sensitive towards other irritants, and such agents would be classed as sternutators. Gaseous irritants, or those dispersed as aerosol particles, penetrate to the deeper recesses of the respiratory tract. Inhalation of a high concentration of a sensory irritant may produce the same degree of damage to the lungs as the lethal lung irritant phosgene.

Skin irritants can also be used to harass, and some pruritogens and algogens (such as dichloroformoxime, also known as phosgene oxime) have been described as possible chemical warfare agents. The more severe skin irritants are also likely to cause damage to the lungs following inhalation which, as in the case of mustard gas, could disqualify them as disabling chemicals. Skin irritation, therefore, is unlikely to be a suitable property for a harassing agent, unless it is combined with other harassing effects, as occurs with some lacrimators and sternutators.

Just as police experience with irritants led to the battlefield use of disabling chemicals on the western front in the First World War in August 1914, so subsequent military experience with harassing agents promoted the use of these compounds for controlling civil disorder. Today, many police forces have access to the lacrimators CN and CS. A number of the military harassing agents are quite unsuited for use by the police, because of the risk of the total incapacitation of exposed individuals or even of death. The principal police requirement is either to incapacitate an individual temporarily in order to effect an arrest or, in the case of a riot, to force individuals out of a particular area.

An appropriate irritant for police use would be one with physical and toxicological properties ensuring that lethal exposures were extremely rare and harassing effects relatively mild. Agents currently employed by police forces around the globe include CS, CN and the active ingredient of red pepper, oleoresin capsicum. Deaths have been recorded following the use of all of these agents. However, apart from uses of CN in large concentrations that have been documented as the cause of lung damage, it is not possible to say whether the other two irritant agents caused death directly or merely contributed to it. A number of individuals died as a result of restraining techniques applied after they had been sprayed with irritant. Some restraining techniques will cause postural asphyxia, resulting in death *(58, 59)*. Where these techniques have been used on individuals who were also sprayed with an irritant, it has proved difficult to assess the contribution of the irritant in causing death. Many irritants employed by police forces are used in quantities significantly greater than those that would constitute an incapacitating dose.

3.2.1 Adamsite

Also known as 10-chloro-5,10-dihydrophenarsazine (CAS Registry Number 578-94-9), diphenylaminechlorarsine, phenarsazine chloride or DM, adamsite is a yellow-to-brown crystalline solid melting at 195 °C that was developed as a sternutator during the First World War. It is intensely irritating to the nose, throat and respiratory tract. Peripheral sensory nerves are affected, and eye, and to a lesser extent, skin irritation may occur. Lower dosages affect the upper respiratory tract; higher dosages cause deeper lung irritation.

Sources

Adamsite was once available commercially as a riot-control agent, in which role it is nowadays generally regarded as obsolete.

Exposure

Injury is normally through inhalation. Harassing effects of military significance occur at dosages of about 10 mg.min/m³. Lethal dosages are estimated to be some 15 000 mg.min/m³.

Latency period and recovery time

Symptoms are apparent 2–3 minutes after initial exposure. Recovery is usually complete in 1–2 hours if exposure is not prolonged.

Main clinical symptoms

Inhalation causes an initial irritant tickling sensation in the nose, followed by sneezing, and a flow of viscous mucus similar to that accompanying a bad cold. Irritation spreads down into the throat causing coughing and choking. Finally, air passages and lungs are also affected. Headache, especially in the forehead, increasing in intensity until almost unbearable, is accompanied by a feeling of pressure in the ears and pain in the jaws and teeth.

In parallel with these symptoms, there is oppressive pain in the chest, shortness of breath, nausea (followed shortly by violent retching and vomiting), unsteady gait, vertigo, weakness in the legs and all-over trembling. Mental depression may occur as symptoms progress. Very high dosages may damage the lungs. Deaths have been reported. Blistering on exposed arms, chest and neck has been reported in factory workers loading adamsite powder into munitions *(60)*.

Detection

Adamsite has no odour. Symptoms are the first indication of exposure.

Rapid detection using GC–MS, the most specific technique, is now available. Many other methods for detecting arsenic in biological samples, including X-ray fluorescence and neutron activation, have been described *(61)*.

Principles of medical management

The patient should be removed from the source of exposure. Clothing may be contaminated and should be removed with care to avoid spreading any powder.

Prophylaxis/treatment

Breathing may be relieved by inhaling low concentrations of chlorine, e.g. from a bottle of bleach. Dust particles in the eye and on the skin should be removed with copious amounts of water. Treatment, by and large, is symptomatic. If the inhaled dose is significant, the patient may require treatment for arsenic poisoning.

Decontamination/neutralization

Oxidation with solutions of hypochlorite (bleach), chloramine or potassium permanganate is effective.

Protection

A military-type gas mask provides protection.

3.2.2   *Agent CN*

CN is 2-chloroacetophenone (CAS Registry Number 532-27-4), a white crystalline solid melting at 59 °C and having an appreciable vapour pressure. It is a lacrimator that was under development at the end of the First World War and soon afterwards was widely used by police forces. It is intensely irritating to the eyes and the mucous membranes in the nose and upper respiratory tract. For police use, it may be disseminated as a pyrotechnically generated aerosol, as a dust cloud or, in solution, as a liquid spray. In spray weapons, carrier/propellant solvents include trichlorofluoroethane, 1,1,1-trichloroethane and kerosene-type hydrocarbons *(62)*.

Sources

CN is widely available commercially as a riot-control agent and in personal-protection devices.

Exposure

Irritation of the nose and respiratory tract occurs following inhalation, and irritation of the skin after direct contact.

Concentrations of 0.5 mg/m³ will cause copious tears in under a minute. Military harassing dosages are in the region of 80 mg.min/m³.

Lethal dosages for humans are estimated to be between 7000 and 11 000 mg.min/m³.

Latency period and recovery time

Symptoms occur almost instantaneously. Direct eye contact at low concentrations causes a copious flow of tears in less than a minute.

Symptoms persist for some 15–30 minutes after exposure ceases. Conjunctival irritation and injection may last 24 hours. Damaged skin may take 3–5 weeks to recover.

Main clinical symptoms

The toxicity of CN may be due to the alkylation and subsequent inhibition of sulfydryl-containing enzymes.

Stinging and burning of the eyes are usually the first symptoms, followed by similar effects on the nose and throat. Copious tears are produced, excess salivation and rhinorrhoea occur, as well as chest tightness, shortness of breath and gasping. Irritation is caused by contact with skin, and exposure to CN is associated with both primary and allergic contact dermatitis. Dermal contact with CN can cause itching, erythema, oedema, induration and necrosis. Necrotic eschars may occur some 5–6 days following contact. Skin recovery may take 3–5 weeks *(63)*.

CN can have severe effects on the eyes including iridocyclitis, hypophyon, keratoconjunctivitis and stromal oedema. Permanent damage to the cornea of rabbits occurs with concentrations greater than 4%.

Lung damage occurs following the use of CN grenades in confined spaces. Injury to the lung may not be immediately apparent, and symptoms may be delayed for several days. Pulmonary oedema and bronchospasm have occurred following accidental, but prolonged exposure *(64)*. Markedly oedematous lungs and intra-alveolar haemorrhage were observed at autopsy of an individual whose death was associated with inhalation of CN *(65)*. Five deaths from lung damage have been reported following exposure to CN in confined spaces.

Long-term health implications

CN is embryotoxic and affects the nervous system of developing chick embryos. The effects are reversible with sulfhydryl compounds. Embryotoxicity occurs at administered concentrations of 0.5–3 mmol, following exposures for 15–120 minutes. The effects of inhaling equivalent concentrations on humans are unknown. There is no evidence of malformations in humans attributable to CN exposure, and available evidence indicates that CN is neither a mutagen nor a carcinogen.

Detection

At low concentrations, CN smells like apple blossom. The odour threshold is 0.1–0.15 mg/m^3. Laboratory confirmation (and in mobile field vehicles) is by GC–MS. GC with thermal-conductivity or flame-ionization detectors may suffice if a well characterized method is used. HPLC methods are also available.

Principles of medical management

The patient should be removed from the source of exposure. Clothing and shoes may be contaminated, and should be removed with care to avoid any powder becoming airborne.

Prophylaxis/treatment

Any particles in the eye should be removed by flushing with copious amounts of water. For relief, the eyes can be washed with a weak solution of boric acid. The airways should be checked. Oxygen may be required if lung injury is evident. Contaminated skin should be washed with a solution of warm sodium carbonate solution. If this is not available, soap and water can be used; water alone is not nearly as effective, but may help if there is a plentiful supply. The affected area should be washed under running water for 20 minutes. Victims should be kept quiet and warm. Soothing lotions such as calamine can be used on injured skin *(29, 63)*.

Stability/neutralization

Data are insufficient to predict the biodegradation of CN in soil, a matrix in which it is likely to have moderate to high mobility.

CN in water may be broken down by UV light (photolysis), but the available data are insufficient to predict the rate of breakdown. Volatilization occurs slowly from water, and reported half-lives range from 13.3 to 159 days. Aquatic bioconcentration and absorption on sediment are minimal.

CN reacts with photochemically produced hydroxyl radicals and has a half-life of some 9.2 days in the vapour phase.

To dispose of CN, the chemical can either be wrapped in paper or some other flammable material, or dissolved in a flammable solvent, and burned in a suitable combustion chamber or well-ventilated area. When heated, CN is degraded to hydrogen chloride.

Protection

A suitable respirator or military-type gas mask should be worn. Skin contact should be avoided. Protective clothing should be worn when clearing a large quantity of chemical arising from a spill.

3.2.3   Agent CS

CS is 2-chlorobenzalmalononitrile (CAS Registry Number 2698-41-1), also known as [(2-chlorophenyl)methylene]propanedinitrile, *o*-chlorobenzylidene malononitrile and ßß-dicyano-*o*-chlorostyrene. It is a white crystalline solid at ambient temperatures. It is a lacrimator that was initially developed to replace CN for police use but was subsequently also widely used on the battlefield. More rapid in action than CN, it is intensely irritating to the eyes and mucous membranes in the nose and upper respiratory tract. It is also a general skin irritant. For police use, it may be disseminated as a pyrotechnically generated aerosol, as a dust cloud, or, in solution, as a liquid spray. In spray weapons, the carrier solvents in use include methylene chloride, acetone and methyl isobutyl ketone, while the propellants include nitrogen, carbon dioxide and butane *(66)*.

Sources

CS is widely available commercially as a riot-control agent.

Exposure

Irritation of the nose, throat and upper respiratory tract occur following inhalation, and of the skin through direct contact. Direct eye contact at low concentrations causes intense eye irritation and copious tears.

Eye and respiratory tract irritation is just detectable in 50% of people after 1-minute exposures to 0.004 and 0.023 mg/m^3 respectively. Harassment is marked at concentrations of 4 mg/m^3, with the eyes and respiratory tract affected almost immediately *(62)*. As a peripheral sensory irritant, CS is about 10 times more potent than CN. Estimates of the human median lethal dosage, based on extrapolation from animal data, are uncertain and range from 25 000 to 150 000 mg.min/m^3. The particle size and method of delivery affect toxicity to the lung. Lethal concentrations cause lung damage, leading either to asphyxia and circulatory failure or to bronchopneumonia secondary to respiratory tract damage.

Latency period and recovery time

Eye and respiratory tract symptoms occur very rapidly at harassing concentrations of 4 mg/m^3. Recovery is usually complete 30 minutes after exposure ceases, but some signs may persist for longer. The usual times for recovery from particular effects are approximately as follows: visual acuity (a few minutes); chest discomfort (5 minutes); coughing and breathing difficulties (10 minutes); lacrimation (up to 15 minutes); salivation (15 minutes); skin sensations (15 minutes); conjunctival injection and subjective sensation of eye irritancy (25–30 minutes); erythema of eyelid margins (1 hour) *(62)*.

Solutions of CS cause skin irritation, often as a two-phase response, with an initial erythema occurring within a few minutes and persisting for about an hour, followed some 2 hours later by a delayed erythema which persists for 24–72 hours. However, the onset of the delayed erythema may be as much as 12 hours–3 days after exposure, with vesicles, blisters and crusts appearing on the skin *(67)*. Recovery of the skin from this more serious damage may take weeks.

Main clinical symptoms

Stinging and burning of the eyes, lacrimation, rhinorrhoea, salivation, blepharospasm, conjunctival injection, sneezing and coughing develop rapidly at harassing concentrations. The chest may feel sore and tight, and some individuals may voluntarily hold their breath. Exposed skin, particularly in moist areas, begins to sting and burn after a few minutes, and erythema may follow. Some individuals may feel nauseous and vomit.

When the CS is delivered in a carrier solvent, exposure to the latter may sometimes further complicate the clinical picture. More CS is likely to be deposited on the skin and in the eyes by this procedure and both eye and skin irritation are more persistent *(63, 67)*.

Apprehension is common, and exposure to CS aerosols may cause a transient increase in both blood pressure and heart rate *(68)*.

Eye damage, other than temporary conjunctival injection, is unlikely.

CS exposure is associated with both primary and allergic contact dermatitis, while reactive airways dysfunction syndrome (RADS) is a risk following exposure to high concentrations *(69)*. Asthmatic symptoms may occur in susceptible individuals. Chronic bronchitics may suffer from a superimposed acute bronchitis and bronchopneumonia.

Authenticated deaths from CS have not been recorded. Deaths following the use of CS have occurred in police custody, and the role of CS in either causing or contributing to such deaths is a cause of concern. High concentrations of CS in confined spaces over a prolonged period would be necessary to achieve lethal dosages. Under these conditions, lung damage could occur, leading to asphyxia and circulatory failure.

CS is an alkylating agent with cyanogenic potential. It undergoes stepwise metabolism to thiocyanate, some of which is then metabolized to cyanide. Any lethal effects of the agent would be mediated by both the alkylating properties and the cyanogenic potential. At harassing concentrations, however, cyanide production would be exceedingly small and of no clinical importance.

Long-term health implications

CS is mutagenic in some in vitro systems. However, it has not been demonstrated to cause mutations in vivo following administration to test animals. No evidence exists that CS is carcinogenic, and 2-year studies in rats and mice provided no evidence of carcinogenicity. Available evidence also indicates that CS is neither embryo-lethal nor teratogenic.

Detection

Symptoms are the first indication of exposure because of the low vapour pressure. Laboratory confirmation (also in mobile field laboratories) is by GC–MS. GC and HPLC methods are also available for CS and its metabolites *(61)*.

Principles of medical management

The patient should be removed from the source of exposure. Clothing and shoes may be contaminated and should be removed carefully to avoid any powder becoming airborne. CS delivered in a solvent spray may become airborne after evaporation of the solvent and abrasion of the CS particles.

Prophylaxis/treatment

Treatment will depend on the way CS is delivered. If a fine powder is dispersed, it is preferable to keep it dry and blow as much of it as possible off the individual by using, for example, a hair dryer.

Spray delivery with a solvent will result in exposure to both CS and the solvent. Irrigation of affected areas with tepid water for at least 15 minutes is then advisable. Any particles deposited in the eye after evaporation of the solvent should be washed out by using copious amounts of tepid water for 15 minutes or more. Brief contact with water hydrolyses CS and may exacerbate burning symptoms. Soap and water can be used to wash the skin, but should be followed by irrigation with tepid water for 15 minutes. CS will dissolve rapidly in a solution of sodium metabisulfite, and such solutions can be used to remove solid particles of the irritant. Sodium metabisulfite solutions will release sulfur dioxide, which may be a hazard for asthmatics *(70)*.

Saline or weak solutions of boric acid may relieve eye symptoms, and soothing lotions such as calamine can be used on injured skin. Wet dressings, which allow evaporation to take place (i.e. are not plastic-backed), may soothe skin. Dressings should be changed every 2–3 hours *(29)*. Any skin infections should be treated with antibiotics. Airways should be checked and patients reassured.

Stability in environment/decontamination/neutralization

Formulations of CS are available that increase its persistence in the environment. Two hydrophobic anti-agglomerative powder formulations, CS1 and CS2, have been developed for explosive burst or fogging machines. CS1 contains 5% hydrophobic silica aerogel and persists for some 2 weeks under normal weather conditions. CS2, a siliconized form of CS1, has greater weather resistance, and may remain active for up to 48 days. Because of their persistence, these two forms of CS are likely to be used only in a military context *(62)*.

CS powder used for riot control and dust derived from it can settle on the ground and remain active for 5 days. Traces of CS may persist for longer than this.

The data available are insufficient for any estimate of biodegradation in soil to be possible. Leaching can occur, but if CS is dissolved in water, hydrolysis is rapid and the agent will be degraded before leaching takes place.

Particle size and surface area affect the rate of dissolution in water, and CS can float and travel considerable distances before it dissolves. Its half-life in seawater is 281.7 minutes and 14.5 minutes at 0 °C and 25 °C, respectively.

At 25 °C, CS has an atmospheric half-life of some 4.9 days.

When heated, CS produces hydrogen chloride, nitrogen oxides and cyanide.

For disposal, particles should be swept on to a flammable material (e.g. paper or card) or dissolved in an organic solvent (such as alcohol) before burning in a suitable combustion chamber or in a well-ventilated area. Spills can be decontaminated by washing with 5% sodium hydroxide solution in 1:1 ethyl alcohol (or isopropyl alcohol)/water mixture, leaving for 20 minutes and flushing with water.

Protection

A suitable respirator with a charcoal filter or a military-type gas mask should be worn. Protective clothing may be necessary to avoid skin contact when sweeping spills.

3.2.4   Agent CR

CR is dibenz-(b,f)1:4-oxazepine (CAS Registry Number 257-07-8), a pale yellow solid first characterized in the early 1960s. It is a sensory irritant some six times more powerful than CS. It is intensely irritating to the eyes and mucous membranes in the nose and upper respiratory tract. Application in liquid solution produces intense irritation of the skin, but the effects are less persistent than those produced by CS or CN. It may be disseminated as a pyrotechnically generated aerosol or as a liquid spray *(62)*. Spray formulations of CR in a 0.1–1% solution in either propylene glycol and water or propylene glycol alone have been approved for riot-control purposes in the United States *(71)*.

Sources

CR is available to internal security forces in a number of countries.

Exposure

Direct eye contact at low concentrations causes intense discomfort and pain and copious tears. The mouth, nose, throat and respiratory tract are irritated following inhalation, and direct contact will cause stinging, burning and occasional erythema of the skin.

Eye and respiratory tract irritation are detectable in 50% of people within 1 minute of exposure to concentrations of 0.004 and 0.002 mg/m^3. Harassment is marked at concentrations of 0.7 mg/m^3 (for aerosol), with effects on the eye and respiratory tract likely to be intolerable. CR has a very low mammalian toxicity, much lower than those of CS and CN. Based on animal data, the estimated acute lethal dosage for pyrotechnically generated CR in humans would be in excess of 100 000 mg.min/m^3 *(62)*. Pyrotechnically generated CR is more toxic than pure (thermally generated) aerosols of the irritant because of the presence of pyrotechnic decomposition products.

Latency period and recovery time

Respiratory tract and eye irritation occur rapidly at harassing concentrations of 0.7 mg/m^3 or above. The principal effects of CR on the eyes and skin are likely to last less than 30 minutes, but some reddening of the eye may persist for hours. Pain and erythema of the skin occur within minutes of contamination. Although the pain usually subsides within 30 minutes, it will occasionally recur every time the skin is washed. Chest discomfort and breathing are likely to return to normal within about 15–30 minutes, as with CS.

The effects of CR on the eye are usually immediate but transitory. Single or multiple applications of CR either as a solid or in a 1% or 5% solution in propylene glycol have been tested on the eyes of rabbits. Solid CR caused only minor lacrimation and irritation of the conjunctivae for

1 hour. After single applications, CR in solution caused mild to moderate inflammatory effects for a few days. At higher concentrations (5% and 10%), a similar duration of effect was observed. After repeat applications over a number of weeks, the effect was a moderate transient conjunctivitis. Solutions of higher concentration (10%) cause detectable keratitis usually of only a few days duration. In humans, a rise in intraocular pressure of short duration is usually seen during the acute phase and may be an additional risk factor for the over-40s.

Solutions of CR (0.001–0.0025% w/v) have been applied as whole-body liquid drenches to the skin of volunteers. The eyes were immediately affected, with skin irritation starting around the eyes about a minute later and then at other sites. The degree of pain and erythema that occurred was related to the thickness of the stratum corneum, with the particularly sensitive areas being the face, back of the neck and trunk, and external genitalia *(68)*.

Main clinical symptoms

Stinging and burning of the eyes, lacrimation, blepharospasm, conjunctival injection, rhinorrhoea, salivation, sneezing and coughing occur rapidly at harassing concentrations. Individuals may complain of difficulty in opening the eyelids and of an unpleasant taste or burning sensation in the mouth and on the skin. There may also be complaints of difficulty in breathing. On examination, the skin will show well demarcated, moderate to marked erythema. Blood pressure may be increased but usually returns to normal within 30 minutes. The inability to see clearly and the severe irritation may cause some subjects to develop anxiety, and this may be the main presenting complaint in some cases *(72)*.

Subjects presenting more than 30 minutes after being splashed may complain of a "gritty" sensation in the eyes and of a mild burning of the skin. Examination may reveal residual conjunctival injection and erythema of the eyelids and contaminated skin.

Long-term health implications

There is no evidence that CR is teratogenic, mutagenic or carcinogenic. Embryo-lethal effects have been seen following intravenous administration; these may have been due to the precipitation of CR from saturated solution on injection *(73)*.

Detection

Symptoms are the first indication of exposure. Laboratory confirmation (and in mobile field laboratories) is by GC–MS. In addition to GC, HPLC methods are also available for the separation of CR. Data on nuclear magnetic resonance and infrared spectra are well characterized and can be used for identification *(61)*.

Principles of medical management

The patient should be removed from the source of exposure. Contaminated clothing should be removed with care by personnel wearing impermeable gloves and placed in suitable containers (e.g. disposable polyethylene bags). The skin should be decontaminated with soap and water. If the hair is contaminated, care should be taken to prevent any material from being washed into the eyes.

Prophylaxis/treatment

The patient should be reassured by stressing that the pain is temporary. Particles should be washed out of the eye with copious amounts of tepid water. Saline or weak boric acid solutions may relieve eye symptoms and can be used to irrigate the eyes. If pain in the eye persists, it may be relieved by instillation of 0.5% tetracaine hydrochloride, appropriate precautions being taken to avoid mechanical trauma. Acute burning sensations of the skin subside after about 10 minutes. Both skin and hair should be washed thoroughly with soap and water and only after washing, if necessary, should a soothing lotion such as calamine be applied to the skin. It is possible that CR will exacerbate the effects of psoriasis or eczema in some patients, and the normal treatment of these conditions should be used. Rhinorrhoea and excessive salivation are transient, and any symptoms in the mouth disappear rapidly. The mouth should be washed if necessary.

Stability/neutralization

Because of its stability, CR may persist in the environment for months. The dibenzoxazepines were stable for several hours when refluxed in concentrated hydrochloric acid and in 20% sodium hydroxide *(74)*. Failure to hydrolyse dibenzoxazepines under these extreme acidic and alkaline conditions demonstrates significant stability. The ether linkage in the molecule has been broken by reduction with sodium and ethanol, but no practical decontaminant is available at present. CR is very toxic to aquatic life *(75)*.

Protection

A suitable respirator with a charcoal filter or a military-style gas mask should be worn. Protective clothing may be necessary to avoid contact when cleaning spills.

3.2.5   Agent OC

OC is oleoresin capsicum, a natural oil of the chilli pepper, *Capsicum annuum* or *C. frutescens* (Solanaceae family) that is almost insoluble in water but soluble in such organic solvents as ether, alcohol or chloroform. The active principles of OC, typically constituting some 60–80% of the oil, are capsaicin, also known as *trans*-8-methyl-*N*-vanillyl-6-nonenamide (CAS Registry Number 8023-77-7), and dihydrocapsaicin, but at least 100 other chemicals are also present in OC. Capsaicin can also be synthesized. The substance was proposed for use as a harassing agent during the First World War, but does not appear to have been used as a disabling chemical until long afterwards, in personal-protection devices. It is now quite widely used by police forces in the form of "pepper spray". Such sprays typically contain 1–10% of OC oil in a solvent/propellant. OC acts rapidly and is an intense irritant to the eyes, nose and respiratory tract. It is also a mild skin irritant. "Pepper spray" is a designation sometimes also used for compositions containing synthetic congeners of capsaicin, such as pelargonic acid vanillylamide (PAVA).

Sources

OC is isolated commercially from paprika and cayenne pepper, and is used as a flavouring agent in some foods. It also has medicinal applications and has been used for centuries for pain relief. It is now used following herpes zoster infections (post-herpetic neuralgia) and for psoriasis, diabetic neuropathy and a range of other conditions (76).

Exposure

Direct eye contact at low concentrations causes intense eye irritation and copious tears. Irritation of the nose, throat and upper respiratory tract occur following direct contact.

Incapacitating dosages in humans are not documented, but 50 mg/litre concentrations applied to the eyes of rats caused obvious pain and blepharospasm. Estimated oral lethal doses in humans range from 0.5 to 5 g/kg (77).

Capsaicin acts on nociceptive afferent nerve fibres, and is thought to deplete Substance P, a neurotransmitter of pain. Topical application of capsaicin desensitizes an area of skin to chemical, thermal and mechanical stimuli in a dose-dependent manner.

Latency period and recovery time
Eye and respiratory tract symptoms occur almost immediately after spraying OC on the face. Severe pain and inflammation last from 45 minutes to several hours. Lingering effects usually disappear in 1–2 days. Deaths have been recorded following the use of OC sprays, but in the majority of cases, other factors such as the use of cocaine, or postural asphyxia (caused by restraining procedures) were considered to be the likely cause of death (58). Pepper spray is documented as contributing to only one death, that of an asthmatic (78).

Main clinical symptoms
The main symptoms are stinging and burning of the eyes, and lacrimation, and burning of the nose and mouth. Inhalation of aerosol will cause sneezing, rhinorrhoea, choking and gasping for breath. Erythema may be present on exposed skin. Bronchoconstriction may occur in subjects with obstructive lung disease.

Long-term health effects
There is some concern about neurotoxic effects, but these have not been documented in humans following topical application. There is equivocal evidence on mutagenicity, and both positive and negative results have been reported for different test systems. The evidence available is not sufficient to evaluate carcinogenicity, but it is unlikely to be of real concern following a single exposure to a relatively low dose of capsaicin in a spray (78).

Detection in the laboratory
GC and HPLC procedures are available (79).

Principles of medical management
Patients should be removed from the source of exposure. Clothing may be contaminated and should be removed. Capsaicin is not volatile and presents no vapour hazard.

Prophylaxis/treatment

A jet of liquid will probably have been sprayed in the face. Irrigation of the eyes with water is the most common treatment described, but capsaicin is practically insoluble in water so that more effective procedures are required. Skin can also be washed with vegetable oils *(78)*.

Patients should be reassured and bronchoconstriction treated, if present.

Stability in environment/decontamination/neutralization

As capsaicin is not volatile, the only risk is from direct contact. Capsaicin should be removed from contaminated clothing with an organic solvent and burned.

Protection

Eyes, nose and mouth should be protected with a military-type gas mask.

REFERENCES

1.   Khateri S. Statistical views on late complications of chemical weapons on Iranian CW victims. *The ASA Newsletter*, No. 85, 31 August 2001, 1: 16–19.

2.   Mazandarani M. Secretary-General of the Association for Helping Victims of Iraq's Chemical Warfare with Iran. Statement reported by the Islamic Republic News Agency, 1 December 1996. Web site: *http://www.irna.com/en/about/ index.shtml.*

3.   Gosden C et al. Examining long-term severe health consequences of CBW use against civilian populations. *Disarmament Forum*, 1999, No. 3:67–71.

4.   *Phosgene*. Geneva, World Health Organization, 1997 (Environmental Health Criteria, No. 193).

5.   Diller WF. Pathogenesis of phosgene poisoning. *Toxicology and Industrial Health*, 1985, 1:7–15.

6.   Diller WF. Early diagnosis of phosgene overexposure. *Toxicology and Industrial Health*, 1985, 1:73–80.

7.   Diller WF. Late sequelae after phosgene poisoning: a literature review. *Toxicology and Industrial Health*, 1985, 1:129–136.

8.   Regan RA. Review of clinical experience in handling phosgene exposure cases. *Toxicology and Industrial Health*, 1985, 1:69–72.

9.   Wells BA. Phosgene: a practitioner's viewpoint. *Toxicology and Industrial Health*, 1985, 1:81–92.

10. *Chloropicrin*. Hamilton, ON, Canadian Centre for Occupational Health and Safety (CHEMINFO No. 2000–2003); available at *http://ccinfoweb.ccohs.ca/ cheminfo/Action.lasso* and *http://www.ccohs.ca/products/databases/ cheminfo.html.*

11. Hayes WJ. *Pesticides studied in man*. Baltimore, MD, Williams & Wilkins.

12. Condie LW et al. Ten and ninety-day toxicity studies of chloropicrin in Sprague-Dawley rats. *Drug and Chemical Toxicology*, 1994, 17:125–137.

13. Berck B. Analysis of fumigants and fumigant residues. *Journal of Chromatographic Science*, 1975, 13:256–267.

14. Spencer EY. *Guide to the chemicals used in crop protection*, 7th ed. Ottawa, Information Canada (Publication 1093).

15. Harris DK. Polymer-fume fever. *Lancet*, 1951, ii:1008–1011.

16. Urbanetti, JS. Toxic inhalational injury. In: Sidell F, Takafuji ET, Franz DR, eds. *Medical aspects of chemical and biological warfare*. Washington, DC, Department of the Army, Office of The Surgeon General and Borden Institute, 1997.

17. Maidment MP, Rice P, Upshall DG. Retention of inhaled hexafluorocyclobutene in the rat. *Journal of Applied Toxicology*, 1994, 14:395–400.

18. Robbins JJ, Ware RL. Pulmonary edema from Teflon fumes. *New England Journal of Medicine*, 1964, 271:360–361.

19. Lewis CE, Kerby GR. An epidemic of polymer-fume fever. *Journal of the American Medical Association*, 1965, 191:103–106.

20. Williams N, Atkinson W, Patchefsky AS. Polymer-fume fever: not so benign. *Journal of Occupational Medicine*, 1974, 16:519–522.

21. Lailey AF. Oral *N*-acetlycysteine protects against perfluoroisobutene toxicity in rats. *Human and Experimental Toxicology*, 1997, 16:212–221.

22. Lailey AF et al. Protection by cysteine esters against chemically induced pulmonary oedema. *Biochemical Pharmacology*, 1991, 42:S47–S54.

23. Isom GE, Way JL. Effects of oxygen on the antagonism of cyanide intoxication: cytochrome oxidase, in vitro. *Toxicology and Applied Pharmacology*, 1984, 74:57–62.

24. *Cyanides*. Washington, DC, United States Environmental Protection Agency, 1980 (EPA# 440/5-80-037). Available at *http://www.epa.gov/ost/pc/ ambientwqc/cyanides80.pdf* and *http://www.epa.gov/waterscience/pc/ ambient2.html*.

25. Marrs TC, Maynard RL, Sidell FR. *Chemical warfare agents: toxicology and treatment*. Chichester, Wiley, 1996.

26. Vedder EB. *The medical aspects of chemical warfare*. Baltimore, MD, Williams & Wilkins, 1925.

27. Sidell FR, Patrick WC, Dashiell TR. *Jane's chem-bio handbook*. Coulsdon, England, Jane's Information Group, 1998.

28. Ellenhorn MD et al. *Ellenhorn's medical toxicology: diagnosis and treatment of human poisoning*, 2nd ed. Baltimore, MD, Williams & Wilkins, 1997:1299–1300.

29. Dreisbach RH. *Handbook of poisoning: prevention, diagnosis and treatment*. Los Altos, CA, Lange Medical, 1980.

30. Warthin AS, Weller CV. *The medical aspects of mustard gas poisoning*. London, Henry Kimpton, 1919.

31. Alexander SF. Medical report of the Bari Harbor mustard casualties. *The Military Surgeon*, 1947, 101:1–17.

32. Willems JL. Chemical management of mustard gas casualties. *Annales Medicinae Militaris Belgicae*, 1989, 3(Suppl.):1–61.

33. Benschop HP et al. Verification of exposure to sulfur mustard in two casualties of the Iran-Iraq conflict. *Journal of Analytical Toxicology*, 1997, 21:249–251.

34. Black RM, Read RW. Biological fate of sulphur mustard, 1,1-thiobis(2-chloro-ethane): identification of ß-lyase metabolites and hydrolysis products in urine. *Xenobiotica*, 1995, 25:167–173.

35. Rice P et al. Dermabrasion – a novel concept in the surgical management of sulphur mustard injuries. *Burns*, 2000, 26:34–40.

36. Fidder A et al. Biomonitoring of exposure to lewisite based on adducts of haemoglobin. *Archives of Toxicology*, 2000, 74:207–214.

37. Morimoto F, Shimazu T, Yoshioka T. Intoxication of VX in humans. *American Journal of Emergency Medicine*, 1999, 17:493–494.

38. Nozaki H et al. A case of VX poisoning and the difference from sarin. *Lancet*, 1995, 346:698–699.

39. Lallement G et al. Review of the value of gacyclidine (GK-11) as adjuvant medication to conventional treatments of organophosphate poisoning: primate experiments mimicking various scenarios of military or terrorist attack by soman. *Neurotoxicology*, 1999, 20:675–684.

40. Grob D. Anticholinesterase intoxication in man and its treatment. In: Koelle GB, ed. *Handbuch der experimentellen Pharmakologie. [Handbook of experimental pharmacology.]* Berlin, Springer Verlag, 1963.

41. Polhuijs M, Langenberg JP, Benschop HP. New method for the retrospective detection of exposure to organophosphorus anticholinesterases: application to alleged victims of Japanese terrorists. *Toxicology and Applied Pharmacology*, 1997, 146:156–161.

42. Minami M et al. Method for the analysis of the methylphosphonic acid metabolites of sarin and its ethanol-substituted analogue in urine as applied to the victims of the Tokyo sarin disaster. *Journal of Chromatography B Biomedical Sciences and Applications*, 1997, 695:237–244.

43. Nagao M et al. Definite evidence for the acute sarin poisoning in the Tokyo subway. *Toxicology and Applied Pharmacology*, 1997, 144:198–203.

44. Shih TS, McDonough JH Jr, Koplovitz I. Anticonvulsants for soman-induced seizure activity. *Journal of Biomedical Science*, 1999, 6:86–96.

45. *NATO handbook on the medical aspects of NBC defensive operations. Part II – Biological*. Brussels, North Atlantic Treaty Organization, 1996 (NATO AMed P-6(B)).

46. *Chemical warfare*. London, Defence Research Policy Committee, United Kingdom Ministry of Defence, 1960 (memorandum DEFE 10/382, held by Public Record Office, Ruskin Avenue, Richmond TW9 4DU, England).

47. Ellenhorn MD et al. *Ellenhorn's medical toxicology: diagnosis and treatment of human poisoning*, 2nd ed. Baltimore, MD, Williams & Wilkins, 1997:387–391.

48. Gilman AG et al., eds. *Goodman & Gilman's pharmacological basis of therapeutics*, 8th ed. New York, Pergamon, 1990.

49. Haddad LM. *Clinical management of poisoning and drug overdose*, 2nd ed. Philadelphia, PA, Saunders, 1990:59–76.

50. Sun J. Lysergic acid diethylamide (LSD) determination by GC–MS. *American Clinical Laboratory*, 1989, 8:24–27.

51. Ketchum JS. *The human assessment of BZ*. Edgewood Arsenal, Aberdeen, MD, US Army Chemical Research and Development Laboratory, 1963 (CRDL Technical Memorandum 20-29).

52. Panel on Anticholinesterase Chemicals, Panel on Anticholinergic Chemicals, Committee on Toxicology, Board on Toxicology and Environmental Health Hazards. *Possible long-term health effects of short-term exposure to chemical agents, Vol. 1.* Washington, DC, National Academy Press, 1982.

53. *Report of the mission dispatched by the Secretary-General to investigate an alleged use of chemical weapons in Mozambique*. New York, United Nations, 1992 (Security Council Report S/24065).

54. Andersson G, Persson SA. *Final report of the experts appointed by ASDI to assist the government of Mozambique in order to investigate the alleged use of chemical warfare agent(s) in the Ngungue incident*. Stockholm, National Defence Research Establishment, 1992.

55. Hay A. Surviving the impossible. *Medicine, Conflict and Survival*, 1998, 14:120–155.

56. *NATO handbook on the medical aspects of NBC defensive operations.* AMedP-6. Washington, DC, Departments of the Army, the Navy and the Air Force, 1973.

57. Olajos EJ, Salem H. Riot control agents: pharmacology, toxicology, biochemistry and chemistry. *Journal of Applied Toxicology*, 2000, 21:355–391.

58. Reay DT et al. Positional asphyxia during law enforcement transport. *American Journal of Forensic Medicine and Pathology*, 1992, 13:90–97.

59. Pollanen MS et al. Unexpected death related to restraint for excited delirium: a retrospective study of deaths in police custody and in the community. *Canadian Medical Association Journal*, 1998, 158:1603–1607.

60. Haber LF. *The poisonous cloud.* Oxford, Clarendon Press, 1986.

61. *Systematic identification of chemical warfare agents. B.3: Identification of non-phosphates.* Helsinki, Ministry for Foreign Affairs, 1982.

62. Ballantyne B. Riot control agents – biomedical and health aspects of the use of chemicals in civil disturbances. *Medical Annual*, 1977:7–14.

63. Gaskins JR et al. Lacrimating agents (CS and CN) in rats and rabbits. Acute effects on mouth, eyes, and skin. *Archives of Environmental Health*, 1972, 24:449–454.

64. Vaca FE, Myers JH, Langdorf M. Delayed pulmonary oedema and broncho-spasm after accidental lacrimator exposure. *American Journal of Emergency Medicine*, 1996, 14:402–405.

65. Stein AA, Kirwan WE. Chloroacetophenone (tear gas) poisoning: a clinico-pathologic report. *Journal of Forensic Sciences*, 1964, 9:374–382.

66. Hu H et al. Tear gas – harassing agent or toxic chemical weapon? *Journal of the American Medical Association*, 1989, 262:660–663.

67. Parneix-Spake A et al. Severe cutaneous reactions to self-defense sprays [letter]. *Archives of Dermatology*, 1993, 129:913.

68. Ballantyne B, Gall D, Robson DC. Effects on man of drenching with dilute solutions of *o*-chlorobenzylidene malonitrile (CS) and dibenz(b,f)-1,4-oxazepine (CR). *Medicine, Science and the Law*, 1976, 16:159–170.

69. Hu J. Toxicodynamics of riot-control agents (lacrimators). In: Somani SM, ed. *Chemical warfare agents.* San Diego, CA, Academic Press, 1992:271–288.

70. Jones GRN. CS sprays: antidote and decontaminant. *Lancet*, 1996, 347:968–969.

71. Biskup RK et al. *Toxicity of 1% CR in propylene glycol/water (80/20)*. Edgewood Arsenal, Aberdeen Proving Ground, Aberdeen, MD, 1975 (Technical Report EB-TR-75009).

72. Ballantyne B, Beswick FW, Thomas DP. The presentation and management of individuals contaminated with solutions of dibenzoxazepine. *Medicine, Science and the Law*, 1973, 13:265–268.

73. Upshall DG. The effects of dibenz(b,f)-1,4-oxazepine (CR) upon rat and rabbit embryonic development. *Toxicology and Applied Pharmacology*, 1974, 29:301–311.

74. Higginbottom R, Suschitzsky H. Syntheses of heterocyclic compounds. Part II: Cyclisation of *o*-nitrophenyl oxygen ethers. *Journal of the Chemical Society*, 1962, 962:2367–2379.

75. Johnson DW, Haley MV, Landis WG. The aquatic toxicity of the sensory irritant and riot control agent dibenz(b,f)-1,4-oxazepine. In: Landis WG, van der Schalie WH, eds. *Aquatic toxicology and risk assessment, Vol. 13*. Philadelphia, PA, American Society for Testing and Materials, 1990:1767–1788.

76. Govindarajan VS, Sathyanarayana MN. Capsicum – production, technology, chemistry, and quality. Part V. Impact on physiology, pharmacology, nutrition, and metabolism; structure, pungency, pain, and desensitization sequences. *Critical Reviews in Food Science and Nutrition*, 1991, 29:435–474.

77. Salem H et al. *Capsaicin toxicology overview*. Edgewood Research Development and Engineering Center, Aberdeen Proving Ground, Aberdeen, MD, 1994 (MD ERDEC-TR-199).

78. Busker RW, van Helden HPM. Toxicologic evaluation of pepper spray as a possible weapon for the Dutch police force: risk assessment and efficacy. *American Journal of Forensic Medicine and Pathology*, 1998, 19:309–316.

79. Govindarajan VS. Capsicum – production, technology, chemistry, and quality. Part III. Chemistry of the color, aroma and pungency stimuli. *Critical Reviews in Food Science and Nutrition*, 1986, 24:245–355.

Further reading

Ballantyne B, Marrs TC, eds. *Clinical and experimental toxicology of organophosphates and carbamates*. London, Butterworth–Heinemann, 1992.

Papirmeister B et al. *Medical defense against mustard gas: toxic mechanisms and pharmacological implications*. Boca Raton, FL, CRC Press, 1991.

Somani SM, ed. *Chemical warfare agents*. San Diego, CA, Academic Press, 1992.

Somani SM, Romano JA, eds. *Chemical warfare agents: toxicity at low levels*. Boca Raton, FL, CRC Press, 2001.

ANNEX 2: TOXINS

1. Introduction

As a category, toxins have recently acquired greater prominence in the literature on biological warfare *(1, 2)*, though not because of any increase in their potential for weaponization, despite their being among the most toxic substances known today. It is, however, true that some toxins are becoming more accessible to quantity production than they once were.

"Toxin" is a word that has no commonly accepted meaning in the scientific literature. This may be of little account to the health authorities of Member States unless they become obliged to seek international assistance because of a toxin-warfare attack, whether actual or threatened. It may then be important to understand how toxins are treated in the Biological and Chemical Weapons Conventions since, to differing degrees, these two international treaties are potential sources of such assistance.

The 1972 Biological and Toxin Weapons Convention covers "toxins whatever their origin or method of production". It does not define toxins, but its *travaux préparatoires* show that the term is intended to mean toxic chemicals produced by living organisms. The actions of the United States are important in this connection. On 14 February 1970, during the negotiation of the Convention, the United States announced that it had decided to renounce offensive preparations for the use of toxins as a method of warfare. Shortly afterwards, it informed the treaty-negotiating body that toxins "are poisonous substances produced by biological organisms, including microbes, animals, and plants" *(3)*, and it has since reiterated and even expanded that definition in the legislation implementing the Convention in United States law. This states that:

> the term "toxin" means the toxic material of plants, animals, micro-organisms, viruses, fungi, or infectious substances, or a recombinant molecule, whatever its origin or method of production, including – (A) any poisonous substance or biological product that may be engineered as a result of biotechnology produced by

a living organism; or (B) any poisonous isomer or biological product, homolog, or derivative of such a substance *(4)*.

The essence of this definition evidently found favour with all the other States Parties to the Convention, for the Final Declaration of the Second Biological Weapons Convention Review Conference states that "toxins (both proteinaceous and non-proteinaceous) of a microbial, animal or vegetable nature and their synthetically produced analogues are covered" by the treaty *(5)*.

Inasmuch as toxins are both toxic and chemical in nature, they also automatically fall within the scope of the 1993 Chemical Weapons Convention, which states that:

> "toxic chemical" means any chemical which through its chemical action on life processes can cause death, temporary incapacitation or permanent harm to humans or animals. This includes all such chemicals, regardless of their origin or of their method of production, and regardless of whether they are produced in facilities, in munitions or elsewhere.

So, although there is no consensus on the term among scientists, international law regards a wide range of substances as "toxins". At one end of the range are the bacterial toxins, such as botulinum toxin and staphylococcal enterotoxin, both of which have in the past been stockpiled for weapons purposes. They are high-molecular-weight proteins that can at present be produced on a significant scale only by the methods of industrial microbiology. In the middle of the range are the snake poisons, insect venoms, plant alkaloids and a host of other such substances, some of which are becoming accessible to chemical synthesis and others, e.g. curare, batrachotoxin and ricin, have been used as weapons. At the other end of the range are small molecules such as potassium fluoroacetate (found in the plant *Dicephalatum cymosum*), which are typically synthesized by chemical processes when they are needed even though they are also produced by certain living organisms, thereby falling within the legal definition of "toxin". Hydrogen cyanide is another such toxin. It occurs in some 400 varieties of plant, in certain animals, and is synthesized by at least one bacterium (*Bacillus pyocyaneus*).

In the sense of the Biological and Toxin Weapons Convention, "toxin" includes substances to which scientists would not normally apply the term. For example, there are chemicals that occur naturally in the human body that would have toxic effects if administered in large enough quantity. Where a scientist might see a bioregulator, say, the treaty would see a poisonous substance produced by a living organism, in other words a toxin – nor is this unreasonable. Wasp venom, for example, is clearly a toxin, yet its active principle is histamine, which is also a human bioregulator. Although histamine might not itself be made into an effective weapon, the same cannot necessarily be said for other bioregulators.

Indeed, now that large-scale production processes for biologically active peptides and similar substances are undergoing rapid commercial development, bioregulators and other toxins constitute a field rich in potential weapons as well as pharmaceuticals, and in particular weapons of intense disabling or incapacitating power. It is fortunate, therefore, that this advance in biotechnology should have coincided with the adoption of the Chemical Weapons Convention, since it places its States Parties under the express obligation to ensure that bioregulators and other toxins, like all other toxic chemicals, are used only for the purposes that the Convention does not prohibit.

Some of the toxins that have been weaponized in the past are described below. Others, such as hydrogen cyanide and its derivative cyanogen chloride, are covered in the annex on chemical agents (Annex 1), as is a toxin that is finding widespread use as a riot-control agent, namely oleoresin capsicum, also known as Agent OC.

The bioregulator that, in the 1960s, initiated consideration of these often complex chemicals as weapons was the endecapeptide known as Substance P *(6)*, a tachykinin. Several other bioregulatory peptides have recently attracted similar attention *(7–11)*, but are not discussed here.

2. Bacterial toxins

2.1 *Staphylococcus aureus* enterotoxins

Staphylococcal enterotoxins are a common cause of diarrhoeal food poisoning after ingestion of improperly handled food. They are proteins ranging in size from 23 to 29 kDa, and are thought to work by stimulating the massive release of a variety of cytokines that then mediate the different toxic effects. The toxins are known in at least five antigenically distinct forms, of which type B is the most studied. It is heat-stable and, in aqueous solution, can withstand boiling. It is active by inhalation, by which route it causes a clinical syndrome markedly different, and often more disabling, than that following ingestion. It has been studied as a warfare agent of the incapacitating type. The median disabling dose for human beings by inhalation has been estimated at 0.4 ng/kg body weight. The corresponding lethal dose is estimated as being 50 times larger *(12)*.

Sources

The toxins are excreted by the Gram-positive coccus *Staphylococcus aureus*, which occurs worldwide. The culturing of some strains can yield large amounts of type B enterotoxin.

Main clinical features

When *Staphylococcus aureus* contaminates food products and the resulting preformed toxin is ingested, symptoms – usually nausea, vomiting and diarrhoea – occur within 1–6 hours of eating the contaminated food.

After inhalation of staphylococcal enterotoxin B (SEB), intoxication is apparent within 3–12 hours with the sudden onset of fever, headache, chills, myalgias and a non-productive cough. More severe cases may develop dyspnoea and retrosternal chest pain. If toxin is swallowed, nausea, vomiting and diarrhoea will occur in many patients, and fluid losses may be substantial. The fever, with variable degrees of chills and prostration, may last up to 5 days, and the cough may persist for as long as 4 weeks.

Diagnosis and detection

The diagnosis of inhalation SEB intoxication is clinical and epidemiological. Patient samples are unlikely to test positive for the toxin following aerosol exposure unless the exposure is large and samples are obtained rapidly. Enterotoxins may be detected in environmental samples using a variety of antibody-based tests.

Medical management

Supportive therapy has proved adequate in cases of accidental respiratory exposure to SEB aerosol. Hydration and oxygenation will require close attention. In severe cases, where pulmonary oedema develops, ventilation with positive and expiratory pressure and diuretics may be necessary. Most patients would be expected to do well after the initial acute phase of the illness, but will remain unfit for normal activities for 1–2 weeks *(13)*. Since the illness is an intoxication, no isolation or other quarantine measures are required.

Prophylaxis

No human vaccine is available, although several are in development, including some that, in animal studies, have been shown to protect against inhalation exposure to SEB. Passive protection has also been demonstrated.

Stability/neutralization

SEB can be detoxified by treatment with 0.5% hypochlorite for 10–15 minutes.

2.2   *Clostridium botulinum* neurotoxins

Clostridium botulinum neurotoxins are the cause of deadly food poisoning from canned foodstuffs that have been improperly prepared. They are proteins of around 150 kDa in size, and in culture are associated with other proteins to form complexes of some 300–900 kDa. There are seven antigenically distinct forms of botulinus neurotoxin, each consisting of two chains, the heavier of which binds to cholinergic synapses. The internalized lighter chain is a zinc protease and acts by cleaving proteins involved in the process of acetylcholine release. Particular substrate specificity varies between the different serotypes and may be correlated with observable differences in speed of onset of botulism and duration of paralysis. Botulinum toxins are the most acutely lethal of all toxic natural substances. As dry powder, they may be stable for long periods. They are active by inhalation as well as ingestion, the clinical picture being much the same by either route. They have long been studied as warfare agents of the lethal type *(14)*, particularly, though not exclusively, types A and B. The median lethal dose of type A for humans by inhalation has recently been estimated at 2 ng per kg body weight. By ingestion, the dose is estimated to be some three times smaller *(12)*.

Sources

The toxins are excreted by the Gram-positive spore-forming bacillus *Clostridium botulinum*, which occurs in soil and aquatic sediments worldwide, and which grows and produces neurotoxin under anaerobic conditions.

Main clinical features

Botulism, in the natural form caused by ingestion of bad food, is a dramatic disease that is frequently fatal for animals and humans alike, causing 60% mortality in reported cases before 1950. It is well described in the medical literature *(15)*. Inhalation botulism, on the other hand, is rare, but efforts have recently been made to describe it systematically *(12, 13, 16)*.

Following inhalation exposure, symptoms may begin within 1–3 days; the smaller the dose, the longer the onset time. At the start, bulbar palsies may be prominent, with eye symptoms such as blurred vision due to mydriasis, diplopia, ptosis and photophobia, as well as other bulbar signs such as dysarthria, dysphonia and dysphagia. Skeletal-muscle paralysis follows, with symmetrical, descending and progressive weakness. This may culminate abruptly in respiratory failure.

Diagnosis and detection

Misdiagnosis of botulism is frequent *(16)*. It may be confused with stroke, for example, Guillain–Barré syndrome or myasthenia gravis. Several diagnostic tests should therefore be performed to rule out these other syndromes, since waiting for the definitive diagnosis of botulism can take days, and patients need to have treatment immediately. Diagnosis depends on identifying the presence of toxin in blood samples, using some form of antigen–antibody reaction. In the natural disease, the bacterium and/or preformed toxin may be identified in unconsumed food samples.

Medical management

The treatment of severe cases of botulism is essentially supportive, with mechanical ventilation. Administration of immune globulin (either human or despeciated equine) to neutralize toxin not already bound to cholinergic synapses can help. The most serious complication, and the most common cause of death in botulism, is respiratory failure secondary to paralysis of the respiratory muscles. Intubation and ventilatory assistance will be needed, and tracheostomy may be required. There is no infection and thus no requirement for isolation or special hygiene measures.

Prophylaxis

Toxoid vaccines against types A–F have been produced and evaluated in animal and human studies. Type A toxoid has a product licence in the United Kingdom. The present toxoid vaccines require several doses over a period of weeks to produce protection. Primate studies have also demonstrated passive protection against inhalation or injection of toxin by equine or human immune globulin *(17)*. The level of protection depends entirely on the stoichiometric relationship between the amount of circulating antibody and the amount of toxin to which an individual may have been exposed.

Stability/neutralization

Botulinum toxins are rather easily inactivated. In food or drink, heating to an internal temperature of 85 °C for more than 5 minutes is sufficient. In the airborne state, the toxin is degraded by extremes of temperature or humidity. The rate of decay of aerosolized toxin has been estimated at 1–4% per minute, depending on the weather conditions *(16)*. Contaminated surfaces should be cleaned with 0.1% hypochlorite solution if they cannot be avoided for the few hours to days that natural degradation would require.

2.3 Aflatoxins and other fungal toxins

Before the 1960s, there was little systematic attention to fungal toxins as important causes of illness; the literature has developed mostly since the conclusion of the Biological and Toxin Weapons Convention. It is now well known that some fungi produce a single toxin, others may produce many, and different fungal genera may produce the same mycotoxin. Many genera, including *Acremonium*, *Alternaria*, *Aspergillus*, *Claviceps*, *Fusarium* and *Penicillium* produce mycotoxins. While the evidence indicates that ingestion of mouldy fodder is the primary route to animal mycotoxicoses, airborne fungal spores and infested/infected plant particulates may also induce disease leading to death in both animals and humans *(18)*. The weapons potential of such airborne toxins has not been disregarded, although, in the 1992 returns of information under the BWC confidence-building measures in which the Russian Federation declared offensive biological research and development programmes during the period since 1946, it is stated that "in the opinion of the experts, mycotoxins have no military significance" *(19)*.

Nevertheless, two categories of mycotoxin have been considered as warfare agents, namely the aflatoxins and the trichothecenes, and will be considered briefly here. The United Nations Special Commission (UNSCOM) on Iraq mentioned weaponization of an aflatoxin in its synoptic report of January 1999, stating that the "question remains open regarding the aims and reasons of the choice of aflatoxin as an agent". However, it went on to report that one Iraqi document "refers to military requirements to produce liver cancer using aflatoxin and the efficacy against military and civilian targets" *(20)*. The trichothecenes were the subject of allegations of weapons use ("yellow rain") in Cambodia and the Lao People's Democratic Republic during 1975–1984 that have since been discredited *(21)*.

Aflatoxicosis in humans is associated with the consumption of aflatoxin from food contaminated with the mould *Aspergillus flavus*. A number of aflatoxins with a range of potency ($B_1 > G_1 > B_2 > G_2$) are produced by *Aspergillus*, the relative proportions depending on the species of mould. Jaundice, fever, ascites, oedema of the feet, and vomiting are the symptoms associated with aflatoxicosis. In 397 patients estimated to have consumed 2–6 mg aflatoxin daily for a month, 106 fatalities occurred. Fatalities also followed estimated intakes of 12 mg/kg of aflatoxin B_1. Five-year follow-up of survivors of acute poisoning (including liver biopsies) showed almost complete recovery. The principal concern with aflatoxin (particularly B_1) is the possibility of liver cancer associated with the chronic consumption of mouldy food.

Aflatoxin chemistry and metabolism are well described. Aflatoxin B_1 is metabolized to a range of metabolites by microsomal systems. The active metabolite is presumed to be aflatoxin B_1 8-9 epoxide. Inactivation is dependent on glutathione conjugation, with susceptibility to acute intoxication dependent on the activity of the enzyme glutathione-S-transferase. The B_1 epoxide binds covalently to a range of proteins that have both structural and enzymic functions. Protein phosphorylation is also altered by aflatoxin B_1. All aflatoxins are genotoxic *(22, 23)*.

Trichothecene mycotoxins are a group of structurally related toxins produced by the *Fusarium* fungi found on many crops, and also by other mould genera such as *Stachybotrys*. They are sesquiterpinoids of low molecular weight, in the range 250–550 Da. Two of the better known toxins are T-2 and deoxynivalenol (or vomitoxin). Symptoms caused by the toxins are wide-ranging and include vomiting, diarrhoea, ataxia and haemorrhaging. The toxins are immunosuppressants and inhibit protein synthesis at the ribosomal level. They bind to the 60S subunit of eukaryotic ribosomes, altering peptidyl transferase activity. Inhibition of enzyme activity depends on toxin structure, and results in the failure either of polypeptide chain initiation or elongation. Toxicity of the toxins in in vitro test systems varies by as much as four orders of magnitude *(24)*.

In animals, the toxicity of T-2 is markedly species-dependent. Vomiting is induced in cats at 0.1–0.2 mg/kg after oral dosing. Guinea-pigs are unaffected at 0.75 mg/kg per day in the diet, but develop irritation and ulceration of the gut at 2.5 mg/kg per day. Immunosuppression is observed in rhesus monkeys at 0.5 mg/kg and in mice at 20 mg/kg. The LD_{50} in mice following intraperitoneal administration is reported to be 5.2 mg/kg. The toxicity of the trichothecenes in comparison with other toxins is therefore relatively low. They are, however, unusual among toxins in their ability to damage the skin, causing skin pain, pruritis, vesicles, necrosis and sloughing of epidermis.

The Joint FAO/WHO Expert Committee on Food Additives assessed the safety of aflatoxins and trichothecenes in food at its 56th meeting in February 2001 *(25)*.

2.4 Algal and other plant toxins

2.4.1   *Saxitoxin*

Saxitoxin is one of the phycotoxins that contribute to paralytic shellfish poisoning. It can also, though with difficulty, be synthesized. Consumption of seafood contaminated with marine algal toxins may cause either paralytic or diarrhoeal shellfish poisoning (PSP or DSP). In addition to their production by marine algae, PSP toxins can also be made by certain bacteria, cyanobacteria and red algae. Depending on the substituent side-groups, these are small molecules of around 300 Da. The parent compound, saxitoxin itself, is a powerful neurotoxin that binds with high affinity to sodium channels on cell membranes, inhibiting influx of sodium ions into cells without altering potassium ion efflux. Cell action potentials are suppressed, and paralysis results, the extent of which is dose-dependent. Saxitoxin binding to sodium channels is reversible. The toxin is soluble in water and stable, and dispersal as an aerosol is feasible. Fatalities in adults have been reported following ingestion of 0.5–12.4 mg. Minimum lethal doses in children are estimated to be 25 μg/kg *(26, 27)*.

Sources
The PSP toxins, including saxitoxin, can be isolated from bivalve molluscs, such as the butterclam, *Saxidona giganteus*, that have accumulated PSP-producing dinoflagellates, such as *Gonyaulax catanella*, during feeding. In one reported experiment, about 8 tonnes of clams were processed to produce a single gram of saxitoxin *(28)*.

Main clinical features
Reported clinical symptoms describe the outcome of ingestion of saxitoxin. Onset of symptoms is typically within 10–60 minutes. Numbness or tingling of the lips and tongue (attributable to local absorption) spreads to the face and neck, followed by a prickling feeling in fingers and toes. With moderate to severe exposure, the paraesthesia spreads to the arms and legs. Motor activity is reduced, speech becomes incoherent and respiration laboured and subjects die from respiratory arrest. The terminal stages may occur within 2–12 hours. No cases of inhalation exposure have been reported in the medical literature, but animal experiments suggest that the entire syndrome is compressed, and that death may occur within minutes

Diagnosis and detection
Diagnosis is confirmed by detection of the toxin, using ELISA or mouse bioassay, in samples of, for example, stomach contents, water or food.

Medical management
No specific antidotes exist, and treatment is symptomatic. The toxin is normally cleared rapidly from the body via the urine, so that victims who

survive for 12–24 hours usually recover. Diuretics may help. Specific antitoxin therapy has been successful in animals.

Prophylaxis

No vaccine against saxitoxin exposure has been developed for human use.

Stability/neutralization

Saxitoxin maintains its activity in water heated to 120 °C.

2.4.2   Ricin

Ricin is a highly toxic glycoprotein (a lectin) of approximately 65 kDa that occurs in the seed of the castor oil plant, *Ricinus communis*. Ricin consists of two protein chains, the larger (B chain, 34 kDa) attaching to cell surface receptors and facilitating entry of the smaller (A chain, 32 kDa), which affects cellular ribosomal activity. It inhibits protein synthesis in eukaryotic cells, and is toxic by all routes, including inhalation, but least so by ingestion. Horses are the animals most susceptible to ricin, cattle and pigs less so, with ducks and hens the least susceptible. In mice, the systemic LD_{50} is 2.7 μg/kg *(12, 13)*.

Sources

Ricin can be extracted relatively easily from castor oil beans, about 1 million tons of which are processed per year in the production of castor oil. Ricin accounts for some 5% by weight of the waste mash.

Main clinical features

A latency period of many hours, sometimes days, follows exposure. After inhalation, significant lung pathology is evident, with increased cytokine concentrations, marked inflammation and pulmonary oedema. Ingestion results in severe gastroenteritis, often haemorrhagic. Convulsions, shock and renal failure may develop. Nerve cells, the heart and spleen are all affected by ricin. Ricin dust exposure will cause local irritation of eyes, nose and throat *(26)*. Sublethal lung pathology has been described in immunized mice following inhalation challenge with aerosolized ricin. Survivors of a ricin aerosol challenge may therefore experience some injury, particularly to the lungs.

Diagnosis and detection

The primary diagnosis is clinical and epidemiological. Specific ELISA testing on serum or immunohistochemical techniques for direct tissue analysis can be used to confirm the diagnosis.

Medical management

Management is supportive and should include maintenance of intra-vascular volume. No antitoxin is yet available.

Prophylaxis

There is no currently approved prophylaxis for human use, though both active immunization and passive antibody prophylaxis are under study. Formaldehyde toxoids against ricin have been used successfully to immunize rats. Toxoid was administered subcutaneously in 3 doses at 3-weekly intervals and prevented deaths in animals exposed to 5 LCt_{50} by inhalation challenge *(29)*.

Stability/neutralization

Ricin is soluble in water, the solution being less stable than the dry product. In the dry state, it is normally stable at room temperature but denatures at elevated temperature, the stability decreasing with increasing moisture content *(30)*.

REFERENCES

1. Madsen JM. Toxins as weapons of mass destruction. *Clinics in Laboratory Medicine*, 2001, 21:593–605.

2. Roberts B, Moodie M. *Biological weapons: towards a threat reduction strategy*. Washington, DC, National Defense University, 2002 (Defense Horizons, No. 15).

3. United States of America. *Working paper on toxins*. Conference of the Committee on Disarmament, 21 April 1970 (document CCD/286).

4. United States Code; Title 18, Crimes and Criminal Procedure; Chapter 10, Biological Weapons; Section 178, Definitions.

5. *Final document: 2nd Review Conference of the Parties to the Convention on the Prohibition of the Development, Production and Stockpiling of Bacteriological (Biological) and Toxin Weapons*. Geneva, United Nations, 1986 (document BWC/CONF.II/13).

6. Koch BL, Edvinsson AA, Koskinen LO. Inhalation of substance P and thiorphan: acute toxicity and effects on respiration in conscious guinea pigs. *Journal of Applied Toxicology*, 1999, 19:19–23.

7. *Novel toxins and bioregulators*. Ottawa, Ministry of External Affairs and International Trade, 1991.

8. *Evaluation of biological agents and toxins: working paper submitted by the Republic of Croatia*. Ad Hoc Working Group of the States Parties to the Convention on the Prohibition of the Development, Production and Stockpiling of Bacteriological (Biological) and Toxin Weapons and on their Destruction. Geneva, United Nations, 19 July 1999 (document BWC/ADHOCGROUP/WP.356/Rev.1).

9. Bokan S, Breen SG, Orehovec Z. An evaluation of bioregulators as terrorism and warfare agents. *ASA Newsletter*, 2002, 90:16–19.

10. Dando M. *The new biological weapons: threat, proliferation, and control*. Boulder, CO, Lynne Rienner, 2001:67–85.

11. Kagan E. Bioregulators as instruments of terror. *Clinics in Laboratory Medicine*, 2001, 21:607–618.

12. Sidell FR, Takafuji ET, Franz DR, eds. *Medical aspects of chemical and biological warfare*. Washington, DC, Department of the Army, Office of The Surgeon General and Borden Institute, 1997.

13. *Handbook: medical management of biological casualties*, 2nd ed. Fort Detrick, MD, United States Army Medical Research Institute of Infectious Diseases, 1996.

14. Patocka J, Splino M. Botulinum toxin: from poison to medicinal agent. *ASA Newsletter*, 2002, 88:14–19.

15. Shapiro RL, Hatheway C, Swerdlow DL. Botulism in the United States: a clinical and epidemiological review. *Annals of Internal Medicine*, 1998, 129:221–228.

16. Arnon SS et al. Botulinum toxin as a biological weapon: medical and public health management. *Journal of the American Medical Association*, 2001, 285:1059–1070.

17. Franz DR et al. Efficacy of prophylactic and therapeutic administration of antitoxin for inhalation botulism. In: Dasgupta BR, ed. *Botulinum and tetanus neurotoxins: neurotransmission and biomedical aspects*. New York, Plenum, 1993:473–476.

18. Malloy CD, Marr JS. Mycotoxins and public health: a review. *Journal of Public Health Management and Practice*, 1997, 3:61–69.

19. *Compilation of declarations of information by BWC States Parties in accordance with the extended confidence-building measures agreed at the Third Review Conference*. New York, United Nations, Office of Disarmament Affairs, 1992 (document DDA/4-92/BW3, Add.1, Add.2, and Add.3: Form F filed by the Russian Federation, as translated by WHO).

20. *Report: disarmament* (as transmitted to the President of the Security Council, 27 January 1999, and subsequently distributed as document S/1999/94, dated 29 January 1999). New York, United Nations, 1999.

21. Tucker JB. The "Yellow Rain" controversy: lessons for arms control compliance. *The Nonproliferation Review*, 2001, 8:25–42.

22. *Some naturally occurring substances: food items and constituents, heterocyclic aromatic amines and mycotoxins*. Lyon, International Agency for Research on Cancer, 1993:245–384 (IARC Monographs on the evaluation of carcinogenic risks to humans, Vol. 56).

23. Eaton DL, Groopman JD, eds. *The toxicology of aflatoxins. Human health, veterinary and agricultural significance*. London, Academic Press, 1994.

24. Rotter BA, Prelusky DB, Pestka JJ. Toxicology of deoxynivalenol (vomitoxin). *Journal of Toxicology and Environmental Health*, 1996, 48:1–34.

25. *Evaluation of certain mycotoxins in food. Fifty-sixth report of the Joint FAO/WHO Expert Committee on Food Additives*. Geneva, World Health Organization, 2002 (WHO Technical Report Series, No. 906).

26. United States National Library of Medicine. Hazardous Substances Data Bank, 1999 (available at *http://toxnet.nlm.nih.gov/cgi-bin/sis/htmlgen?HSBD)*.

27. Aune T. Health effects associated with algal toxins from seafood. *Archives of Toxicology Supplement*, 1997, 19:389–397.

28. Schantz EJ. Biochemical studies on paralytic shellfish poison. *Annals of the New York Academy of Sciences*, 1960, 90:843–855.

29. Griffiths GD et al. Protection against inhalation toxicity of ricin and abrin by immunisation. *Human and Experimental Toxicology*, 1995, 14:155–164.

30. Cope AC, Dee D, Cannan RK. Ricin. In: Renshaw B, ed. *Summary Technical Report of Division 9, NDRC. Vol. 1: Chemical warfare agents and related chemical problems, parts I–II*. Washington, DC, National Defense Research Committee, 1946:179–203.

ANNEX 3: BIOLOGICAL AGENTS

1. Introduction

Extensive research, development and testing by military establishments have shown that large-scale production of certain infective agents and their incorporation into weapons for atmospheric dispersal of pathogens is feasible in suitably designed facilities with specialized equipment and appropriate precautions to protect the workers and prevent accidental release to the environment. The selection of the agent and strain, its large-scale growth and its further processing present numerous technical problems and require specialized technologies and associated effort in research, development and testing. Several modes of delivery have received attention in military offensive programmes but by far the greatest emphasis has been placed on methods of disseminating biological agents as inhalable aerosols. Numerous additional technical difficulties must be overcome in order to develop munitions or other devices that produce stable aerosols, and specific delivery and atmospheric conditions must be met if the aerosol is to reach the target population. Throughout all these steps, including that of aerosol cloud travel, special techniques and conditions are required to maintain the inhalability, infectivity and virulence of the agent. Nevertheless, despite the fact that the development of strategic biological weapons within military establishments historically required large-scale efforts over several years, some infective agents could be produced and used as weapons of terror on a smaller scale using relatively simple techniques. Pathogens variously cited as possible agents of biological warfare or terrorism are listed in Table A3.1 below.

This annex presents information about the 11 particular infective agents, all of them listed in Table A3.1, that were selected in Chapter 3 for inclusion in the representative group of agents. All but one continue to cause naturally occurring human disease, especially in endemic regions and among populations without access to adequate sanitation, public health, veterinary and medical systems, and proper nutrition. The only exception is the variola virus, the agent of smallpox, declared by the 1980 World Health Assembly to have been eradicated.

Table A3.1. Biological agents variously cited as possible weapons for use against humans

Biological agent and WHO alphanumeric code for the disease[a] it can cause	United Nations[b] (1969)	WHO[c] (1970)	BWC[d] CBM-F (1992)	Australia Group[e] (1992)	NATO[f] (1996)	CDC[g] category A (2000)	BWC[h] draft Protocol (2001)
BACTERIA (including RICKETTSIA and CHLAMYDIA)							
Bacillus anthracis, A22 (anthrax)	X	X	X	X	X	X	X
Bartonella quintana, A79.0 (trench fever)				X			
Brucella species, A23 (brucellosis)	X	X	X	X	X		X
Burkholderia mallei, A24.0 (glanders)	X	X	X	X			X
Burkholderia pseudomallei, A24 (melioidosis)	X	X	X	X	X		X
Franciscella tularensis, A21 (tularaemia)	X	X	X	X	X	X	X
Salmonella typhi, A01.0 (typhoid fever)	X	X		X	X		
Shigella species, A03 (shigellosis)	X				X		
Vibrio cholerae, A00 (cholera)	X	X		X	X		
Yersinia pestis, A20 (plague)	X	X	X	X	X	X	X
Coxiella burnetii, A78 (Q fever)	X	X	X	X	X		X
Orientia tsutsugamushi, A75.3 (scrub typhus)					X		
Rickettsia prowazekii, A75 (typhus fever)	X	X	X	X	X		
Rickettsia rickettsii, A77.0 (Rocky Mountain spotted fever)	X	X		X	X		X
Chlamydia psittaci, A70 (psittacosis)	X				X		
FUNGI							
Coccidioides immitis, B38 (coccidioidomycosis)	X	X			X		
VIRUSES							
Hantaan/Korean haemorrhagic fever, etc., A98.5		X		X	X		
Sin nombre, J12.8							X
Crimean-Congo haemorrhagic fever, A98.0		X		X	X		X
Rift Valley fever, A92.4		X		X	X		X
Ebola virus disease, A98.3				X			X
Marburg virus disease, A98.4		X		X	X	X	X
Lymphocytic choriomeningitis, A87.2				X		X	X

Agent	a	b	c	d	e	f	g	h
Junin haemorrhagic fever, A96.0 (Argentine haemorrhagic fever)	X			X		X	X	X
Machupo haemorrhagic fever, A96.1 (Bolivian haemorrhagic fever)	X			X		X		X
Lassa fever, A96.2	X			X		X	X	X
Tick-borne encephalitis/Russian spring–summer encephalitis, A84.0/A84	X	X		X		X		X
Dengue, A90/91	X	X		X		X		
Yellow fever, A95	X	X		X		X		X
Omsk haemorrhagic fever, A98.1					X			
Japanese encephalitis, A83.0	X	X		X				
Western equine encephalomyelitis, A83.1	X	X		X			X	
Eastern equine encephalomyelitis, A83.2	X	X		X		X		X
Chikungunya virus disease, A92.0	X	X		X		X		
O'nyong-nyong, A92.1	X							
Venezuelan equine encephalitis, A92.2	X	X	X	X		X		X
Variola major, B03 (smallpox)	X	X		X		X	X	X
Monkeypox, B04				X				X
White pox (a variant of variola virus)				X		X		
Influenza, J10, 11	X	X		X				

PROTOZOA

Agent	a	b	c	d	e	f	g	h
Naeglaeria fowleri, B60.2 (naegleriasis)								X
Toxoplasma gondii, B58 (toxoplasmosis)	X							
Schistosoma species, B65 (schistosomiasis)	X							

Notes

a Diseases are identified by the alphanumeric code assigned by the WHO *International Statistical Classification of Diseases and Related Health Problems*, 10th Revision (ICD-10).

b United Nations, *Chemical and bacteriological (biological) weapons and the effects of their possible use: Report of the Secretary-General*, New York, 1969.

c World Health Organization, *Health aspects of chemical and biological weapons: Report of a WHO group of consultants*, Geneva, 1970.

d UN Office of Disarmament Affairs, compilation of declarations of information by BWC States Parties in accordance with the extended confidence-building measures agreed at the Third Review Conference, DDA/4-92/BW3 plus Add.1, Add.2 and Add.3, data from Section 2, *Past offensive biological R&D programmes*, of Form F as filed by Canada, France, Russian Federation, UK, and USA in 1992.

e Australia Group document AG/Dec92/BW/Chair/30 dated June 1992.

f *NATO Handbook on the Medical Aspects of NBC Defensive Operations*, AmedP-6(B), Part II – Biological, 1996.

g Centers for Disease Control and Prevention: Biological and Chemical Terrorism: Strategic Plan for Preparedness and Response. Recommendations of the CDC Strategic Planning Workgroup. *Morbidity and Mortality Weekly Report*, 2000; 49 (No.RR-4):1–14.

h Ad Hoc Group of the States Parties to the Convention on the Prohibition, Development, Production and Stockpiling of Bacteriological (Biological) and Toxin Weapons and on their Destruction, document BWC/AD HOC GROUP/56-2, at pp 465–466, which is in Annex A of the Chairman's Composite Text for the BWC Protocol.

1.1 Recognizing deliberate release

Although all of the listed agents are known because of the diseases they cause naturally, there are aspects important for response planning in which their effects if used as weapons, particularly as aerosols, are likely to differ from their effects in naturally occurring infections.

Suddenness. Individual exposures in natural outbreaks affecting groups of people caused by animal or insect carriers or by person-to-person transmission are usually spread over a period of many days or longer. In contrast, inhalatory exposures to a pathogen contained in an aerosol in a single attack would be mainly confined to the passage or dispersal time of the aerosol. This is because the limited deposition of aerosol particles and the inefficiency of their resuspension as particles small enough to be inhaled would generally make subsequent exposures much less than those from the initial aerosol. The time course of an outbreak following such an attack would therefore be expected to exhibit a more sudden rise and probably, except for contagious disease, a more rapid fall-off than is characteristic of the same disease in a natural outbreak. It is also possible, however, that deliberate release could be spread out over time, as would be the case for repeated attacks.

Severity of disease following inhalatory infection. Disease initiated by inhalatory infection may follow a course and exhibit symptoms differing from and more severe than those characteristic of other routes of entry. For some diseases that are ordinarily of low lethality for healthy adults, such as Venezuelan equine encephalitis, normally acquired from the bite of infected mosquitoes, it is possible that atypical infection of humans through the respiratory tract, which may bypass such normal protective mechanisms as local inflammatory processes, would be less susceptible to vaccine protection and/or would have increased virulence and lethality. By analogy with other infections of humans where inhalatory infection is associated with particularly high lethality, such as pneumonic plague and inhalational anthrax, this should be regarded as a strong possibility.

Number of cases. If a large-scale attack on a population centre were attempted and if the many technical difficulties in its preparation and execution were overcome, large numbers of people could become infected.

Unusual geographical or demographic distribution. An unusual geographical distribution of persons or animals at the time of their probable exposure could point to deliberate use. Aerosol release resulting in an airborne cloud, for example, would give a distribution consistent with meteorological conditions at the time. Other unusual distributions or association with suspicious objects or activities may also be indicative of deliberate use.

Rareness. Although natural or inadvertent introduction of an exotic pathogen is not an uncommon occurrence, the unexplained appearance of an infectious disease of humans or animals that is ordinarily very rare or absent in a region may indicate deliberate use.

1.2   Prevention, protection and therapy

The unprecedented case-load, the sudden nature of the outbreak and the severe and possibly unfamiliar course of the illness resulting from a biological attack could place demands on even a reasonably well prepared emergency response and health care system beyond its ability to cope. As in ordinary public health matters, therefore, emphasis must be placed on measures for prevention in all its aspects, a subject addressed in Chapters 4 and 5.

Exposure to aerosolized biological agents can be greatly reduced by a properly fitted military gas mask, by a high-efficiency particulate arresting (HEPA)-type microbiological mask or by a shelter or building provided with suitably filtered or disinfected air. The safe and effective use of masks requires training in their use. Timely masking and unmasking or entry and exit from shelters depend on advance warning of an impending attack and notification of when the inhalation hazard has passed. Some aspects of protection are discussed in Chapters 3 and 4.

Vaccines affording various degrees of protection for various periods of time against a few of the agents of concern have been approved by national regulatory authorities as effective and sufficiently safe for general use against naturally occurring infection. Information on a number of vaccines and their sources of supply will be posted on the WHO web site, so that the information can be regularly updated. It should be noted, however, that the availability of some vaccines may be restricted.

Because individual vaccines are specific for individual pathogens, a decision to engage in widespread vaccination as prophylaxis against biological attack must be based on a judgement that there is a serious risk to a particular population, that the probable identity of the threat agent is known, and that the vaccine would be effective against it. A further complexity is that naturally occurring strains of a given agent may differ in their susceptibility to vaccine prophylaxis, and strains not amenable to vaccine prophylaxis might be produced artificially. Also, the cost and resources required by any large-scale vaccination programme must be balanced against other needs and, depending on the vaccine, its administration may entail health risks in the form of adverse reactions and may be subject to contraindications for specific population groups. Finally, for most of the agents of concern, vaccines approved for general use do not exist.

Post-exposure vaccination for the agents described here is of proven value only in the case of smallpox, where its timely administration to persons who may have been exposed would probably be of major importance in helping to halt epidemic spread.

Antimicrobial drugs for prophylaxis in cases of anticipated or suspected exposure and for therapy of those already infected can be effective for many bacterial and fungal diseases. Proper choice, procurement and use of the antimicrobials most likely to be effective requires timely identification of the agent and its sensitivity to specific antimicrobials. As the initial signs of many of the diseases of concern are nondescript, rapid diagnostic procedures should be immediately instituted whenever there is a sudden appearance of cases of unexplained illness. Advance preparations should therefore be made for rapid access to local, regional, national and international reference laboratories, should they be needed. In this regard, encouragement should be given to the adoption, as they become available, of rapid, reliable and specific DNA-based, immuno-based and other newer methods of laboratory diagnosis in order to facilitate the timely and effective treatment and prophylaxis of both natural and, should it occur, deliberately caused infectious disease.

1.3 Specific agents

The information that follows is intended to provide only a general description of the characteristics, diagnostic procedures and medical and public health measures relevant to each listed agent. Additional information may be found in the specific references given at the end of the section for each agent and in the more general works cited at the end of this annex. The information given below includes the following categories:

- *Name of the agent/disease.* The name of the pathogen and the disease it causes. Each disease is also designated by its alphanumeric code assigned by ICD-10.
- *Description of the agent.* Classification and description of the agent.
- *Occurrence.* Places where the disease is prevalent.
- *Reservoirs.* Principal animal and environmental sources of human infection.
- *Mode of transmission.* Principal modes of transmission to humans: vector-borne, person-to-person, waterborne, foodborne, airborne, etc.
- *Incubation period.* The time between exposure and the first appearance of symptoms. This will vary from individual to individual and for some pathogens is highly variable. Incubation periods also depend on the route of entry and on dose, generally being shorter for higher doses.
- *Clinical features.* Principal signs and symptoms characteristic of the disease. For many of the listed agents the initial symptoms are nondescript, resembling those of influenza and making early clinical identification difficult.
- *Laboratory diagnosis.* Laboratory methods for identification of pathogens in clinical and environmental specimens. Biosafety recommendations for laboratory workers.
- *Medical management and public health measures.* Isolation requirements, protection of caregivers, disposal of contaminated materials and, where applicable, quarantine and hygienic measures.
- *Prophylaxis and therapy.* Vaccines, antimicrobials and antisera, where applicable.
- *Other information.*
- *Selected references.*

2. Bacteria

2.1 *Bacillus anthracis* /Anthrax (A22)

The vegetative form of *B. anthracis* is a non-motile, rod-shaped, Gram-positive, aerobic or facultatively anaerobic bacillus measuring 1–1.2 μm x 3–5 μm. The vegetative bacillus multiplies readily in infected animals and in laboratory media. Under nutrient-limiting conditions in the presence of free oxygen, an egg-shaped spore forms within the vegetative cell and is released upon lysis. In contrast to the fragile vegetative form, mature anthrax spores are highly resistant to drying, heat, ultraviolet and ionizing radiation and other forms of stress and can remain infective in the environment for years. When introduced into the body of a susceptible host and if not inactivated by host defence mechanisms, the spore may germinate to become a vegetative bacillus, restarting the cycle.

Occurrence

Anthrax is mainly a disease of mammals, most commonly encountered in grazing animals. Until the introduction and widespread use of effective veterinary vaccines, it was a major cause of fatal disease in cattle, sheep, goats, camels, horses and pigs throughout the world. Anthrax continues to be reported from many countries in domesticated and wild herbivores, especially where livestock vaccination programmes are inadequate or have been disrupted. Human anthrax, acquired from diseased animals and animal products, is most frequent in Africa, the Middle East and central and southern Asia.

Reservoirs

Anthrax spores are a contaminant of soil where animals have died of the disease. Depending on temperature and soil conditions, vegetative cells in blood and other secretions spilt on the ground from newly dead or dying animals form spores upon exposure to air, creating foci of contaminated soil. These may persist for years as a source of further infection. Additional foci may be created by the scavenged remains of dead animals. Infective spores can also persist for long periods in hides, hair and bonemeal from infected animals. A number of large outbreaks in livestock have been traced to the introduction of animal feed containing contaminated bonemeal. Vegetative cells remaining within the carcass of a diseased animal, however, are rapidly destroyed by putrefaction.

Mode of transmission

It is the spore rather than the vegetative form that is generally the agent by which the disease is transmitted and it is doubtful that the vegetative form ever proliferates significantly outside the animal body. The vegetative form is infective, however, and is presumed to be responsible at times for infection by fly bites. Although definitive studies are lacking, infection of animals is thought mainly to result from entry of ingested spores through epithelial lesions, with inhalation of contaminated dust and transmission by biting flies as less frequent possibilities.

The most common mode of transmission to humans is by the entry of spores from infected animal products through lesions of the skin, especially on exposed parts of the body such as the arms, face and neck. Less frequently, infection is by ingestion of meat of infected animals or by inhalation of spores, as from contaminated wool, hair or hides. The disease is generally regarded as being non-contagious. Records of person-to-person spread exist, but are rare. Evidence from animal experiments, including experiments in non-human primates, suggest that the introduction of only a few spores through a lesion may induce cutaneous or gastrointestinal infection but that a much larger number of spores is required to produce a high probability of infection by inhalation. Nevertheless, the possibility cannot be excluded that inhalation of even a single spore can initiate infection by any of the routes, although with very low probability in the case of inhalation or ingestion anthrax.

Incubation period

Symptoms of human cutaneous and gastrointestinal anthrax generally appear between 1 and several days after exposure. The incubation period for inhalational anthrax, derived from limited data, is reported to range from 1 to 7 days. Longer times, possibly extending up to several weeks, may occur in rare cases. As with other pathogens, average incubation period may be inversely associated with dose.

Clinical features

Cutaneous infection starts as a painless, non-scarring, pruritic papule progressing over a period of about a week to a black depressed eschar with swelling of adjacent lymph glands and localized oedema, which may become extensive. Although usually self-limiting, untreated cutaneous anthrax can become systemic and is fatal in 5–20% of cases. With proper antimicrobial therapy, the death rate in cutaneous anthrax is less than 1%.

Inhalational anthrax begins with nondescript or influenza-like symptoms that may elude correct diagnosis. These may include fever, fatigue, chills, non-productive cough, vomiting, sweats, myalgia, dyspnoea, confusion, headache, and chest and/or abdominal pain, followed after 1–3 days by the sudden development of cyanosis, shock, coma and death. Nasal congestion and rhinorrhoea, common in influenza and other viral respiratory illnesses, are rare in patients with inhalational anthrax. Chest X-rays usually show a widened mediastinum, marked pleural effusions and mediastinal lymphadenopathy. During terminal stages, blood levels of vegetative bacilli may reach 10^8/ml or more. Late administration of antimicrobials may sterilize the blood while not preventing death from the action of anthrax toxin already released. The average time between onset and death is typically 1–4 days. Reported case-fatality rates without treatment are 90% and higher. Meningitis is not uncommon and is a dangerous potential sequel to any of the forms of anthrax. Pneumonia may be present but is not a regular feature, and the lungs usually remain clear of growing bacteria until late stages.

Gastrointestinal and oropharyngeal anthrax result from the ingestion of contaminated meat. Gastrointestinal anthrax may be accompanied by fever, nausea, vomiting, abdominal pain and bloody stools. Oropharyngeal infection is characterized by oedematous swelling of the neck, often massive and accompanied by fever and lymphoid involvement. Mortality in gastrointestinal anthrax is variable, depending on the outbreak, but in some outbreaks it is reported to approach that of inhalational anthrax. However, in both gastrointestinal and inhalational forms, mild or subclinical infections may occur and be undetected.

Laboratory diagnosis
Confirmation of clinical diagnosis may be made by direct visualization of the vegetative bacilli or by culturing. Microscopic identification of the vegetative bacilli in fresh smears of vesicular fluid or blood may be done using the McFadyean staining method or the indirect immunofluorescence assay. On blood agar plates, *B. anthracis* forms white or

greyish white, coherent, non-haemolytic colonies in which chains of vegetative bacilli are present together with spore-containing cells. In blood and infected tissues and also under anaerobic conditions in the presence of bicarbonate, but not on ordinary culture plates, the vegetative cell forms a prominent poly-γ-d-glutamic acid capsule. If the patient has been treated with antimicrobials, however, it may be difficult or impossible to demonstrate the bacilli in blood or tissue specimens. For identification in sterile fluids and other sterile samples, methods have been developed for rapid detection based on monoclonal antibodies and on polymerase chain reaction (PCR). Seroconversion may be detected using enzyme-linked immunosorbent assay (ELISA).

Biosafety Level 2 practices, equipment and facilities are recommended for manipulations involving clinical specimens. Biosafety Level 3 practices, equipment and facilities are recommended for manipulations involving culturing or activities with a significant potential for aerosol production.

Medical management and public health measures

Patient isolation is not required and there are no quarantine requirements. Cadavers should be cremated. Dressings, discharges from lesions, and other contaminated materials should be disinfected, preferably by incineration or by deep burial with quicklime. Sterilization or disinfection may also be achieved by autoclaving, soaking with aqueous formaldehyde, glutaraldehyde, hypochlorite, hydrogen peroxide or peracetic acid. Fumigation with ethylene oxide, formaldehyde vapour or chlorine dioxide may be employed to inactivate spores in contaminated rooms or buildings.

Prophylaxis and therapy

Live spore vaccines based on attenuated strains are produced for human use in China and in the Russian Federation. In other countries, live spore vaccines are restricted to veterinary applications and are not licensed for human use. Cell-free vaccines containing anthrax-protective antigen (see below) are produced and licensed for human use in the United Kingdom and the USA. The use of such vaccines has been associated with a major reduction of anthrax in individuals whose occupations place them at risk.

With respect to protection against infection by the aerosol route, experimental immunization with live spore vaccines and cell-free vaccines containing anthrax-protective antigen has been shown to be capable of protecting laboratory animals (guinea-pigs, rabbits, monkeys) against inhalational anthrax. Evidence regarding the degree and duration of protection that existing vaccines may afford to humans against inhalationally acquired anthrax is based to some extent on epidemiological analyses of at-risk occupations but, for the purpose of bioaggression scenario modelling, is heavily dependent on extrapolation from such animal experiments and on indirect measures of human immune parameters. Efficacy of these vaccines as part of a post-exposure prophylaxis programme has not been determined.

Antimicrobial therapy is effective in treating cutaneous anthrax and is likely to be effective against human inhalational anthrax provided that it is begun before or very soon after symptoms appear. Once high levels of toxin are produced by anthrax bacilli in the body, antimicrobial therapy becomes ineffective. If available, specific human gamma globulin may be effective in cases where otherwise lethal levels of anthrax toxin have already accumulated. Antimicrobial therapy should also be used for prophylaxis in asymptomatic patients with suspected exposure to anthrax spore aerosol. Prolonged treatment is needed to allow time for clearance or inactivation of spores deposited in the lungs, as spores are not affected by antimicrobials. Because of the possibility of extended incubation periods in rare instances, continuation of antimicrobial treatment for up to 60 days has been recommended in the USA.

Penicillin is generally effective against human cutaneous anthrax. Tests in non-human primates indicate that penicillin, doxycycline and ciprofloxacin are effective for prophylaxis and for early treatment of inhalational anthrax. The use of cell-free vaccine for post-exposure prophylaxis in combination with antimicrobials has been suggested on the basis of limited studies on non-human primates.

Other information

The disease is associated with the action on mammalian cells of a toxin composed of three protein components produced by the vegetative bacillus. One of the components, protective antigen (PA), binds to receptors on the cell surface and mediates the entry into the cell of the other two components, oedema factor (EF) and lethal factor (LF).

The other principal anthrax virulence factor, in addition to the toxin, is the polypeptide capsule of the vegetative bacillus, which affords protection against phagocytosis. The symptoms of anthrax infection in experimental animals can be produced by the administration of the purified toxin.

Reported estimates of the dose required to infect 50% of a population of non-human primates in experimental studies of inhalational anthrax vary enormously, from 2500 to 760 000 spores, apparently reflecting differences in the many variables involved in such experiments. While doses lower than the LD_{50} produce correspondingly lower rates of infection, the very large number of experimental animals that would be required makes it impractical to determine doses that would infect only a small percentage of those exposed.

The largest reported outbreak of human inhalational anthrax took place in 1979 in Sverdlovsk (Ekaterinburg), former Soviet Union. Of 66 documented fatal cases, all were more than 23 years in age, suggesting that adults may be more susceptible to inhalational anthrax than younger individuals. The concomitant infection of sheep and cattle as far as 50 kilometres down wind of the apparent source points to the hazard of long-distance aerosol travel of infective spores.

An outbreak of inhalational anthrax and cutaneous anthrax in the United States during October and November 2001 was caused by *B. anthracis* spores intentionally placed in envelopes sent through the post. Of the total of 11 reported inhalational cases, the probable date of exposure could be determined in six, and for these the median incubation period was 4 days (range 4–6 days). Prolonged antimicrobial prophylaxis administered to persons thought to be at greatest risk may have prevented cases from occurring later. All 11 inhalational cases received antimicrobial and supportive therapy and six survived. As in the Sverdlovsk outbreak, there was a lack of young persons among the inhalational cases, whose ages ranged from 43 to 94.

Selected references

Abramova FA, Grinberg LM. Pathologic anatomy of anthracic sepsis: macroscopical findings during the infectious outbreak in 1979, Sverdlovsk. *Arkhiv Patologii*, 1993, 55:12–17 (in Russian).

Abramova FA, Grinberg LM. Pathology of anthracic sepsis: materials of the infectious outbreak in 1979, Sverdlovsk. *Arkhiv Patologii*, 1993, 55:18–23 (in Russian).

Abramova FA et al. Pathology of inhalational anthrax in 42 cases from the Sverdlovsk outbreak of 1979. *Proceedings of the National Academy of Sciences*, 1993, 90:2291–2294.

Brachman PS. Anthrax. In: Evans AS, Brachman PS, eds. *Bacteriological infections of humans: epidemiology and control*, 2nd ed. New York, Plenum, 1991:75–86.

Bryskier A. *Bacillus anthracis* and antibacterial agents. *Clinical Microbiology and Infectious Disease*, 2002, 8:467–468.

Dixon TC et al. Anthrax. *New England Journal of Medicine*, 1999, 341:815–826.

Friedlander AM et al. Postexposure prophylaxis against experimental inhalation anthrax. *Journal of Infectious Diseases*, 1993, 167:1239–1242.

Hanna P. Anthrax pathogenesis and host response. *Current Topics in Microbiology and Immunology*, 1998, 225:13–55.

Inglesby TV et al. Anthrax as a biological weapon: medical and public health management. *Journal of the American Medical Association*, 1999, 281:1735–1745.

Inglesby TV et al. Anthrax as a biological weapon, 2002: updated recommendations for management. *Journal of the American Medical Association*, 2002, 287:2236–2252.

Jerningan JA et al. Bioterrorism-related inhalation anthrax: the first 10 cases reported in the United States. *Emerging Infectious Diseases*, 2001, 7:933–944.

Meselson M et al. The Sverdlovsk anthrax outbreak of 1979. *Science*, 1994, 266:1202–1208.

Mourez M et al. 2001: a year of major advances in anthrax toxin research. *Trends in Microbiology*, 2002, 10:287–293.

Pile JC et al. Anthrax as a potential biological warfare agent. *Archives of Internal Medicine*, 1998, 158:429–434.

Swartz MN. Recognition and management of anthrax – an update. *New England Journal of Medicine,* 2001, 345:1621-1626.

Turnbull PCB. Current status of immunization against anthrax: old vaccines may be here to stay for a while. *Current Opinion in Infectious Diseases*, 2000, 13:113–120.

Turnbull PCB et al. *Guidelines on surveillance and control of anthrax in humans and animals*. Geneva, World Health Organization, 1998 (document WHO/EMC/ZDI/ 98.6; also available at *www.who.int/emc-documents/zoonoses/whoemczdi986c.html*).

Turnbull PCB. Guidance on environments known to be or suspected of being contaminated with anthrax spores. *Land Contamination and Reclamation*, 1996, 4:37–45.

Watson A, Keir D. Information on which to base assessments of risk from environments contaminated with anthrax spores. *Epidemiological Infection*, 1994, 113:479–490.

2.2 *Brucella abortus, Brucella suis* and *Brucella melitensis* / Brucellosis (A23)

Brucella species, which may also be regarded as different strains of *B. melitensis*, are non-motile, Gram-negative, aerobic, unencapsulated cocci or short rods measuring approximately 0.5–0.7 μm x 0.6–1.5 μm. The bacteria are able to grow intracellularly in infected hosts. Infective cells can persist in the environment for weeks and dried preparations can retain virulence for years.

Occurrence
Worldwide.

Reservoirs
Diverse domesticated and wild mammals, especially cattle, goats, sheep, pigs, camels, buffaloes and marine mammals. Preferred hosts exist for each species: *B. abortus* commonly infects cattle; *B. suis* commonly infects pigs; and *B. melitensis* commonly infects goats, sheep and camels. *B. melitensis* and biovars 1 and 3 of *B. suis* are particularly virulent for humans.

Mode of transmission
Most human infections result from ingestion of raw animal products, especially unpasteurized dairy products. Infection may also result from entry of the bacteria from diseased animals through skin lesions or mucous membranes or from inhalation of contaminated dust or aerosols. Inhalation of only a few organisms is sufficient to cause a significant

likelihood of infection. Laboratory infection is common, especially by inhalation of aerosols. Person-to-person transmission occurs very rarely, if ever. Many countries are now essentially free of animal brucellosis, owing to control and eradication programmes based on test-and-slaughter programmes and/or vaccination of cattle, sheep and goats.

Incubation period

The incubation period is highly variable, usually 5–60 days but can be as long as several months, with shorter periods expected after severe exposure.

Clinical features

Onset may be gradual or acute, with variable symptoms, consisting most frequently of undulating fever, chills, exhaustion, depression, back and leg pains, sweating, headaches and loss of appetite. Cutaneous and soft tissue manifestations may include contact lesions, rash and soft tissue abscesses. Splenomegaly and hepatomegaly with associated organ tenderness occur in some patients. Without treatment, patients usually recover within 2–3 months but there may be cycles of relapse and remission extending over years, accompanied by liver, spleen, bone, genito-urinary, central nervous system and cardiac complications. Fatality among untreated patients is approximately 2% or less, although somewhat higher for *B. melitensis*, and is usually from endocarditis. All age groups are susceptible, although children may be somewhat less so.

Laboratory diagnosis

Laboratory identification to the genus level, sufficient for treatment of patients, may be made in acute cases by microbiological and bio-chemical identification of the pathogen isolated from venous blood, bone marrow and other tissues. Serological tests, particularly serum agglutination and ELISA, are useful during acute infection, although antibody titres tend to be low in chronic or recurrent cases. Reliable identification of individual strains by PCR with genus-specific primers has been demonstrated. Biosafety Level 3 practices, equipment and facilities are recommended for manipulations involving clinical specimens and for all manipulations of cultures.

Medical management and public health measures

As there is no evidence of person-to-person transmission, patient isolation is not required. Standard precautions should be observed against infection from splashes or other direct contact with draining lesions and contaminated discharges or other contaminated materials. Exudates and dressings should be disinfected by autoclaving, incineration or treatment with standard disinfectants.

Prophylaxis and therapy

Veterinary vaccines protect animals to a substantial but not unlimited extent. No human vaccine is available. A 6-week course of oral doxycycline concomitant with either 6 weeks of oral rifampin or 3 weeks of intramuscular streptomycin is usually successful if begun early. Even prolonged antimicrobial treatment is only moderately effective in cases of chronic infection.

Selected references

Alton GG et al. *Techniques for the brucellosis laboratory*. Paris, France, INRA, 1988.

Bovine brucellosis. In: *The OIE manual of standards for diagnostic tests and vaccines*, 4th ed. Paris, France, Organisation mondiale de la Santé animale (OIE), 2000:328–345.

Caprine and ovine brucellosis. In: *The OIE manual of standards for diagnostic tests and vaccines*, 4th ed. Paris, France, Organisation mondiale de la Santé animale (OIE), 2000:475–489.

Crespo León F. *Brucelosis ovina y caprina*. [Ovine and caprine brucellosis.] Paris, France, Organisation mondiale de la Santé animale (OIE), 1994.

Joint FAO/WHO Expert Committee on Brucellosis. Sixth report. Geneva, World Health Organization, 1986 (WHO Technical Report Series, No. 740).

Nielsen K, Duncan JR, eds. *Animal brucellosis*. Boca Raton, FL, CRC Press, 1990.

Porcine brucellosis. In: *The OIE manual of standards for diagnostic tests and vaccines*, 4th ed. Paris, France, Organisation mondiale de la Santé animale (OIE), 2000:623–629.

Young EJ, Corbel MJ, eds. *Brucellosis: clinical and laboratory aspects*. Boca Raton, FL, CRC Press, 1989.

2.3 *Burkholderia mallei* / Glanders (A24.0)

Formerly classified as *Pseudomonas mallei*, the organisms are Gram-negative rods with rounded ends, 1.5–3.0 μm long and 0.3–0.6 μm wide, which often stain irregularly. They have no flagellae and are therefore non-motile. The organism is not highly resistant to environmental conditions.

Occurrence

The disease in humans is rare or absent in most parts of the world. Enzootic foci exist in Asia, some eastern Mediterranean countries and parts of the Middle East and central and south America.

Reservoirs

Primarily a disease of equines, including horses, donkeys and mules, for which it is highly contagious.

Mode of transmission

The disease is acquired by humans by direct contact with infected animals or contaminated animal tissue, the agent entering the body through skin lesions or through conjunctival, oral or nasal mucous membranes. The disease is not considered to be very contagious from person to person. It is likely to be infectious by aerosol exposure.

Incubation period

Although most cases appear 1–14 days after exposure, the disease can remain latent for many years.

Clinical features

Glanders infection can present in several forms, depending on the route of entry and the site of infection. Initial symptoms may include fever, malaise, myalgia and headache. Localized infection may become apparent a few days after exposure, with pus-forming ulcerations on the skin that may spread over most of the body, or as purulent ulcerations of the mucosa of the nose, trachea, pharynx and lungs. Pulmonary infection is associated with pneumonia, pulmonary abscesses and pleural effusion. Localized infection in the lobes of the lungs may be apparent in chest X-rays. Untreated bloodstream infections are usually fatal within a few days. Chronic infections are associated with multiple abscesses in the muscles of the arms and legs, or in the spleen or liver. Subclinical infections are sometimes detected at autopsy.

Laboratory diagnosis

Identification may be made by isolation of the microorganism from skin lesions, pus, sputum or blood, followed by direct fluorescent antibody staining or by PCR. Serological tests include complement fixation, agglutination tests and ELISA. Biosafety Level 2 practices, equipment and facilities are recommended for manipulations involving clinical specimens or experimentally infected laboratory rodents. Biosafety Level 3 practices, equipment and facilities are recommended for manipulations involving the concentration of cultures or activities with a high potential for aerosol production.

Medical management and public health measures

Standard precautions should be observed against infection from splashes or other direct contact with draining lesions, blood and contaminated discharges or other contaminated materials. Exudates and dressings should be disinfected by autoclaving, incineration or treatment with standard disinfectants.

Prophylaxis and therapy

No vaccine is available. Owing to the rareness of the disease, the medical literature regarding its therapy is sparse. Sulfadiazine and ceftazidime are recommended for therapeutic use. The organism is also sensitive to tetracyclines, ciprofloxacin, streptomycin, novobiocin, gentamicin, sulfonamides, or a combination of imipenem and doxycycline. There may be relapses even after prolonged antimicrobial therapy.

Selected references

Howe C, Miller WR. Human glanders: report of six cases. *Annals of Internal Medicine*, 1947, 26:93–115.

Jennings WE. Glanders. In: Hull TG, ed. *Diseases transmitted from animals to man*, 5th ed. Springfield, IL, Charles C. Thomas, 1963:264–292.

Kenny DJ et al. In vitro susceptibilities of *Burkholderia mallei* in comparison to those of other pathogenic *Burkholderia* spp. *Antimicrobial Agents and Chemotherapy*, 1999, 43:2773–2775.

Loeffler F. The etiology of glanders (in German). *Arbeiten aus dem Kaiserlichen Gesundheitsamte*, 1886, 1:141–198.

Neubauer H, Meyer H, Finke EJ. Human glanders. *Revue Internationale des Services de Santé des Forces Armées*, 1997, 70:258–265.

Popov SF et al. Capsule formation in the causative agent of glanders (in Russian). *Mikrobiolohichnyi zhurnal*, 1991, 53:90–92.

Robins GD. A study of chronic glanders in man. *Studies from the Royal Victoria Hospital*, 1906, 2:1–98.

Srinivasan A et al. Glanders in a military microbiologist. *New England Journal of Medicine*, 2001, 354:256–258.

van der Schaaf A. Malleus. In: Hoeden J, ed. *Zoonoses*. Amsterdam, Elsevier, 1964:184–193.

Woods DE et al. *Burkholderia thailandensis* E125 harbors a temperate bacteriophage specific for *Burkholderia mallei*. *Journal of Bacteriology*, 2002, 184:4003–4017.

2.4 *Burkholderia pseudomallei* /Melioidosis (A24)

Formerly classified as *Pseudomonas pseudomallei*, the organism is an aerobic, motile, Gram-negative rod 1.5 μm x 0.8 μm. The organism is not highly resistant to environmental conditions.

Occurrence

The disease is prevalent in South-East Asia, particularly in wet, rice-growing areas, and in northern Australia. A number of cases have also been reported from central and south America.

Reservoir

B. pseudomallei is found in soil and water in tropical and subtropical regions and infects many species of mammals, including marine mammals.

Mode of transmission

Humans become infected through skin lesions as a result of contact with contaminated soil or water. Infection can also occur by aspiration or ingestion of contaminated water or by inhalation of contaminated dust. Person-to-person transmission may occasionally occur but is rare.

Incubation period

The incubation period may range from a few days to years.

Clinical features

Clinical features resemble those of glanders and are highly variable. Cutaneous infection may give rise to subcutaneous infected nodules with acute lymphangitis and regional lymphadenitis, generally with fever. Inhalation or ingestion or haematogenous spread from cutaneous lesions may result in internal involvement, with chronically infected suppurating abscesses in lungs, liver, spleen, lymph nodes, bone or joints. Pulmonary involvement is associated with consolidation and necrotizing pneumonia, and may vary from mild to fulminant. The disease can resemble tuberculosis or typhoid fever. A fulminant septicaemia with shock may occur and is probably invariably fatal. Asymptomatic infection has been detected serologically and may cause disease long after exposure.

Laboratory diagnosis

Identification may be made by isolation of the organism from sputum or purulent exudates, followed by microbiological identification. Serological testing may be done by ELISA. Biosafety Level 2 practices, equipment and facilities are recommended for manipulations involving clinical specimens. Biosafety Level 3 practices, equipment and facilities are recommended for manipulations involving the concentration of cultures or activities with a high potential for aerosol production.

Medical management and public health measures

Standard precautions should be observed against infection from splashes or other direct contact with draining lesions, blood and contaminated discharges or other contaminated materials. Exudates and dressings should be disinfected by autoclaving, incineration or treatment with standard disinfectants.

Prophylaxis and therapy

No vaccine is available. Current recommendations for therapy of severe melioidosis include intravenous ceftazidime or imipenem for 10 days to 4 weeks, followed by maintenance therapy with oral amoxicillin–clavulanic acid or a combination of trimethoprim–sulfamethoxazole and doxycycline for 10–18 weeks.

Selected references

Chaowagul W et al. Melioidosis: a major cause of community-acquired septicemia in northeastern Thailand. *Journal of Infectious Diseases*, 1989, 159:890–899.

Dance DAB. Melioidosis. In: Guerrant RL, Walker DH, Weller PF, eds. *Tropical infectious diseases: principles, pathogens, and practice*. Philadelphia, PA, Churchill Livingstone, 1999:430–437.

Mays EE, Ricketts EA. Melioidosis: recrudescence associated with bronchogenic carcinoma twenty-six years following initial geographic exposure. *Chest*, 1975, 68:261–263.

Rajchanuvong A et al. A prospective comparison of co-amoxiclav and the combination of chloramphenicol, doxycycline, and co-trimoxazole for the oral maintenance treatment of melioidosis. *Transactions of the Royal Society of Tropical Medicine and Hygiene*, 1995, 89:546–549.

Sookpranee T et al. *Pseudomonas pseudomallei*, a common pathogen in Thailand that is resistant to the bactericidal effects of many antibiotics. *Antimicrobial Agents and Chemotherapy*, 1991, 35:484–489.

White NJ et al. Halving of mortality of severe melioidosis by ceftazidime. *Lancet*, 1989, ii:697–701.

Whitmore A. An account of a glanders-like disease occurring in Rangoon. *Journal of Hygiene*, 1913, 13:1–35.

Woods ML II et al. Neurological melioidosis: seven cases from the Northern Territory of Australia. *Clinical Infectious Diseases*, 1992, 15:163–169.

Wuthiekanun V et al. Value of throat swab in diagnosis of melioidosis. *Journal of Clinical Microbiology*, 2001, 39:3801–3802.

Yabuuchi E, Arakawa M. *Burkholderia pseudomallei* and melioidosis: be aware in temperate area. *Microbiology and Immunology*, 1993, 37:823–836.

2.5 *Francisella tularensis* /Tularaemia (A21)

The organism is a small, non-motile, Gram-negative, facultatively intracellular, aerobic coccobacillus, measuring 0.2 μm x 0.3–0.7 μm. Within the species, there are two predominant sub-species: *F. tularensis tularensis* or Type A is more virulent than *F. tularensis palaearctica* or Type B. The organism can survive for up to several weeks in the natural environment.

Occurrence

F. tularensis tularensis is found in North America, while *F. tularensis palaearctica* occurs in Asia, Europe and North America.

Reservoirs

Many wild animals, especially rabbits, hares, voles, muskrats and beavers, as well as some hard ticks. The disease has been reported in many other animals, including various rodents, birds, reptiles, amphibians and marine mammals. It is also found in soil and water.

Mode of transmission

Tularaemia is primarily a disease of a wide variety of wild mammals and birds. Humans become infected mainly through the bite of arthropods, particularly ticks and mosquitoes, and through the skin, conjunctival sac or oropharyngeal mucosa, by direct contact with infected animals or animal materials and by ingestion of contaminated food or water or inhalation of contaminated dust or aerosols. *F. tularensis* is easily transmitted by aerosols and inhalation of only a few organisms is likely to cause infection. Person-to-person transmission has not been documented.

Incubation period

The incubation period varies from 1 to approximately 14 days, averaging 3–5 days.

Clinical features

Clinical manifestations depend on the route of entry and the virulence of the agent. Infection through the skin or conjunctiva usually produces an ulceroglandular form, with an indolent ulcer at the site of entry and painful swelling of local lymph glands, which may suppurate. In some cases the site of entry is inconspicuous, there being only local lymph gland involvement. Infection resulting from ingestion is characterized by a painful pharyngitis and associated cervical lymphadenitis. Rarely, an intestinal form may develop with infection of the mesenteric nodes, and characterized by abdominal pain, diarrhoea and vomiting. Both forms are usually accompanied by an abrupt onset of fever, accompanied by chills, malaise and joint and muscle pain. Ulceroglandular tularaemia caused by virulent strains, if untreated, has a case-fatality rate of about 5% and lasts 2–4 weeks, with a convalescent period of up to 3 months.

Depending on the site in the respiratory system at which infection occurs, inhalational tularaemia may take the form of a primary pneumonia or of tracheitis and bronchitis. The initial manifestation, however, may be influenza-like without evident signs of respiratory involvement. Pleuropulmonary tularaemia with a virulent strain has a high case-fatality rate (40–60%) if untreated.

The organism may enter the bloodstream, causing systemic illness, often severe. Untreated sepsis with the more virulent Type A strain is often fatal. Systemic illness without apparent site of primary infection is commonly termed "typhoidal tularaemia".

Laboratory diagnosis

Direct microscopic examination of clinical specimens showing small, poorly staining Gram-negative bacteria may suggest the diagnosis, and be supported by direct fluorescent antibody staining. Other supportive tests include PCR and antigen-capture ELISA methods. Confirmation is obtained by culturing the organism in cysteine-rich media, such as cysteine-enriched broth, thioglycolate broth, or cysteine heart blood agar, and by detecting diagnostic antibody titres to *F. tularensis*. Confirmatory tests, however, do not provide rapid results, and treatment should not be delayed if the diagnosis is clinically suspected.

The organism is extremely infectious and poses a substantial risk of laboratory-acquired infection unless handled according to stringent safety guidelines. Biosafety Level 2 practices, equipment and facilities are recommended for routine handling of clinical specimens from humans or animals. Biosafety Level 3 practices, equipment and facilities, including the use of a negative pressure biosafety cabinet, are recommended for all manipulations of cultures and any procedures posing a risk of aerosolization, such as centrifugation.

Medical management and public health measures

There is no requirement for quarantine of patients or immunization of contacts. Standard precautions are indicated where there are open lesions and discharges from ulcers, including autoclaving, incineration or disinfection of discharges and contaminated materials.

Prophylaxis and therapy

Live attenuated vaccines applied intradermally have proved effective in preventing or attenuating infection by the cutaneous and inhalatory routes. Vaccines of this type have been used to reduce the risk of tularaemia in populations living in endemic regions of the former Soviet Union and, although not approved or available for general use in the USA, among at-risk employees at Fort Detrick, Maryland. At present, tularaemia vaccine supplies are available in the Russian Federation only, but the vaccine may be available outside the Russian Federation in the future, if necessary. Attempts to develop improved vaccines are under way in a number of countries.

For antimicrobial prophylaxis, oral administration of doxycycline or ciprofloxacin is recommended for a 14-day period following the last day of exposure. For therapy, streptomycin is the recommended antimicrobial of choice, and is administered parenterally at 15 mg/kg twice daily for 10 days, but not to exceed 2 g per day. Parenteral gentamicin, doxycycline or ciprofloxacin are recommended alternatives to streptomycin. Patients beginning treatment with parenteral doxycycline or ciprofloxacin can switch to oral antimicrobial administration when clinically indicated. Recommended duration of administration of gentamicin or ciprofloxacin for treatment of tularaemia is 10 days. Doxycycline, however, is bacteriostatic, and treatment should continue for 14–21 days to avoid relapse. Chloramphenicol has been used to treat tularaemia, but there is a higher rate of primary treatment failure and relapse with its use than with the antimicrobials noted above.

Selected references

Bell JF. Tularemia. In: Steele JH, ed. *CRC Handbook series in zoonoses, Vol 2.* Boca Raton, FL, CRC Press, 1980:161–193.

Cross JT, Penn RL. *Francisella tularensis* (tularemia). In: Mandell GL et al., eds. *Principles and practice of infectious diseases.* Philadelphia, PA, Churchill Livingstone, 2000:2393–2402.

Dennis DT. Tularemia as a biological weapon: medical and public health management. *Journal of the American Medical Association*, 2001, 285:2763–2773.

Enderlin G et al. Streptomycin and alternative agents for the treatment of tularemia: review of the literature. *Clinical Infectious Diseases*, 1994, 19(1):42–47.

Evans ME et al. Tularemia: a 30 year experience with 88 cases. *Medicine*, 1985, 64:251–269.

Feldman KA et al. Outbreak of primary pneumonic tularemia on Martha's Vineyard. *New England Journal of Medicine*, 2001, 345:1601–1606.

Grunow R et al. Detection of *Francisella tularensis* in biological specimens using a capture enzyme-linked immunosorbent assay, an immunochromatographic handheld assay, and a PCR. *Clinical and Diagnostic Laboratory Immunology*, 2000, 7:86–90.

Johansson A et al. Ciprofloxacin for treatment of tularemia. *Clinical Infectious Diseases*, 2001, 33:267–268.

Reintjes R et al. Tularemia investigation in Kosovo: case control and environmental studies. *Emerging Infectious Diseases*, 2002, 8:69–73.

Saslaw S et al. Tularemia vaccine study. II. Respiratory challenge. *Archives of Internal Medicine*, 1961, 107:134–146.

Sawyer WD et al. Antibiotic prophylaxis and therapy of airborne tularemia. *Bacteriological Reviews*, 1966, 30:542–548.

Syrjälä H et al. Airborne transmission of tularemia in farmers. *Scandinavian Journal of Infectious Diseases*, 1985, 17:371–375.

Tärnvik A. Nature of protective immunity to *Francisella tularensis*. *Review of Infectious Diseases*, 1989, 11:440–451.

2.6   *Yersinia pestis* / Plague (A20)

Yersinia pestis is a Gram-negative non-motile, non-spore-forming coccobacillus measuring approximately 1.5 μm x 0.75 μm, capable of both aerobic and anaerobic growth. The pathogen can remain viable for days in water or moist soil and can resist drying if protected by mucus or other substances but is killed by a few hours of direct exposure to sunlight.

Occurrence

During the 1990s there were human outbreaks in Africa, Asia, and south America and sporadic cases in many countries, including the USA. Known historically as the Black Death and still a serious problem, it is limited to sporadic cases where adequate surveillance and modern public health measures are practised.

Reservoirs

The pathogen is present in animal reservoirs, particularly in wild rodents, in endemic foci worldwide, with the exception of Australia.

Mode of transmission

Plague is transmitted between rodents and to other animals via fleas, consumption of infected animal tissues or, possibly, contaminated soil or respiratory droplet exposures. In endemic rural areas, plague typically occurs sporadically among persons who come in contact with wild rodent hosts of *Y. pestis* and their fleas. Outbreaks affecting large numbers of people can occur in cities when plague infects populations of urban rodents, particularly the black rat, *Rattus rattus*, and the brown rat, *Rattus norvegicus*. The most common form of the disease in humans, bubonic plague, is spread mainly by the bite of fleas regurgitating plague bacteria from infected rodents or by entry of the pathogen from infected fleas through a skin lesion. If the lungs become infected, as may occasionally occur in patients with the bubonic form, a much more virulent form, pneumonic plague, ensues and can be transmitted directly from person to person by droplet infection.

Incubation period

The incubation period is 2–6 days in bubonic plague and somewhat less for the pneumonic form.

Clinical features

Initial symptoms may be nonspecific, with sudden onset of fever, chills, malaise, myalgia, nausea, sore throat and headache. Cases acquired by aerosol inhalation would probably present as primary pneumonia, possibly accompanied by bloody cough. Infection spreads from the inoculation site via the lymphatics to regional nodes, which become swollen and painful (buboes). In a minority of cases, the pathogen enters the bloodstream giving rise to plague septicaemia. Haematogenous spread of the pathogen to the lungs causes the pneumonic form of the disease, which then can spread directly from person to person by droplet infection. As the disease progresses, patients experience shock, delirium and coma. Untreated bubonic plague has a case-fatality rate as high as 60%, while untreated pneumonic plague is almost always fatal. Less common forms are plague meningitis and plague pharyngitis.

Laboratory diagnosis

Strong suggestive evidence of Y. *pestis* in sputum, blood or material aspirated from a bubo is provided by observation of Gram-negative ovoidal bacilli that stain preferentially at their ends with Giemsa or Wayson's stains, although such bipolar distribution of stain may not always be clearly evident or specific. The bacillus may be identified by direct fluorescent antibody stain for the Y. *pestis* capsular antigen, by lysis by specific bacteriophage and by PCR. Various serological methods are also available. Biosafety Level 2 practices, equipment and facilities are recommended for all activities involving infective clinical materials and cultures. Biosafety Level 3 should be used for activities in which there is a high potential for aerosol or air droplet production or for work with antimicrobial-resistant strains and infected fleas.

Medical management and public health measures

Emphasis must be placed on preventing epidemic spread. For patients with pneumonic plague, strict precautions against airborne droplet spread are essential, including patient isolation and wearing of surgical masks by patients and caregivers. Patients with confirmed pneumonic plague may be placed together in shared rooms if private rooms are not available. For patients with any type of plague, standard precautions must be taken against contamination from discharges and contaminated articles, including hand washing and the wearing of gloves, gowns and face protection. If indicated, flea control measures should be instituted.

Prophylaxis and therapy

Plague vaccines are available worldwide but are not recommended for immediate protection in outbreak situations. Vaccination is recommended only for high-risk groups, e.g. health workers and laboratory personnel who are constantly exposed to the risk of contamination.

Preventive vaccination with killed or live attenuated Y. *pestis* is moderately effective against bubonic but not against pneumonic plague. With killed vaccine, protection is relatively short-lived (3–12 months) and periodic revaccination is necessary. Vaccination is of little use during a plague outbreak, as at least a month is needed for immunity to build up and recommendations for administration of killed bacteria vaccines include an initial injection and two booster injections over a period of 6 months. As with various other pathogens, massive infection can overcome vaccine-conferred immunity. Persons in close contact with pneumonic plague patients or who are likely to have been exposed to infected fleas, have had direct contact with body fluids or tissues of an infected mammal, or for any other reason are suspected to have been exposed to the pathogen should receive antimicrobial prophylaxis for a week after the last suspected exposure. Doxycycline and ciprofloxacin are recommended for such use.

Antimicrobial therapy is effective if begun early in the disease and continued for at least 3 days after body temperature returns to normal. Streptomycin is the historical drug of choice but is not immediately available everywhere. Gentamicin is considered to be an acceptable alternative to streptomycin, based on in vitro and animal experiments, and on limited clinical observations in humans. Tetracyclines are effective against plague, and are widely used for treatment and prophylaxis. Doxycycline, administered twice daily, is preferred for oral treatment because of its ready gastrointestinal absorption. Chloramphenicol has been used to treat various forms of plague, including plague pneumonia, and is recommended for treatment of plague meningitis because of its ability to cross the blood–brain barrier. Fluoroquinolones have demonstrated efficacy in treating plague in animal experiments. Ciprofloxacin was observed to be at least as efficacious as aminoglycosides and tetracyclines in studies of mice with pneumonic plague. In vitro studies show activity of several fluoro-quinolones to be equivalent to or greater than that of the aminoglyco-sides or tetracyclines. Several sulfonamides (sulfathiazole, sulfadiazine, sulfamerazine and trimethoprim–sulfamethoxazole) have been used successfully for the treatment and prophylaxis of plague. Data indicate, however, that sulfonamides are less effective than streptomycin or tetracycline, particularly for pneumonic plague. Sulfisoxazole should not be used because of its rapid renal excretion. Penicillins, macrolides and cefalosporins are thought not to be clinically efficacious and are not recommended for treatment of plague. Multidrug resistance imparted by a transferable plasmid has been reported in a single clinical isolate, as has plasmid-mediated streptomycin resistance. Antimicrobial-resistant strains have been developed in the laboratory.

Selected references

Chu MC. *Laboratory manual of plague diagnostic tests.* Atlanta, GA, Centers for Disease Control and Prevention, 2000.

Dennis DT et al. *Plague manual: epidemiology, distribution, surveillance and control.* Geneva, World Health Organization, 1999 (document WHO/CDS/CSR/EDC/99.2).

Galimand M et al. Multidrug resistance in *Yersinia pestis* mediated by a transferable plasmid. *New England Journal of Medicine*, 1997, 337:677–681.

Inglesby TV et al. for the Working Group on Civilian Biodefense. Plague as a biological weapon: medical and public health management. *Journal of the American Medical Association*, 2000, 283:2281–2290.

Titball RW et al. In: Plotkin S, Mortimer EA, eds. *Vaccines*, 3rd ed. Philadelphia, PA, WB Saunders, 1999:734–742.

2.1   *Coxiella burnetii* / Q Fever (A78)

Coxiella burnetii is a pleomorphic, Gram-negative obligate intracellular coccobacillus measuring approximately 0.2 μm x 0.7 μm. The spore-like form, produced in infected host cells, is resistant to drying and environmental influences and can survive for months in water and food. It is extremely infective to humans.

Occurrence

Worldwide.

Reservoirs

The zoonotic pathogen exists in a wide range of animal hosts, including domesticated livestock (especially cattle, sheep, goats) cats, dogs, rodents, baboons and wild birds. The enzootic cycle includes numerous species of ixodid and argasid ticks. Arthropod vectors, however, do not play a significant role in transmission to humans.

Mode of transmission

Transmission to humans occurs primarily by inhalation of dust, droplets or aerosols from parturient fluids and excreta of infected livestock. Contaminated droplets and dust may also infect the conjunctivae and abraded skin. Inhalation of only a few organisms is sufficient to cause infection. Contaminated aerosols released to the atmosphere may cause infection at distances up to several kilometres from their source. Sporadic human infections may also result from ingestion of unpasteurized dairy products. High-temperature pasteurization is sufficient to kill the organism. Person-to-person transmission has been reported but is rare.

Incubation period
The incubation period is usually 18–21 days, but can be less if large doses of the organism are inhaled.

Clinical features
The onset may be sudden, with chills, fever, sweating, headache, loss of appetite, malaise, and muscle and chest pains. There may also be nausea, vomiting and diarrhoea. In severe cases the disease progresses to extreme stiffness of the neck and back, disorientation and pneumonia. The fatality rate is usually less than 1%, although somewhat higher rates have been reported in some outbreaks. Weakness and fever may continue for months. Long-term complications are uncommon but may include endocarditis. Asymptomatic infections routinely occur and may be revealed by serology.

Laboratory diagnosis
Isolation and microbiological identification of the organism from blood or other clinical materials is a valid diagnostic test but is hazardous to personnel. Specific and relatively rapid identification of the organism in blood or paraffin-embedded tissue may be accomplished by PCR assays. Serological diagnosis may be performed by complement fixation, indirect immunofluorescent antibody test or ELISA. Biosafety Level 2 practices, equipment and facilities are recommended for activities not involving propagation of the pathogen and involving only limited manipulation of infected materials, such as microscopic and serological examinations. Biosafety Level 3 is recommended for activities involving the handling of infected human or animal tissues or isolation of the pathogen.

Medical management and public health measures
Patient isolation is not required. Patient materials and contaminated articles should be autoclaved, incinerated or disinfected with solutions containing hypochlorite, peroxide, 70% ethanol, phenol or a quatenary ammonium compound.

Prophylaxis and therapy
A formalin-inactivated vaccine, commercially available in Australia, has been developed for laboratory workers and others at high risk.

Tetracyclines, particularly doxycycline, are effective if given early and may abort the infection if administered before symptoms appear.

Selected references

Ackland JA, Worswick DA, Marmion BP. Vaccine prophylaxis of Q fever: a follow-up study of the efficacy of Q-Vax (CSL) 1985–1990. *Medical Journal of Australia*, 1994, 160:704–708.

Dasch GA, E Weiss E. The rickettsiae. In: Collier L, Balows A, Sussman M, eds. *Topley and Wilson's microbiology and microbial infections, Vol. 2*, 9th ed. New York, Oxford University Press, 1998: 853–876.

Dupont HT et al. Epidemiologic features and clinical presentation of acute Q fever in hospitalized patients: 323 French cases. *American Journal of Medicine*, 1992, 93:427–434.

Dupuis G, Petite J, Vouilloz M. An important outbreak of human Q fever in a Swiss alpine valley. *International Journal of Epidemiology*, 1987, 16:282–287.

Fiset P, Woodward TE. Q fever. In: Evans AS, Brachman PS, eds. *Bacterial infections of humans: epidemiology and control*, 3rd ed. New York, NY, Plenum Medical Book Company, 1998:583–595.

Fournier PE, Marrie TJ, Raoult D. Diagnosis of Q fever. *Journal of Clinical Microbiology*, 1998, 36:1823–1834.

Levy PY et al. Comparison of different antibiotic regimens for therapy of 32 cases of Q fever endocarditis. *Antimicrobial Agents and Chemotherapy*, 1991, 35:533–537.

Marrie TJ, Raoult D. Coxiella. In: Murray PR et al., eds. *Manual of clinical microbiology*, 7th ed. Washington, DC, ASM Press, 1999:815–820.

Maurin M, Raoult D. Q fever. *Clinical Microbiology Reviews*, 1999, 12:518–553.

Peter O et al. Evaluation of the complement fixation and indirect immunofluorescence tests in the early diagnosis of primary Q fever. *European Journal of Clinical Microbiology*, 1985, 4:394–396.

Raoult D. Treatment of Q fever. *Antimicrobial Agents and Chemotherapy*, 1993, 37:1733–1736.

Raoult D et al. Treatment of Q fever endocarditis: comparison of 2 regimens containing doxycycline and ciprofloxacin or hydroxychloroquine. *Archives of Internal Medicine*, 1999, 159:167–173.

Raoult D et al. Diagnosis of endocarditis in acute Q fever by immunofluorescence serology. *Acta Virologica*, 1988, 32:70–74.

Raoult DH et al. Q fever 1985–1998: clinical and epidemiologic features of 1383 infections. *Medicine*, 2000, 79:109–123.

Scott GH, Williams JC. Susceptibility of *Coxiella burnetii* to chemical disinfectants. *Annals of the New York Academy of Sciences*, 1990, 590:291–296.

2.8 *Rickettsia prowazekii* / Epidemic typhus (A75)

Rickettsia prowazeki is a small obligately intracellular Gram-negative bacterium measuring approximately 0.4 μm x 1.5 μm.

Occurrence
The great epidemics of typhus that plagued humans since ancient times ceased shortly after the Second World War with the widespread application of insect control procedures and other hygienic measures. Endemic foci exist in certain regions where louse infestation is common, including parts of Mexico, central and south America, central and east Africa and various regions of Asia. Epidemics may reappear during times of war or famine.

Reservoirs
Humans, flying squirrels (United States only).

Vectors
Transmitted from person to person by lice; fleas may play a role in transmission of flying-squirrel-associated typhus.

Mode of transmission
The disease is transmitted particularly by the body louse *Pediculus humanus corporis*. Infection of humans occurs by contact of mucous membranes or abraded skin with the faeces of lice or fleas that have bitten a person with acute typhus fever. Infection probably also occurs by inhalation of dust contaminated with infected insect faeces or body parts. Patients are infective for lice during the febrile phase of the disease and perhaps for 2–3 days afterwards. Direct person-to-person transmission does not occur.

Incubation period
The incubation period is usually 1–2 weeks.

Clinical features

The disease has a variable onset, often sudden, with chills, body aches, fever, headache and weakness. During the first week a macular rash appears, initially on the upper trunk, and then spreads. The symptoms grow progressively more severe, with the critical period in the second or third week. Stupor and coma may be interrupted by attacks of delirium. Recovery is marked by abrupt cessation of fever, usually in the second febrile week, but, if untreated, mortality ranges from 10% to 40%, increasing with age. The disease may reappear years after the initial infection, usually in a milder form known as Brill-Zinsser disease.

Laboratory diagnosis

Specific antibodies appear about 2 weeks after infection, when diagnosis may be obtained by immunofluorescent antibody test. More rapid diagnosis may be obtained by immunohistological demonstration of the organism or by PCR, using blood collected during the acute phase of the disease. Biosafety Level 2 practices, equipment and facilities are recommended for activities not involving propagation of the pathogen, such as microscopic and serological examinations. Biosafety Level 3 is recommended for activities involving the handling of infected human or animal tissues.

Medical management and public health measures

Isolation of patients is not necessary. If lice are present, insecticide should be applied to clothing, bedding, living quarters and patient contacts in order to prevent spread of the disease. Louse-infested individuals likely to have been exposed to typhus fever should be deloused and placed under quarantine for 15 days after insecticide application and close patient contacts should be kept under fever watch for 2 weeks. Reapplication of insecticide may be needed as previously laid eggs hatch.

Prophylaxis and treatment

Antimicrobials including doxycycline are effective in prophylaxis and treatment and should be given if typhus is suspected.

Selected references

Duma RJ et al. Epidemic typhus in the United States associated with flying squirrels. *Journal of the American Medical Association*, 1981, 245:2318–2323.

Eremeeva ME, Dasch GA. Rickettsia and Orientia. In Sussman M, ed. *Molecular medical microbiology*. London, Academic Press, 2001:2175–2216.

Lutwick LI. Brill-Zinsser disease. *Lancet*, 2001, 357:1198–1200.

Perine PL et al. A clinico-epidemiological study of epidemic typhus in Africa. *Clinical Infectious Diseases*, 1992, 14:1149–1158.

Raoult D, Roux V. The body louse as a vector of reemerging human diseases. *Clinical Infectious Diseases*, 1999, 29:888–911.

Raoult D et al. Survey of three bacterial louse-associated diseases among rural Andean communities in Peru: prevalence of epidemic typhus, trench fever, and relapsing fever. *Clinical Infectious Diseases*, 1999, 29:434–436.

Raoult D et al. Jail fever (epidemic typhus) outbreak in Burundi. *Emerging Infectious Diseases*, 1997, 3:357–359.

Tarasevich I, Rydkina E, Raoult D. Outbreak of epidemic typhus in Russia. *Lancet*, 1998, 352:1151.

Wisseman CL Jr. Concepts of louse-borne typhus control in developing countries: the use of the living attenuated E strain typhus vaccine in epidemic and endemic situations. In: Kohn A, Klingberg MA, eds. *Immunity in viral and rickettsial diseases*. New York, NY, Plenum, 1972:97–130.

3. Fungi

3.1 *Coccidioides immitis* and *Coccidioides posadasii* / Coccidioidomycosis (B38)

These agents are species of dimorphic fungi that propagate as mycelial moulds in soil and as spherules bearing endospores in mammalian tissue. Mature hyphal filaments of the mycelial form develop arthroconidia which detach and may then become airborne. Arthroconidia are lightweight, barrel-shaped cells measuring approximately $3\,\mu m \times 6\,\mu m$ that are stable to drying.

Occurrence

The fungus occurs in soil, especially in arid and semi-arid regions of south-western United States, northern Mexico and focal areas of central and south America. A substantial percentage of cattle, swine, sheep, dogs and humans in endemic regions have had asymptomatic infections, as revealed by skin testing.

Reservoirs

Soil, in particular arid regions of the western hemisphere.

Mode of transmission

Infection usually takes place by inhalation of arthroconidia. A dust storm originating in an endemic region of California in 1977 caused an elevated incidence of the disease over an area of thousands of square kilometres. Mammals, including humans, inhaling even a single arthroconidium may become infected. Once within the host, arthroconidia undergo a morphological change into spherules. These are round, segmented structures of 30–60 μm. Within these are hundreds of 2–3 μm ovoidal endospores which themselves may develop into endospore-bearing spherules, spreading the disease throughout the body.

Incubation period

The incubation period is usually 1–3 weeks.

Clinical features

In endemic areas, the majority of infections are asymptomatic, but may be detected by skin tests. The percentage of persons residing in endemic areas found to react positively to skin tests ranges from 5% to more that 50%.

For those developing clinical disease, the initial symptoms resemble those of other upper respiratory infections, and include cough, fever, night sweats, chills, chest pain, sputum production and headache. Less often, there may also be various skin manifestations, including erythema nodosum or erythema multiforme with or without joint aches. The initial form of the disease usually resolves without therapy within several weeks, although occasional patients have a more protracted convalescence.

Persistent symptomatic coccidioidomycosis of the lungs occurs in a small percentage of patients and is more frequent in patients with diabetes mellitus. It is characterized by progressive destructive pulmonary disease with continuous low-grade fever, weakness, cough with sputum production, dyspnoea, haemoptysis and pleuritic chest pain. Extrapulmonary dissemination is seen in approximately 1% of all infected persons, and usually becomes evident weeks to months after primary disease. It is characterized by involvement of the skin, subcutaneous tissues, bones, joints and the central nervous system Patients with AIDS or other deficiencies in cellular immunity are especially susceptible to these complications. Without treatment, the disseminated form, which may follow a rapid or a prolonged course, has a mortality rate of more than 50%, approaching 100% if meningitis develops.

Recovery from clinical disease appears usually to be accompanied by lifelong immunity, and most individuals with asymptomatic infection also develop lifelong immunity.

Laboratory diagnosis

Spherules and endospores may be visualized with calcafluor, Papanicolaou, haematoxylin–eosin and Gomori methenamine staining in sputum samples, pus and biopsy tissue. The organism is rarely identified in cerebrospinal fluid. Direct microscopic examination of sputum samples placed in 10% potassium hydroxide reveals spherules and endospores in fewer than 30% of cases and may be complicated by the presence of spherule-like artefacts, such as pollen. Skin tests for hypersensitivity to preparations derived from the fungal mycelia (with coccidioidin) or from spherules (with spherulin) have been useful for epidemiological studies but may give false-negative results in individual cases, especially if the disease is advanced. Skin testing reagents are not currently commercially available.

Medical management and public health measures

As the disease is not contagious, quarantine and patient isolation are not indicated. As the arthroconidia easily become airborne and are highly infective, manipulation of clinical specimens and sporulating cultures should be conducted under Biosafety Level 3 conditions. Contaminated specimens and materials may be sterilized by autoclaving or by treatment with iodine or glutaraldehyde-based disinfectants.

Prophylaxis and therapy

No vaccine against coccidioidomycosis is available at the present time. Recombinant coccidioidal antigens have been identified as protective in experimental infections and efforts are under way to develop them as vaccine candidates for clinical studies. For serious or persistent cases, prolonged therapy with amphotericin B or oral azole antifungal agents (ketoconazole, fluconazole, itraconazole) is moderately effective. Lifelong administration of fluconazole is recommended for coccidioidal meningitis.

Selected references

Barnato AE, Sanders GD, Owens DK. Cost-effectiveness of a potential vaccine for Coccidioides immitis. *Emerging Infectious Diseases*, 2001, 7:797–806.

Blair JE, Logan JL. Coccidioidomycosis in solid organ transplantation. *Clinical Infectious Diseases*, 2001, 33:1536–1544.

Cairns L et al. Outbreak of coccidioidomycosis in Washington State residents returning from Mexico. *Clinical Infectious Diseases*, 2000, 30:61–64.

Desai SA et al. Coccidioidomycosis in non-endemic areas: a case series. *Respiratory Medicine*, 2001, 95:305–309.

Dixon DM. *Coccidioides immitis* as a Select Agent of bioterrorism. *Journal of Applied Microbiology*, 2001, 91:602–605.

Fisher MC et al. From the cover: biogeographic range expansion into South America by *Coccidioides immitis* mirrors New World patterns of human migration. *Proceedings of the National Academy of Sciences of the United States of America*, 2001, 98:4558–4562.

Fisher MC et al. Molecular and phenotypic description of *Coccidioides posadasii* sp nov., previously recognized as the non-California population of *Coccidioides immitis*. *Mycologia*, 2002, 94:73–84.

Galgiani JN et al. Comparison of oral fluconazole and itraconazole for progressive, nonmeningeal coccidioidomycosis. A randomized, double-blind trial. Mycoses Study Group. *Annals of Internal Medicine*, 2000, 133:676–686.

Galgiani JN et al. Practice guidelines for the treatment of coccidioidomycosis. *Clinical Infectious Diseases*, 2000, 30:658–661.

Pappagianis D. Epidemiology of coccidioidomycosis. *Current Topics in Medical Mycology*, 1988, 2:199–238.

Pappagianis D. Seeking a vaccine against *Coccidioides immitis* and serologic studies: expectations and realities. *Fungal Genetics and Biology*, 2001, 32:1–9.

Pappagianis D, Zimmer BL. Serology of coccidioidomycosis. *Clinical Microbiology Reviews*, 1990, 3:247–268

Rosenstein NE et al. Risk factors for severe pulmonary and disseminated coccidioidomycosis: Kern County, California, 1995–1996. *Clinical Infectious Diseases*, 2001, 32:708–715.

4. Viruses

4.1 Venezuelan equine encephalitis (A92.2)

The agent is a member of the genus *Alphavirus* of the family Togaviridae. The virion is about 70 nm in diameter, consisting of a positive single-stranded RNA enclosed in an icosahedral capsid, surrounded by a lipid bilayer membrane in which surface glycoproteins are embedded. Subtypes IAB and IC are pathogenic for equines and are responsible for major outbreaks in humans. Other variants do not normally cause encephalitis in equids and, although sometimes encountered in humans, have not been isolated from major outbreaks.

Occurrence

Epidemics were first registered in the 1930s in the northern part of south America and then spread to central America. Sizeable epidemics were registered in Mexico in 1969, in Texas in 1971, and in Venezuela in 1995. The disease is endemic in central and northern parts of south America. Enzootic Venezuelan equine encephalitis (VEE) virus is endemic in Mexico and Florida. The Florida virus is Everglades virus, a distinct species.

Reservoirs

The virus is maintained in a rodent–mosquito–rodent cycle. During major outbreaks affecting humans, the disease is transmitted in a cycle involving mosquito vectors and horses or other equines as hosts. For this reason, natural outbreaks are normally preceded by equine epizootics. Humans also may develop sufficient viraemia to serve as hosts in human–mosquito–human cycles. Epidemic and non-epidemic strains may be distinguished antigenically.

Mode of transmission

Humans become infected from the bite of infected mosquitoes. The major species of mosquito that transmit epidemic VEE are *Psorophora confinnis, Aedes sollicitans, Aedes taeniorhynchus* (recently revised to *Ochlerotatus taeniorhynchus)* and *Deinocerites pseudes*. There is no evidence of direct person-to-person transmission or of direct transmission from horses to humans. Although natural aerogenic transmission is not documented in humans, primary aerosol infection in laboratories is well known and inhalation of only a few infective organisms is sufficient to cause a significant likelihood of infection. The VEE virus can initiate infection via the nasal mucosa and the olfactory epithelium of the upper respiratory tract. Virus-containing airborne droplets too large to penetrate more deeply into the respiratory system can therefore constitute a hazard.

Incubation period

The incubation period in natural or aerogenic infection is usually 1–6 days.

Clinical features

Clinical manifestations of the naturally occurring disease are influenza-like, with abrupt onset of severe headache, high fever, chills, myalgia in the legs and lumbosacral area and retroorbital pain. There may also be photophobia, sore throat, nausea, diarrhoea and vomiting. Conjunctival and pharyngeal congestion are the only external signs. Most infections are fairly mild, with symptoms usually lasting 3–5 days. The overall case-fatality rate in the 1962–1963 epidemic in Venezuela, among some 30 000 cases, was approximately 0.6%. In some patients there is a second wave of fever and, particularly in children, CNS involvement ranging from somnolence and disorientation to personality change, convulsions, paralysis and death.

The initial symptoms of respiratory infection are like those of insect-borne infection but CNS involvement appears to be more frequent.

Laboratory diagnosis

The disease exhibits leukopenia during a period usually limited to 1–3 days after onset. During this time, the virus may be sampled from serum or nasopharyngeal swabs and propagated in cell culture or in newborn mice. A variety of serological tests are applicable, including specific IgM ELISA, haemagglutination inhibition, immunofluorescence and complement fixation. PCR has been successfully used to distinguish strains. It may be applied to serum and cerebrospinal fluid without prior propagation of the pathogen. Neutralizing antibodies first appear in convalescent sera from the fifth day up to 2 weeks after onset of symptoms.

Biosafety Level 3 practices, equipment and facilities are recommended for activities using infective clinical materials.

Medical management and public health measures
Persons caring for infected patients should wear gloves, caps, gowns and surgical masks. Infective virus may be present in fresh or dried blood, exudates, cerebrospinal fluid and urine. Such materials should be decontaminated by autoclaving or by chemical disinfection, as with hypochlorite or chloramine. If mosquito vectors are present, patients should be kept in screened or insecticide-treated rooms to prevent mosquito transmission to healthy persons and general mosquito control measures should be instituted.

Prophylaxis and treatment
Attenuated cell-culture propagated live vaccine TC-83, produced but not licensed in the USA, is moderately effective against both natural infection and aerosol challenge but is somewhat reactogenic and fails to induce a minimum neutralizing antibody response in approximately one-fifth of persons receiving it, presumably leaving them unprotected. Two other attenuated live virus vaccines, strains 15 and 230, reported to offer good protection against aerosol challenge, were developed in the Russian Federation. An inactivated vaccine designated C-84, prepared by formalin-inactivation of the TC-83 strain, is currently used to immunize TC-83 non-responders and as a booster for individuals who have declining titres after TC-83 vaccination.

Selected references

Oberste MS et al. Association of Venezuelan equine encephalitis virus subtype IE with two equine epizootics in Mexico. *American Journal of Tropical Medicine and Hygiene*, 1998, 59:100–107.

Rivas F et al. Epidemic Venezuelan equine encephalitis in La Guajira, Colombia, 1995. *Journal of Infectious Diseases*, 1997, 175:828–832.

Rodríguez G, Boshell J. Encefalitis equina Venezolana. [Venezuelan equine encephalitis.] *Biomédica* (Bogota), 1995, 15:172–182.

Tsai TF, Monath TP, Weaver SC. Alphaviruses. In: Richman DD, Whitley RJ, Hayden FG, eds. *Clinical virology*. New York, Churchill Livingstone, 2001:1217–1255.

Walton TE, Grayson MA. Venezuelan equine encephalomyelitis. In: Monath TP, ed. *The arboviruses: epidemiology and ecology, Vol. IV*. Boca Raton, FL, CRC Press, 1988:203–231.

Weaver SC. 2001. Venezuelan equine encephalitis. In: Service MW, ed. *Encyclopedia of arthropod-transmitted infections of man and domesticated animals*. Wallingford, CABI Publishing, 2001:539–464.

Weaver SC et al. Re-emergence of epidemic Venezuelan equine encephalomyelitis in South America. *Lancet*, 1996, 348:436–440.

4.2   Variola virus/Smallpox (B03)

Variola virus is a member of the genus *Orthopoxvirus*, subfamily Chordopoxvirinae of the family Poxviridae. Other members of the genus include *Cowpox virus*, *Camelpox virus*, *Ectromelia virus*, *Vaccinia virus* and *Monkeypox virus*. Since the eradication of variola, the monkeypox virus is regarded as the cause of the most serious poxvirus infections in humans. The vaccinia virus, the best studied poxvirus, measures 370 nm x 270 nm and contains a double-stranded DNA molecule of about 190 000 nucleotide pairs, one of the largest viral genomes known, putatively coding for some 200 different proteins. Variola virus has a slightly smaller genome and the size of the virions has not been determined accurately. There are at least two epidemiological strains of variola virus, the more virulent designated variola major and the milder variola minor or alastrim.

Reservoir

The only known host of the virus was humans, facilitating the worldwide eradication campaign conducted by WHO. The last naturally acquired case occurred in Somalia in 1977 and there was a laboratory-acquired case in England in 1978. The global eradication of smallpox was certified by the World Health Assembly in 1980.

Pending its possible ultimate destruction, all stocks and work with variola virus are authorized only in maximum containment Biosafety

Level 4 laboratories at the CDC in Atlanta, GA, USA, and at VECTOR, Koltsovo, Novosibirsk Region, Russian Federation.

Mode of transmission

The most frequent mode of transmission is by person-to-person spread from deposit of droplets of saliva or nasal secretion from infected persons onto the oropharyngea. Transmission is mainly by direct face-to-face contact via infective saliva deposited onto the oropharyngeal, nasal or respiratory mucosa of a susceptible person. The virus may also be conveyed to the nose or oropharynx by contaminated fingers or other objects contaminated with infective saliva or nasal exudate. Contaminated clothes, bedding or clothing and other fomites may also present a risk of infection.

Incubation period

The first clinical symptoms appear between 7 and 19 days after exposure, commonly 10–14, with rash appearing 2–5 days afterwards.

Clinical features

Onset is sudden, with a 2–4-day prodromal period with influenza-like symptoms including fever, malaise, headache, prostration, severe back pain, and, less often, abdominal pain and vomiting. Fever may then drop and a maculopapular rash appears, first on the oral mucosa, face, hands and forearms and then after a few days progressing to the trunk. Such centrifugal distribution of lesions is an important diagnostic feature. Lesions progress from macules to papules and to pustular vesicles and all lesions in a given area progress together through these stages. From 8 to 14 days after onset, the pustules form scabs which fall off after 3–4 weeks and leave depressed depigmented scars upon healing.

Variola major and variola minor are characterized by similar lesions but variola minor is accompanied by milder symptoms and a case-fatality rate of less than 1%, while the fatality rate of variola major is 20–40%.

Variola is sometimes confused with chickenpox, caused by the *varicella-zoster virus* (human(alpha)herpesvirus3), a member of the family Herpesviridae. Chickenpox is a worldwide infection, especially of children, that is seldom lethal. It is distinguished from variola by its much more superficial lesions, their presence more on the trunk than on the face and extremities and by the development of successive crops of lesions in the same area.

There are two rare forms of smallpox, haemorrhagic and malignant. In the former, invariably fatal in both vaccinated and nonvaccinated patients, the rash is accompanied by haemorrhage into the mucous membranes and the skin. Malignant smallpox is characterized by lesions that do not develop to the pustular stage but remain soft and flat. It is almost invariably fatal for nonvaccinated patients and often fatal even for vaccinated ones.

Laboratory diagnosis

Confirmation of clinical diagnosis may be accomplished by immuno-fluorescent microscopy or negative stain electronmicroscopic observation of the virus. Definitive confirmation and discrimination of variola major from other pox viruses may be accomplished by sequencing of amplicons from PCR with viral DNA extracted from clinical specimens. If virus-containing specimens are not available, anti-smallpox antibodies may be detected in serum by various tests, including virus neutralization, haemagglutination inhibition, Western blot, ELISA or complement fixation. Scabs, vesicular or pustular fluids and other specimens for diagnosis should be collected only by vaccinated persons. So long as there is no recurrence of smallpox, laboratory manipulations with infective materials must be done in maximum containment facilities at Biosafety Level 4, authorized only at the two WHO-designated laboratories in the USA and the Russian Federation.

Medical management and public health measures

Emphasis must be placed on preventing epidemic spread. It should be kept in mind that smallpox patients are not infectious during the incubation stage of the disease but become so from the onset of rash and remain so until all scabs have detached (approximately 3 weeks). Patients are most infectious during the first week of rash, when lesions in the mouth and pharynx release large amounts of virus into the saliva and nasal exudate. As scabs form, patients become less infectious. Immunity develops rapidly after vaccination against smallpox, so that even post-exposure vaccination can prevent or ameliorate the disease so long as it is done within approximately 4 days after exposure and before rash appears.

Patients diagnosed with smallpox should be physically isolated and all persons who have or will come into close contact with them should be vaccinated. As hospitals have proved to be major sites of epidemic magnification during smallpox outbreaks, patient isolation preferably at home or at dedicated facilities with strict limitation of contacts to the essential minimum is advisable. Isolation at home also reduces the risk of infecting persons incorrectly diagnosed with smallpox during an outbreak. Patients who developed rash before their isolation should be asked to recount all recent contacts and, if feasible, these should either be vaccinated or placed on daily fever watch for at least 2 weeks after contact and isolated if fever appears. All specimen collectors, caregivers, attendants, family members and others coming into close contact with patients should be vaccinated as soon as smallpox is diagnosed, and all other known contacts not previously vaccinated should be placed on daily fever watch and vaccinated if fever appears. If there is an outbreak of smallpox, people in the surrounding community should be advised to avoid crowded places, to report any definitely elevated fever and to observe hygienic precautions such as frequent hand washing.

Medical caregivers, attendants and mortuary workers, even if vaccinated, should wear gloves, caps, gowns and surgical masks. All contaminated instruments, excretions, fluids and other materials should be decontaminated chemically or by heat or incineration. Contaminated clothing and bedding, if not incinerated, should be autoclaved or washed in hot water containing hypochlorite bleach. Cadavers should be cremated whenever possible and all persons coming in contact with them should be vaccinated and placed on daily fever watch. Any presumptive case of smallpox should be regarded as a potential international public health emergency and immediately notified to national health authorities and to WHO.

Prophylaxis and treatment

Most existing vaccine stocks and the vaccine used in the WHO eradication campaign consist of pulp scraped from vaccinia virus-infected animal skin, mainly calf or sheep, with phenol added to a concentration sufficient to kill bacteria but not so high as to inactivate the vaccinia virus. This is then freeze-dried and sealed in ampoules for later re-suspension in sterile buffer and intradermal inoculation by jet injector or multiple puncture inoculation with a bifurcated needle. More recent vaccine production is from vaccinia virus-infected human cell-culture or from cultured monkey kidney (Vero) cells.

Vaccination usually prevents smallpox for at least 10 years and, even if symptoms appear, they are milder and mortality is less than in nonvaccinated persons.

Vaccination is contraindicated for certain groups, including pregnant women and persons with immune disorders or under immunosuppression, with HIV infection or with a history of eczema. Nevertheless, if there is danger of epidemic spread it may be advisable to vaccinate such persons and to attempt to limit adverse effects by intramuscular administration of vaccinia immune globulin, if available, from vaccinia-infected sheep or calves. A vaccinia virus-based vaccine, produced in cell culture, is expected to become available within a few years and there is interest in developing monoclonal anti-variola antibody for passive immunization of exposed and infected individuals.

The smallpox vaccine emergency reserve maintained by WHO currently consists of some 600 000 doses, held in Geneva and regularly tested for potency. WHO conducts surveys to estimate country-held smallpox vaccine stocks for civilian purposes, whether retained from the eradication era or recently produced. WHO has no information on possible additional reserves held for military purposes. At the request of Member States, WHO is increasing the size of the existing emergency reserve of smallpox vaccine as part of global preparedness. The emergency reserve would be used only in response to a smallpox outbreak, confirmed clinically and epidemiologically, and only in cases where the vaccine supplies held by the affected country are inadequate.

A number of antiviral drugs are under investigation as chemotherapeutic agents against variola infections. One of these, cidofovir, a broad-spectrum inhibitor of viral DNA polymerase, appears to protect mice against cowpox and cynomolgous monkeys against monkeypox and inhibits variola virus replication in vitro.

Selected references

Breman JG, Henderson DA. Diagnosis and management of smallpox. *New England Journal of Medicine*, 2002, 346:1300–1308.

Esposito JJ, Fenner F. Poxviruses. In: Knipe DN et al., eds. *Field's virology*, 4th ed. Philadelphia, PA, Lippincott Williams & Wilkins, 2001:2885–2921.

Fenner F, Wittek R, Dumbell KR. *The orthopoxviruses*. San Diego, CA, Academic Press, 1989.

Fenner F et al. *Smallpox: its eradication*. Geneva, World Health Organization, 1988.

Henderson DA et al. Smallpox as a biological weapon: medical and public health management. *Journal of the American Medical Association*, 1999, 281:2127–2137.

Herrlich A, Mayr A. *Die Pocken: Erreger, Epidemiologie und klinisches Bild*. [Smallpox: etiology, epidemiology and clinical presentation.] Stuttgart, Georg Thieme Verlag, 1967.

Mack T. A different view of smallpox and vaccination. *New England Journal of Medicine*, 2003, 348:460–463.

Moss B. Poxviridae: the viruses and their replication. In: Knipe DN et al., eds. *Field's virology*, 4th ed. Philadelphia, PA, Lippincott Williams & Wilkins, 2001:2849–2883.

Internet: *http://www.cdc.gov.smallpox*

General references (including web sites)

Acha PN, Szyfres B, eds. *Zoonoses and communicable diseases common to man and animals*, 2nd ed. Washington, DC, Pan American Health Organization/World Health Organization, 1980.

Centers for Disease Control and Prevention. Biological and chemical terrorism: strategic plan for preparedness and response. Recommendations of the CDC strategic planning workgroup. *Morbidity and Mortality Weekly Report*, 2000, 49:No. RR-4:1–14.

CDC Public Health Emergency Preparedness and Response *http://www.bt.cdc.gov/HealthProfessionals/index.asp*

Chin J, ed. *Control of communicable diseases manual*, 17th ed. Washington, DC, American Public Health Association, 2000.

Collier L et al, eds. *Topley and Wilson's microbiology and microbial infections*, 9th ed. London, Arnold, 1998.

Collins CH. *Laboratory acquired infections*, 2nd ed. London, Butterworths, 1988.

Garner JS. Guidelines for isolation precautions in hospitals. *Infection Control and Hospital Epidemiology*, 1996, 17:51–80.

Hoeprich PD, Jordan MC, Ronald AR, eds. *Infectious diseases*, 5th ed. Philadelphia, PA, Lippincott, 1994.

Khan AS, Morse S, Lillibridge S. Public health preparedness for biological terrorism in the USA. *Lancet*, 2000, 356:1179–1182.

Murray PM et al., eds. *Manual of clinical microbiology*, 7th ed. Washington, DC, American Society for Microbiology, 1999.

Richmond JY, McKinney RW. *Biosafety in microbiological and biochemical laboratories*, 4th ed. Washington, DC, US Department of Health and Human Services, 1999 (GPO 017-040-00547-4).

Sidell FR, Takafuji ET, Franz DR, eds. *Medical aspects of chemical and biological warfare*. Washington, DC, Walter Reed Army Medical Center, Office of the Surgeon General, 1997.

WHO recommended strategies for the prevention and control of communicable diseases. Geneva, World Health Organization, 2001 (document WHO/CDS/CPE/SMT/2001.13).

ANNEX 4: PRINCIPLES OF PROTECTION

1. Introduction

A variety of technologies and strategies can be used to protect individuals physically against contamination by chemical and biological agents. In fact, individual protection is often the measure that comes to mind first in considering methods to counter chemical and biological threats. However, protection is achieved only at a price. The use of protective clothing is always a trade-off between the protection achieved and the problems caused by the protective equipment itself, as discussed in Appendix A4.1 below. It is consequently a mistake to consider protection in isolation. It must always be seen as an integral part of the risk-management process, after consideration of the strategies that may be able to reduce the risk and eliminate the need for protection altogether.

This annex describes the role of physical protection in the risk-management process, and highlights the advantages and disadvantages of different risk-control mechanisms. It concludes with a practical example illustrating the application of the principles that have been introduced.

2. Risk-reduction measures

The level of risk posed by a hazard is a function of the probability of exposure to that hazard and the extent of the harm that would be caused by that exposure. Application of risk-control measures, as part of the risk-management process, seeks to reduce or eliminate the probability and/or the severity of harm. Various risk-reduction mechanisms can be introduced for dealing with chemical or biological agents:

1. Administrative controls
2. Engineering controls
3. Physical protection

These should be understood as integral parts of a system, and a risk-control strategy should never be restricted to one method alone. The strategy should preferably begin to take effect as close to the hazard itself as possible. The best way to prevent casualties from a deliberate release of biological or chemical agents is to make the use of such agents impossible, or at least to reduce the probability of their use. If this fails, the objective of risk control is to minimize human suffering and reduce the loss of assets. Every method has its own advantages and disadvantages.

2.1 Administrative controls

In their application to biological and chemical agents, administrative controls include risk communication (including a warning system), and the evacuation and cordoning off of potentially contaminated areas. This simply reduces the possibility of exposure by avoiding the hazard. The hazard itself is not affected, and no physical protection is introduced. Administrative controls are usually relatively easy to apply and are less costly than other risk-control methods. Since the risk is avoided (reduction of probability), risk reduction through other measures is less important. However, people may choose not to follow administrative instructions (e.g. may leave their homes). The setting up of cordons needs resources that cannot then be used elsewhere. Restricted areas or buildings cannot be used for some time, and certain personnel, such as responders, will still need to enter the area. This means that administrative controls can usually only supplement, but not eliminate, the need for other risk-control mechanisms.

2.2 Engineering controls

Engineering controls involve the use of technologies such as airstream control, filters, and various forms of containment, normally used to contain or limit the spread of a hazard. Unlike administrative controls, engineering controls function independently of human decisions. They can, of course, be bypassed, but usually only by a deliberate action, and for technical reasons are limited to specific locations. Since engineering controls prevent contact with the harmful substance without forcing personnel to use individual protective equipment (thereby shifting the preventive measures towards the hazard and away from personnel), they are a preferred method of risk control. An example of engineering control is the use of a biosafety cabinet for the handling of mail suspected of containing a hazardous substance. This example will be explained in more detail below. Buildings with air-filtration systems also constitute a form of engineering control.

2.3 Physical protection

When physical protection is used, the hazard is not contained, as with engineering controls, nor are personnel kept away from the hazard, as with administrative measures. As explained in Appendix A4.1 below, protection can also cause hazards of its own. For these and other reasons, protection is the least desirable method of risk control. While protection is primarily a supplementary measure, it may sometimes be the only practicable method. When it is necessary to rely on physical protection, the objective should be to limit the number of persons exposed, and to expose them to the lowest possible concentration of contaminant for the shortest possible time. The level of protection selected should also be appropriate for the degree and type of hazard. It is not always necessary to use full protection, e.g. a respirator alone may be adequate to protect against a volatile substance that neither damages the skin nor is absorbed through it. Protection can be achieved via:

1. Individual protection
2. Collective protection

Individual protection covers all types of equipment worn by individuals to reduce the possibility of inhalation of and/or skin exposure to chemical and biological weapons (e.g. respirators and protective suits). Collective protection is in fact a special form of engineering control, reducing the risk of exposure for a group of individuals without containing the hazard, e.g. in filter-ventilated buildings and command centres, shelters or vehicles. Wherever possible, collective protection is preferred to individual protection since it does not cause the problems normally associated with individual protection.

3. Individual protection

As usual, risk-management principles should be used in selecting suitable individual protective equipment. With the introduction of protective barriers between the individual and the hazardous substance, a temporary reduction in the exposure can be achieved. However, it must be remembered that, sooner or later, all chemicals and some biological agents will pass through or permeate the protective barriers. Depending on the type of material used, the protection time can range from seconds to days, but no protective equipment protects the wearer against anything indefinitely. In addition, the protection factor[1] depends largely on the seal or tightness that the overall system can achieve. A respirator that does not fit properly will have a low protection factor. In industrial health and safety, two protection factors are often used, namely the theoretical protection factor, which is purely material-related, and the practical or applied protection factor that is actually achieved in the field (which depends on factors such as the seal and fit of the individual protective equipment). Normally, the protection actually achieved with any protective equipment is much lower than the theory would suggest. The individual protective equipment must be chosen in the light of the type and concentration of the agent, other expected hazards (such as oxygen deficiency in confined spaces), and the activity that the wearer is required to perform. Depending on the nature of the threat agent, there are two main components of individual protection that can be used alone or in combination, namely respiratory protection and skin protection.

3.1 Respiratory protection

Most biological and chemical agents are capable of entering the body through the respiratory system, while some, but not all, can penetrate intact skin. Of the two, the respiratory system is more vulnerable than the skin. From a risk-management perspective, therefore, protection of the respiratory system has priority. There are two major types of respiratory-protection equipment:

1. Air-purifying devices (such as military gas masks).
2. Air-supplying devices (such as self-contained breathing apparatus) (SCBA).

---

[1] Concentration of a substance outside the individual protective equipment divided by the inside concentration.

3.1.1 Air-purifying devices

Air-purifying devices (such as filtering masks), remove gases, vapours and/or aerosols from the inhaled air. Clearly, they cannot protect against oxygen deficiency, and their protective ability depends on the filter capacity[2] and selectivity[3] for various contaminants. For biological weapons any aerosol filter will physically retain the contaminants (although not always sufficiently), but filters for chemical agents may require adsorptive materials specifically designed for a certain chemical or group of chemicals.[4] Canisters[5] produced according to military specifications will usually remove known biological and chemical agents from the inhaled air, but industrial canisters may not be suitable for all types of chemical agents. In modern canisters, an aerosol filter is combined with an activated charcoal filter, thereby removing dusts, mists, and vapours or gases. Two major problems may arise with filtering respirators:

1. The filtration capacity may not be adequate for the type and amount of the contaminant.
2. The facial seal may not be tight enough.

The problem of selectivity can be overcome by the use of military-specification canisters, which are suitable for the majority of potential chemical and biological agents. Still, even the best canister can be overwhelmed by very high concentrations of gases and vapours, or even mechanically clogged by otherwise harmless dust, thus increasing the breathing resistance of the canister to unbearable levels. A more serious problem is the effectiveness of the seal of the respirator against the wearer's face. Even the best filter will not protect a person when unfiltered air bypasses the canister via an inadequate facial seal. In industrial health and safety, therefore, the protection factor is often, in practice, orders of magnitude lower than the theoretical (or even tested) protection factor of the canister. Not only the type of respirator (mouthpiece, half-mask, full-face mask or hood), but also the competence of the wearer, facial hair, and other practical factors can significantly reduce the protection level.

---

2   The amount of contamination that a filter can hold back without a break-through.

3   The ability of a filter to protect against one or more different chemicals.

4   The problems with adsorption of certain toxic chemicals, such as hydrogen cyanide or perfluoroisobutene (PFIB), are well known.

5   The filtering cartridge attached to a mask or respirator.

Even when the wearer is well trained and has no facial hair, and the respirator is well fitted, increased breathing will cause an under-pressure inside the mask during inspiration, potentially decreasing the protection. The use of power-assisted respirators, in which an electrically powered fan (blowing unit) is used to produce a slight over-pressure inside the respirator, can partially solve this problem. Power-assisted respirators can also be designed as hoods, covering the head of the wearer completely and not needing a tight face seal, thus ensuring that "one size fits all". However, extremely deep inhalation can still cause an under-pressure, and the air passage through the canister can be increased only to a certain extent without diminishing the filtering effect. In addition, the logistic problems (batteries, maintenance, etc.) and the relatively high cost of power-assisted respirators render them more suitable for specific groups of personnel, such as medical personnel treating potentially contaminated patients. It should also be remembered that the noise from the fan, in some designs, may make communication difficult and put an additional strain on the wearer.

3.1.2   Air-supplying devices

As the name implies, air-supplying devices act independently of the ambient atmosphere and supply the wearer with uncontaminated air. The air supply may be obtained via a stationary system (e.g. a wall-connected air hose), or via transportable systems like the SCBA or the Rebreather.[6] While both types share the advantages of reduced breathing resistance and very high protection factors, they also have certain limitations. The higher protection factors result from the over-pressure inside the respirator facepiece, and the fact that air from a contained and uncontaminated source is being inhaled. In so-called positive-demand devices, the air pressure inside the facepiece is always greater than the outer air pressure. Stationary systems are sometimes equipped with a hood or helmet (constant-flow), and can be used by people who are unable to wear a mask. Stationary systems can provide clean air almost indefinitely, but limit the mobility of the wearer, which will depend on the length of the air hose. In some situations, e.g. in unstable structures or in fire fighting, air hoses cannot be used at all. SCBAs are then more useful, but they provide air for a limited time only. Rebreathers solve this problem to some extent by prolonging the air supply (by a factor of up to four, depending on the model), but not

---

6   A system in which the exhaled air is recirculated, with removal of carbon dioxide and enrichment with oxygen.

completely. Since air-supplying systems are heavy even when made from modern materials such as carbon fibres, they add significantly to the physical burden of the wearer.

Air-supplying systems require a highly skilled wearer if maximal protection is to be achieved. In fact, an untrained person could die from the incorrect use of an otherwise fully functional device. Specialized training and certification of users of air-supplying devices is required by law in a number of countries. Any air-supplying device should undergo regular maintenance and inspection.

It should be clear from the foregoing that correct choice of equipment, proper maintenance, and comprehensive training will all be required if protection is to be adequate. Many organizations have found that a successful approach to respiratory protection requires a formal written Respiratory Protection Programme, which both guides users and draws attention to the many factors that are involved.

3.2 Skin protection

Although the respiratory system is the primary point of vulnerability to chemical and biological agents, the skin may sometimes need protection as well. Depending on the nature of the threat and the required activities, such protection can be provided by coveralls or ponchos, overboots and gloves, or fully encapsulating suits which combine full-body, head, hand and foot protection. Depending on the design and the material used, single or multiple use is possible. The protection factor achieved with body protection depends on:

1. The permeability of the material to chemical and biological agents.
2. The "tightness" of the equipment.

As explained earlier, no material is impermeable to all contaminants for an indefinite period. Both the material's specific resistance to certain chemicals, and abrasions, micro-holes and cuts can reduce the effectiveness of skin protection. Even an "impermeable" material does not provide unlimited protection. Some widely used materials do not protect against certain chemical agents at all: natural rubber is penetrated by sulfur mustard within minutes. On the other hand, almost all materials will provide sufficient protection against biological agents. Most modern military equipment is designed to provide protection against both chemical and biological agents. Suits can be made from air-permeable materials in order to reduce the heat load for the wearer and to allow them to be used for longer periods. Since these air-permeable materials are essentially a charcoal filter on cloth (acting like an air-purifying respirator), they purify the ambient air to a certain extent, thus providing the wearer with limited ventilation. This should not be confused with the undesired ventilation of the "bellows effect" described below.

Movement of the wearer causes air to be pumped through the hood, sleeves and jacket openings – the so-called "bellows effect". This provides cooling and ventilation to the wearer and may be subjectively very welcome, but it also significantly reduces the protection factor. With relatively tight sealing around the mask facepiece, the sleeves and the leg openings, and a one-piece coverall design, the "bellows effect" can be reduced, but not completely eliminated. For extremely high concentrations of chemical and biological agents it is therefore necessary to use a sealed over-pressurized suit. In addition, in the selection of individual protective equipment, it must be remembered that masks and suits are often designed as an ensemble. Using a different mask or donning the ensemble in a different way can reduce the protection factor significantly. As with all individual protective equipment, the use of protective suits requires trained and physically fit personnel. This is especially important in warm or hot environments, where the physiological strain of wearing protective clothing can be considerable, as is discussed further in Appendix A4.1 below.

3.3 Special cases

Certain groups of people cannot wear standard individual protective equipment at all. Small children (under 7 years) and people with lung dysfunction cannot normally overcome the breathing resistance of an air-purifying respirator. Casualties with head or facial injuries may not be able to wear a mask, and a certain percentage of people cannot be provided with properly fitting masks because of their unusual facial dimensions or structure.[7] Special equipment is then needed, such as casualty bags with a power-assisted respirator, childrens' filtrating jackets, or over-pressurized hoods for prams. The psychological problems associated with the wearing of individual protective equipment can make proper use impossible for some individuals, particularly children.

---

7 Respirators are usually designed to fit 95% of the adult population of the country concerned.

4. Collective protection

With collective protection, a group of people are provided with un-contaminated air and protected from skin contact with chemical or biological agents without having to cope with the difficulties associated with individual protective equipment. Collective protection is not affected in any way by the physical and mental condition of the users. It also depends less on the level of training than individual protective equipment. Collective protection can therefore be seen as a special form of engineering control and, when the situation allows, is preferable to individual protection. It can be achieved by means of:

1. Shelters and/or vehicles not specifically designed for protection against chemical and biological weapons.

2. Specially designed units.

Generally, any building or vehicle can be used to provide some protection against chemical and biological weapons by making it airtight, thus preventing agents from entering it. This can be achieved by applying chemically resistant sheets and adhesive tape to all openings, such as windows, doors and ventilation openings. Unfortunately, this not only keeps chemical and biological agents outside, but also the oxygen needed to replenish what is being breathed, and traps carbon dioxide inside. However, a makeshift solution can at least provide some level of temporary protection. Two factors limit the protection factor of makeshift adaptations of conventional buildings or shelters to counter the threat of chemical and biological weapons:

1. The tightness and resistance of the seal.

2. The volume of air per person.

As stated previously, it is extremely difficult, if not impossible, to produce an absolutely airtight system. Contaminating agents will penetrate sooner or later. The paradoxical situation may arise that, after a certain time, the concentration of agent outside the shelter will have naturally decreased to a safe level, while those inside the shelter are still exposed to low concentrations. This can lead to a long period of low-level exposure inside the shelter compared with a short high-level exposure outside for the same dosage.[8] It is important for those inside the shelter to know when it is safe to break the shelter seal. In tightly

---

8   The dosage for vapours and aerosols is the amount of a substance per unit volume per unit time, e.g. mg.min/m³. Depending on the toxicology of a substance, 100 mg/m³ over 1 min can be the same as 1 mg/m³ for 100 min.

sealed shelters, monitoring of the dosage both inside **and** outside the shelter will therefore be necessary. With the wrong sealing material (one not resistant to chemical and biological agents) or inadequate seals, the level of exposure inside the shelter might actually be higher than outside.

Another problem with makeshift airtight shelters is the accumulation inside them of carbon dioxide and the using up of the available oxygen. As a minimum, an airtight shelter should have a volume of 10 m³ per person and per hour (assuming that the occupants will be at rest, or at most, that they undertake only occasional light activities). A somewhat longer period of occupation could be achieved by placing open trays containing quicklime on the floor (to absorb carbon dioxide), but this, of course, does not provide any additional oxygen.

Specifically designed units or shelters are normally fitted with airtight seals and/or over-pressurized with uncontaminated air. The performance of the air-purifying system must be appropriate for the volume of the room and the planned capacity, and a slight over-pressure should preferably be maintained to make airtight seals unnecessary. The system as a whole needs regular inspection and maintenance. Modern buildings are often built with air-conditioning systems. Depending on the capacity of these systems, it may be possible to equip them with high-efficiency particle air (HEPA) and charcoal filters, thus providing an (over-pressurized) shelter. Excellent guidance is available on the protection of building environments.[9]

While a number of factors make the use of collective protection preferable to individual protection, there are also the following disadvantages:

1. Cost
2. Availability in case of need
3. Restriction of mobility

Only a few countries in the world can afford to provide all – or even most – of the population with shelters that will adequately protect against chemical and biological agents. Sweden and Switzerland are two examples of countries that have done so. The costs are determined not only by the building and maintenance costs alone, but also by the loss

---

[9] See, for example, *Guidance for protecting building environments from airborne chemical, biological, or radiological attacks,* published by the Centers for Disease Control and Prevention in the United States, available online at *http://www.cdc.gov/niosh/bldvent/2002-139E.html.*

of rooms for other purposes. In Sweden, therefore, shelters must be built in a way that allows them to be used for other purposes in peacetime (e.g. as music rooms in schools or playrooms in nurseries). People must be able to reach the shelter within a reasonable time after a warning has been given. If they are caught in the open, the procedures to allow them to enter the shelter without introducing contamination can be very complicated, requiring both time and resources (e.g. airlocks, decontamination facilities, clothing to change into, etc.). It is also clear that personnel will not be able to move in and out of the shelter freely to carry out tasks in the open unless the shelter has the necessary facilities. Consequently, protected shelters will usually be suitable only for personnel who do not have outside tasks. Another form of collective protection is provided by vehicles protected against chemical and biological weapons. These vehicles have their own filtered ventilation systems. However, those using them will need lengthy training in the procedures for leaving and re-entering such vehicles to prevent the spread of contamination to the inside.

5. An example of the application of risk-management principles: the problem of potentially contaminated mail

After the "anthrax letters" episode in the USA in 2001[10], a number of organizations and companies all over the world have assessed the risk of such an incident on their premises as significant enough to require action. One way of dealing with the situation that might be suitable for a smaller organization is described here. It is presented as an illustration of the role that protection plays in the risk-management approach, and should not be regarded as a method that would be suitable for all organizations or circumstances.

After a thorough risk assessment, a company producing industrial safety equipment (with around 500 employees) concluded that they

---

10 See Appendix 4.3 to Chapter 4.

might become a target for anthrax hoaxes or an actual attack. They were aware that even a hoax or false alarm would shut down production for at least two days (before an all-clear could be given), and would also reduce the productivity of the employees for an extended period for psychological reasons. The company receives approximately 150 letters and small packages every day, plus a number of letters addressed to individual employees. These were normally opened in the mailroom by a clerk, before registration and distribution.

To reduce the risk to personnel and possible loss of company assets to an acceptable level, the company introduced a system of measures, including administrative and engineering controls, and the limited use of individual protective equipment.

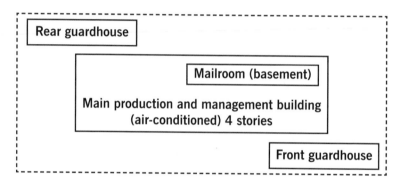

Figure 1. **Schematic facility plan**

Before the "anthrax letters" incident, mail was delivered and visually scanned in the front guardhouse, then received by the mail clerk, opened in the mailroom and distributed to the different parts of the company. Under that system, the opening of an "anthrax letter" would expose the mail clerk to a potentially lethal concentration of anthrax spores, and the air-conditioning system would spread the spores inside the building, thus forcing evacuation and the closing down of production. The company introduced a number of measures to reduce this risk (Figure 1):

1. All employees were requested not to receive any private mail at the company address, thus reducing the amount of mail to be checked by the mail clerk (administrative control).

2. The site for the opening of envelopes was moved from the main building to the rear guardhouse, which has an independent air-conditioning system. In an anthrax scare or hoax, the potentially contaminated area will be restricted to this guardhouse. The production building will not be affected (administrative control).

3. All mail is transported in a tightly sealed plastic bag to the rear guardhouse to prevent any possible cross-contamination (engineering control).

4 All mail is still visually scanned, but now in the rear guardhouse (administrative control).

5. Since the company works with toxic chemicals for testing respirators, several portable chemical fume hoods were available. After assessing the technical specification of these fume hoods, the company safety department recommended that they should be used as biosafety cabinets[11] (engineering control).

6. One fume hood was moved to the rear guardhouse for use as a biosafety cabinet (engineering control).

7. The mail clerk and security personnel were briefed and trained in the opening of the mail inside the biosafety cabinet before carrying out a standard operating procedure requiring that all mail must be opened and screened inside the cabinet (administrative control).

8. Protective gloves and decontamination solution for cleaning the gloves inside the biosafety cabinet were given to the mail clerk (individual protection).

9. As a confidence-building and risk-communication measure, all personnel were informed about the decisions and the process.

The company subsequently experienced two false alarms, both of which were successfully managed without any disruption of daily activity or loss of production.

This is, of course, a simplified example of a logically ordered approach to dealing with a special form of bioterrorism. It illustrates how the use of individual protective equipment can be restricted to the absolutely necessary minimum, preference being given to administrative and engineering controls. The result is not only safer than that achieved by

---

11   A biosafety cabinet is an enclosure with internal under-pressure (ensuring that no air leaks to the outside), equipped with a HEPA filter through which a pumped stream of outgoing air is directed. Such cabinets are commonly used in laboratories where work with potentially harmful organisms is carried out.

the more obvious actions taken by many other organizations (provision of masks and gloves to staff handling mail, i.e. protection alone), but also results in minimal disruption to normal activity, even if a false alarm, hoax, or actual threat materializes.

Further reading

Forsberg K, Mansford SZ. *Quick selection guide to chemical protective clothing*, 3rd ed. New York, Van Nostrand Reinhold, 1997.

The selection, use and maintenance of respiratory protective equipment – a practical guide, 2nd ed. Suffolk, Health and Safety Executive, 1998.

Ridley J. *Safety at work*, 3rd ed. Oxford, Butterworth-Heinemann, 1990.

APPENDIX A4.1: PROBLEMS RELATED TO PROTECTION

Modern biological and chemical protective equipment has made it possible to survive in many types of toxic environment. Such protection, however, may be achieved at the cost of a significantly reduced ability to function. In selecting protective equipment for biological and chemical preparedness, a balance should be struck between the degree of protection necessary for the potential hazard concerned and the resultant increase in difficulty of the functions to be carried out by those wearing such equipment. There may, of course, be considerable differences between the protection requirements of response teams dealing with civil incidents and those of military personnel, who may need to operate for long periods in a toxic biological or chemical environment.

The key to the successful use of protective equipment, whether by civil incident-response teams or the military, is familiarity through repeated training in using the equipment. In extended operations in which protective equipment is required, the following problems need to be carefully considered.

Heat stress

When protective clothing is worn, insulation is increased, evaporation of sweat from body surfaces is reduced, and the body consequently suffers a significant decrease in its natural ability to lose heat. This decrease can be so large, especially if impermeable protective clothing is being worn, that potentially fatal heatstroke is a possibility after less than an hour. Supervisors of responders or emergency services must be aware of the need for careful monitoring of those wearing protective clothing and of the methods of avoiding this problem, e.g. by planned work/rest cycles, or the use of specialized cooling equipment. A further problem associated with the wearing of a respirator is the effort required to breathe against the resistance of the filter canister. This can severely limit the work rate possible, and also significantly increase the psychological stress experienced (see below).

Psychological stress

Apart from the physiological stresses mentioned above, individuals wearing protective clothing can experience great psychological stress. This may even be more important in limiting performance than physiological problems. Stress results from fear of the chemically or biologically contaminated environment, the claustrophobic effects of protective clothing (especially the respirator), the potential impairment of the ability to communicate with colleagues, the general discomfort of wearing the often bulky clothing, perceptions of the increasing physiological stresses (heat and breathing stress), and of the reduced ability to function and perform tasks that may be necessary for survival. As a result, decision-making may be impaired.

Ergonomic difficulties

The nature of chemical protective clothing creates many ergonomic problems that may interfere with the performance even of simple tasks. Thick rubber gloves cause problems with any task requiring fine touch (computer operation, medical examination, etc.), and bulky clothes hamper movement in restricted spaces (e.g. in ambulances). The lenses of the masks may be incompatible with optical equipment, and medical personnel may experience extreme difficulty in carrying out even basic procedures of patient management (cardiopulmonary resuscitation, airway management, etc.).

Side-effects of medication

Certain medications commonly used to counter the effects of biological and chemical agents can create problems of their own. Pyridostigmine is frequently used as a pretreatment drug for nerve-gas poisoning. It is intended to be taken before exposure in order to improve the chances of survival if a nerve-gas attack actually materializes. Pyridostigmine can, however, have side-effects of its own, such as diarrhoea, intestinal cramps and visual problems. The most common item of medical equipment used in chemical defence worldwide is the autoinjector. Although the contents of the different types may vary, the medication generally used is atropine, which is the antidote required after nerve-gas exposure. However, if atropine is injected in the absence of nerve-gas poisoning, it can have significant side-effects, such as increased heart rate, disturbances of the heart rhythm, dry mouth and decreased sweating (causing even more severe heat stress), and blurred vision.

Logistic problems

The logistics associated with the issue of protective equipment to the personnel needing it can also be a problem. Some equipment, once removed from its sealed packaging or contaminated, cannot be readily decontaminated, and consequently is unsuitable for reuse. If large numbers of personnel require protective equipment, this can be extremely costly.

Conclusions

Response teams dealing with civil incidents may be less affected by the problems described above since they are likely to be deployed for shorter periods, and are better able to allow personnel to rest outside the contaminated area without loss of efficiency. If the military are involved, however, some of the problems associated with the use of protective equipment for long periods might arise even when biological or chemical agents have not been released, e.g. when preparations are being made in anticipation of an attack. Such preparations may in themselves be a significant disadvantage for the defending party, and may even be the reason that the threat was introduced by the aggressor. However, a state that elects not to defend or protect itself from biological and chemical weapons might be vulnerable to the full effects of such weapons and to the mass casualties that they produce. It is instructive to note that no major military attack with biological or chemical weapons has yet been made on countries with forces that are well equipped and trained for biological or chemical warfare.

Successful preparedness, including biological and chemical threat assessment, contingency planning and preparation for a biological or chemical incident, calls for a strategy that is both justified by, and relevant to, the potential threat. Overreaction to a threat could be the very effect sought by an aggressor.

ANNEX 5:
PRECAUTIONS AGAINST THE SABOTAGE OF DRINKING-WATER, FOOD, AND OTHER PRODUCTS

1. Introduction

Civilian drinking-water and food supplies have been sabotaged throughout recorded history, usually during military campaigns. More recently, however, in situations not associated with open warfare, such sabotage has been used to terrorize or otherwise intimidate civilian populations *(1)*. Terrorists may have a variety of motives, from settling grudges to political destabilization. It is not necessary to inflict mass casualties to cause widespread panic and disruption, particularly economic. While the deliberate contamination of drinking-water can cause human illness, the long-term disruption of drinking-water supplies will have catastrophic consequences for public health and confidence. Although the deliberate contamination of all food supplies in a given area is unlikely, pre-existing food shortages could be considerably worsened by such contamination. All populations are vulnerable to such attacks.

Governments as well as commercial and other organizations in the private sector should be aware of the need to prevent and respond to deliberate contamination. While threats aimed at extorting money, particularly from organizations in the commercial sector, are usually not considered terrorism, they are far more common than is generally believed. Their economic and social impacts can be the same as those of acts that are clearly terrorism. Security and safety precautions should therefore be evaluated to make sure that they can respond to threats of deliberate contamination. Providers of water supplies, manufacturers, and other private sector organizations must therefore be involved in the development and implementation of safety assurance plans designed to prevent, detect, and respond to deliberate contamination. Such plans must include consumer education and active means of communicating with the press and the public. An improved climate of vigilance will reduce vulnerability to both deliberate and accidental contamination. The threat of terrorism should not, however, mean that other pressing safety concerns, such as the prevention of unintentional contamination of drinking-water and foods, are ignored, nor should it be allowed to cause panic.

Since drinking-water, food, and medicines are consumed by the population, they probably provide the easiest way to deliver lethal or debilitating amounts of toxic chemicals or biological agents. Drinking-water systems and those for manufacture and distribution of food and other consumer products present many opportunities for deliberate contamination. Although globalization and the complex production and delivery systems for many foods and medicines have increased vulnerability, this diversity of sources also reduces the likelihood that all supplies of food and medicines will be contaminated. For water, the lack of alternative sources in most areas creates a more serious problem and increases the potential for panic and hysteria.

Widespread human illnesses have been associated both with a variety of food- and waterborne microorganisms and with drinking-water and food products contaminated with toxic chemicals. Large-scale disruption of food supplies caused by diseases of farm animals has also occurred. Such outbreaks have strained or overwhelmed public services, and given rise to intense media coverage, with consequent adverse economic, social, and political effects. They have also resulted in a loss of public confidence. Where terrorists are successful in spreading contamination or otherwise disrupting services, the same effects are likely to occur.

Programmes designed to prevent the sabotage of drinking-water, food and other consumer products, such as cosmetics and medicines, are based on:

1. Prevention
2. Detection
3. Response

In all of these, *preparedness* plays an essential role.

There is no way of preventing all contamination, whether accidental or the result of the deliberate introduction of chemical, biological, and radioactive agents. A determined terrorist with access to the required resources can penetrate virtually any system. However, the risk of human exposure can be reduced by increasing security and the ability to detect contamination or disruption. Early detection of contamination or attempts to contaminate would prevent or significantly reduce the magnitude of any resulting disease outbreak. While systems that rapidly and effectively detect and respond to disease outbreaks resulting from contamination and other causes are essential, those available are often not rapid enough to prevent all human exposure.

Given the large number of potential threat agents, it is impossible to monitor all of them all of the time. However, adopting sensible precautions is an effective approach to safeguarding public health, whether in areas with complex modern production and distribution systems for water and food or in those where drinking-water is obtained from a catchment and most food is locally produced, stored, and consumed. Proactive risk analysis can reduce vulnerability in the same way as for accidental contamination. Available resources should be allocated based on threat and vulnerability assessments, and should be appropriate to the nature and likelihood of the threats, whether accidental or deliberate.

The purpose of this annex is to increase public awareness of the threat of the deliberate sabotage of drinking-water, food, and other consumer products and services, and to provide general guidance on actions that can be taken to prevent, detect, and respond to this threat. Most multinational and other large commercial organizations and service providers have the resources to develop appropriate security and detection systems. Emphasis should therefore be placed on assisting small or less-developed businesses and utilities to develop and implement systems for the prevention and detection of deliberate contamination.

Worker safety is important in all activities. While not directly covered in this annex, the physical and mental health of workers should be major considerations in the development of security and safety plans.

2. Prevention

2.1 Security

Organizations involved in the supply of drinking-water and food production, processing, and distribution, as well as in the manufacture and distribution of other consumer products should:

- develop security and response plans, including establishing and maintaining up-to-date points of contact, internally and externally, with the public health and law-enforcement authorities, in case an incident is suspected or detected;
- safeguard sources of raw materials, including storage facilities and transport systems;
- restrict and document access to all critical areas, such as processing, storage, and transport;
- screen employees to ensure that their qualifications and background are appropriate to their work and responsibilities;
- screen other personnel (including sanitation, maintenance, and inspection personnel) with access to critical areas;
- minimize opportunities to contaminate the final product in the supply chain;
- for food and other consumer products, increase the ability to trace where any product is and where it has been in the supply chain and to remove it from that chain if it is believed or shown to be contaminated; and
- report threats and suspicious behaviour and activities to the proper authorities, and take appropriate action to make certain that security is maintained.

Preventive approaches do not necessarily require high technology. Increased awareness of potential problems and greater vigilance are among the most effective measures that can be taken. The wax seal is a tamper-evident device that has been used for several thousand years. A variety of such devices can be used to provide evidence of unauthorized access to critical areas and materials. While these precautions are primarily concerned with security and not directly with safety, they can increase safety from deliberate contamination. Increasing security measures will not, however, guarantee safety. Threats, both inadvertent and deliberate, will change. Nevertheless, a culture of secure operations and quality control will deter contamination by creating robust proactive systems that are harder to penetrate and where the likelihood of detection will be increased.

2.2   Reducing the availability of potential threat agents

International efforts to eliminate chemical and biological weapons should be strongly supported. While some of the agents that have been developed as weapons by the armed forces can be used to contaminate food and water, significant threats are also posed by toxic pesticides and industrial chemicals, as well as microbiological pathogens, such as those that are often inadvertent contaminants of food and water. In addition, certain highly toxic pharmaceuticals could be diverted for terrorist use. While most radioactive materials that are widely available for medical use would not cause serious injury if used to contaminate food or water, their presence would cause considerable public alarm. For the purposes of this annex, non-fissionable radioactive materials are considered to be chemical contaminants. Highly toxic pesticides and industrial chemicals, including chemical wastes, are widely available. Information on the preparation and use of chemicals for purposes of terrorism is also readily accessible, particularly on the Internet. Pathogenic microbiological agents are present in clinical and other laboratories, including those concerned with water and food control. A university-level knowledge of chemistry or microbiology is sufficient to produce many agents. Governments and commercial organizations must therefore increase the security of stores of toxic drugs, pesticides, radioactive materials, and other chemicals, and immediately report to the proper authorities any theft or other unauthorized diversion. Increased efforts must also be made to prevent the use of microbiological pathogens in terrorist activities. It is vitally important that clinical, public health, research, and water and food laboratories are aware of this potential and that appropriate security measures are taken to minimize the risk that dangerous materials are diverted for such purposes.

2.3 Screening of employees

Opportunities for the deliberate contamination or sabotage of drinking-water supplies exist at many points in water-supply systems, particularly for those with experience of such systems. Opportunities for the deliberate contamination of food exist from pre-farm to the table, and for other consumer products from pre-production to the consumer. Employers should screen staff to ensure that their qualifications and background are appropriate to their work and responsibilities. All staff should be strongly encouraged to report all suspicious behaviour and activities to the appropriate authorities, but care should be taken to prevent the use of false or unwarranted reports as a means of harassment.

3. Detection

The possibility of the contamination and interruption of water and food supplies should be taken into account in the assessment of safety-assurance systems, such as water safety plans, good manufacturing practices (GMP), and the Hazard Analysis and Critical Control Point (HACCP) system. This is a scientific and systematic way of increasing safety from primary production to final consumption through the identification, evaluation, and control of hazards that are significant for safety *(2)*. However, HACCP systems are designed to control specifically identified hazards. Some HACCP requirements, such as record keeping, may not be necessary or appropriate when the aim is to detect deliberate contamination. Safety-assurance systems should be designed for the specific operation concerned. Proactive risk analysis is needed to reduce vulnerability in the same manner as risks of inadvertent contamination. The resources allocated for this purpose should be proportional to the likelihood of the threat, the magnitude and severity of the consequences, and the vulnerability of the system. The possibility of deliberate contamination must be an integral part of safety planning, and efforts to prevent sabotage should complement, not replace, other essential safety activities.

Early detection of contamination or attempted contamination is essential in reducing the likelihood or magnitude of human exposure. The effects of pathogens are often delayed, so that exposure to contaminated products will continue until the contamination or the outbreak is detected. The failure of disease-surveillance systems, even in more advanced countries, to detect large-scale waterborne outbreaks emphasizes the importance of the prevention or early detection of contamination. Monitoring for contamination in all drinking-water systems and the production of food and other consumer products should be an integral part of routine quality control. Monitoring programmes can include a number of activities, ranging from careful visual examination to high-technology, in-line detection systems. As for inadvertent contamination, it is impossible, both technically and economically, to test for all possible agents all of the time. There may often be indicators of nonspecific variations in product quality, such as appearance, smell, or taste. Allocation of available resources for routine monitoring should therefore be appropriate to the specific product, process, and distribution situation. Rapid follow-up is essential when variations in product quality or in water service indicate the possibility of contamination. Public health officials should work closely with utilities and commercial and other private sector organizations and, where possible, assist in the development of appropriate monitoring programmes.

Individual consumers have a significant role to play in detecting both deliberate and inadvertent contamination. Consumers are often the first to detect differences in water quality, e.g. in taste, odour, or colour, and to become aware of health problems caused by water. If the packaging of a food or other consumer product is not intact, e.g. when anti-tamper seals have been broken, or if the product has an abnormal appearance, odour, or taste, it should not be consumed. If tampering is suspected, the retailer or supplier and the appropriate public health and law-enforcement authorities should be notified.

4. Response

4.1 Surveillance of water, food and other consumer products

Activities carried out in response to outbreaks of illness associated with infectious diseases and food- and waterborne pathogens are also appropriate to the identification of outbreaks associated with deliberate chemical and biological contamination. In general, separate systems should not be developed specifically for dealing with terrorism or other concerns, such as food safety. Public health surveillance should be strengthened to respond to disease outbreaks and other adverse public health events, whatever their cause. Questionnaires used for the surveillance of disease outbreaks should include questions designed to identify the route (for example, air, water, or food), the levels and the source of the contamination. Public health authorities should coordinate their activities with those of drinking-water suppliers and manufacturers and suppliers of food and other consumer products to ensure that appropriate measures, such as trace-back and market recall of foods and other consumer products, are taken as rapidly as possible. If deliberate contamination is suspected, the appropriate law-enforcement authorities should be advised.

4.2 Monitoring of contamination

In response to suspected contamination, threats, or disease outbreaks, the public health authorities and the industry concerned should ensure that all available analytical and investigative resources are called upon to prevent contaminated products from reaching consumers. Response plans should include mechanisms for notifying the appropriate government officials and private sector organizations that monitoring is necessary to determine the extent of the contamination. Public health authorities should prepare inventories of the analytical resources and skilled personnel available in international organizations and governmental, commercial, and academic laboratories. With drinking-water, the time between the end of processing and consumption is often only a few hours. It is therefore important to ensure that monitoring is effective and can give early warning of contamination.

4.3 Trace-back and market recall

Trace-back and market recall of food and other consumer products are needed in the investigation of incidents associated with these products, and should be included in response plans. The rapid determination of the source of the contamination and the location of contaminated products will greatly reduce the number of casualties by facilitating the rapid removal of contaminated products from the market.

Recall is not usually required with drinking-water. Arrangements should be made to notify rapidly all parts of the water-supply system that may be involved, together with consumers. Advance planning and a thorough understanding of the distribution system dynamics and the flow from different sources in the system are extremely important.

Trace-back and market recall are essential in responding to food contamination, whether deliberate or inadvertent. However, neither trace-back of problems nor trace-forward of contaminated products is always simple, as shown by the Belgian dioxin crisis *(3)*, and cannot be used in many agricultural production systems. Where small quantities of raw agricultural products are produced on small farms, they are usually combined, and these lots are then combined with other mixed lots to form larger shipments. It is therefore very important to link a contaminated shipment with an individual producer. With raw materials, the extent of recall will depend on the resources required for trace-back and market recall compared with those required for analysis and other measures for determining the safety of the raw materials at the critical control point of entry into the processing stream. Many foods are produced at centralized plants and distributed over large geographical areas, often globally. Contamination at such plants has affected large numbers of people and has often spread very widely before the outbreak was detected. Rapid determination of the source of the contamination and the location of contaminated products would greatly reduce the number of casualties by facilitating the rapid removal of contaminated products from the market. Market recall from the point of processing is essential.

4.4 Communications

Preparedness must include methods of communicating with the press and the public in order to manage fear and avoid unfounded rumours. Panic and hysteria may result in far more serious consequences to public health, as well as to industry and commerce, than the threat itself. Social and political dislocation and a sense of vulnerability are likely to persist long after the incident, whether or not an outbreak resulted. Some perpetrators of terrorist attacks may therefore regard the resulting publicity and social disruption as more effective in spreading their "message" than the number of people infected or killed, as in the planting of bombs in busy places but giving warnings to avoid injuries and deaths. Accordingly, it is unwise to regard the terrorist threat of the release of biological, radioactive, and chemical agents as one that is purely intended to cause numerous injuries or illnesses. This makes water-supply systems and food supplies attractive targets for deliberate contamination. Achieving sufficient contamination to cause ill health may be less important than ensuring that some physical evidence of a contaminating agent is present and discovered, and that the public is made aware of this.

Public health, safety and law-enforcement authorities, commercial and other private sector organizations, and the media must develop and use methods of communication that provide the information necessary for public safety but that do not contribute to panic. They must communicate actively with the public. Methods must include providing information on incidents that do not result in outbreaks. Such incidents are common and can contribute to public concern. Withholding information from the public can lead to a loss of confidence in the authorities, so that the public must be given the appropriate information, including advice on avoiding exposure and medical advice relevant to the nature of the incident. Cultural aspects should also be taken into account in communications associated with threats and the response to them. For this reason, some types of communication may not be universally applicable.

A systems approach has been taken in the sections below on drinking-water, food, and other consumer products. This can be used to assess vulnerability and the precautions that can be taken to improve safety.

5. Drinking-water supplies

The effects of deliberate contamination of water-supply systems are usually limited by dilution, disinfection, and filtration, nonspecific inactivation (hydrolysis, sunlight, and microbial degradation/predation), and the relatively small amount of water to which individuals are usually exposed compared with the total supply. However, with determination and the necessary resources, any part of the system can be penetrated. Outbreaks of cryptosporidiosis, including the large outbreak in Milwaukee,

Wisconsin, USA (which was not due to deliberate contamination), demonstrate that water-supply systems are vulnerable *(4)*. Water sources in many parts of the world are generally insecure and therefore more vulnerable to deliberate contamination by chemical or biological agents and the sabotage of equipment and facilities. The level of security at treatment plants varies widely.

Deliberate contamination can have not only the direct effects of injury or illness, but also the indirect effects of denial of the supply of drinking-water. A successful terrorist attack, whether by contamination or by other forms of sabotage, such as the use of explosives or other physical means, can disrupt the drinking-water supplies of a large city for months, with serious consequences not only to public health but also to industry and commerce. The sabotage of wastewater-treatment facilities could likewise cause public health problems and similar disruption, particularly downstream, but not of the same magnitude as those caused by the sabotage of drinking-water treatment plants or distribution systems.

Recreational water areas, such as swimming pools, that are not intended for use as sources of drinking-water, are also potential targets for deliberate contamination, but this will not be considered here. However, much of what is said here about drinking-water systems will also apply to water used for recreation.

Drinking-water supply systems consist, in general, of the following components:

- *a water source,* such as a lake, reservoir, river intake, spring catchment tank, or groundwater borehole;
- *a raw water main,* which connects the drinking-water source via a pipeline or aqueduct to a water-treatment plant;
- *a treatment plant,* in which processes such as coagulation, sedimentation, filtration, active carbon treatment, ozonization, and chlorination are carried out;
- *a piped distribution* system in which drinking-water is transported to end-users or, more commonly, to water tanks or water towers elevated above the end-users;
- *water tanks and towers,* which can provide a steady supply of drinking-water at a more constant pressure; and

– *a local piped distribution* system in which pumped or gravity-fed water under pressure is provided to residential water tanks and taps or other end-users.

A large distribution zone in a well-monitored drinking-water supply system can be relatively difficult to penetrate and contaminate effectively. There is often only one supplier of drinking-water in each locality, and drinking-water produced in one place is not normally transported to large areas of a country, so that, for each water system, surveillance and security measures can be concentrated on protecting key local installations. Access to points in the system where chemical or biological agents could be introduced in sufficient quantities to cause a large-scale health threat to water ready for end-use is usually limited. In addition, where disinfection with a residual disinfectant is practised, the range of chemical and biological agents that a terrorist might use to cause illness or injury is restricted to those that are resistant to disinfection and stable in water for more than a few hours. However, a massive biological contamination might not be neutralized by the residual disinfectant.

Nevertheless, there are very few water systems that are not potentially vulnerable to contamination at many points. The distribution system can be the most vulnerable part of the water-supply system, particularly to an experienced water services technician. Commercially available pumps could be used to inject relatively large quantities of contaminants into the system. It may not be necessary to contaminate a large part of the system in order to cause considerable damage and panic.

Most water-supply systems differ in their operational requirements and practices. In areas that rely on the transport of drinking-water, often over considerable distances, greater security may be required, so that the vulnerability and the actions required to reduce it may vary from system to system. The action needed to reduce the threat of deliberate contamination at specific points in the system will therefore depend on the extent of the vulnerability and the potential impact of contamination at any particular point in the system.

The complicity of the staff of the water-supply system, or their coercion, in introducing chemical or biological agents into the water or compromising the water-treatment process, is a possibility that cannot be neglected. Staff should be screened to ensure that their qualifications and experience are appropriate to the work for which they will be responsible. All staff should be encouraged to report suspicious behaviour to the appropriate authorities, but care should be taken to prevent false or unwarranted reports for purposes of harassment.

5.1 Water sources

The possibility of serious human health effects as a result of the contamination of water sources can range from low, as with large reservoirs and rivers, because the water will be diluted and treated before reaching the end-user, to high, as in catchment systems and open shallow wells where treatment is not provided.

The security of the source will depend on:

- the ease of access to the source and the ability of the terrorist to deliver to it quantities of chemical or biological agents sufficient to cause injury or illness in end-users;
- the nature of subsequent water treatment and analysis, and the time available after the detection of a potential problem for a suitable response to be made.

To minimize the risk of unauthorized access to water sources, intakes, inspection points and pump houses, various physical measures, such as fencing and locks, are commonly used. These can be supplemented with on-site security personnel, intrusion detectors, and silent alarms linked to the police and the water-supply company or authority. If resources permit, remote-controlled television surveillance can also be introduced. Local citizens should be strongly encouraged to report suspicious activities to the proper authorities. Certain water sources, such as rivers, can be vulnerable to large-scale contamination, e.g. from the discharge of large quantities of industrial chemicals and the sabotage of wastewater-treatment facilities upstream.

5.2 Raw water mains

Raw water mains carrying water to a treatment plant may be vulnerable to contamination. However, their position upstream of the treatment plant in the overall water-supply system means that subsequent inactivation of toxic chemicals and pathogens or their detection is more likely. However, it will be difficult to detect certain types of chemicals or radioactive materials. In addition, certain microbial agents cannot be detected immediately. Most chemicals and radioactive materials, and certain microbial agents, will not necessarily be removed or inactivated by conventional treatment.

Physical security measures, such as those suggested above for water sources, can also be applied in pipelines and pumping stations.

5.3 Treatment plants

Water-treatment plants are of vital importance in water-supply systems. Reducing or eliminating disinfection, in combination with the deliberate introduction of pathogenic organisms, will greatly increase the likelihood that an infectious dose containing a large number of organisms will be delivered. Some recent outbreaks of waterborne diseases have resulted from the interruption of disinfection operations *(5)*.

For the traditional reasons of protecting public health from communicable diseases and industrial chemicals, access to water-treatment plants in large water-supply systems is usually closely controlled, and on-site laboratory staff analyse samples for a wide range of potential pollutants. Small to medium systems may be more vulnerable. Undetected access to a treatment plant to introduce a contaminating agent should be made more difficult by introducing multi-barrier security and access. These can be supplemented by other measures, such as patrols at irregular intervals, closed-circuit television, and anti-tamper locks and alarms on important equipment and inspection covers.

Chlorination is effective against many, but not all, pathogenic biological agents, and can easily be overwhelmed. In addition, the presence of large chlorine-gas storage tanks, especially in areas with large populations, poses its own terrorist risk. Ozonization is a more expensive form of disinfection, but is generally more effective against contaminating agents, pathogens, and toxins. However, it does not provide any residual protection, such as that provided by chlorination.

5.4 Piped distribution systems

Treated water is usually distributed to end-users through piped distribution systems under pressure and below ground. While the main function of pressurized piped distribution systems is to convey water to people, the pressurized nature of the network can prevent surface water, groundwater, and sewage from coming into contact with treated drinking-water. This makes the deliberate introduction of contaminating agents more difficult, but not impossible. An experienced technician can easily gain access to these systems. Since the water has already gone through the treatment process, any contamination will most likely remain undetected until it reaches the end-user.

5.5 Water tanks and water towers

In many systems, most end-users do not receive their drinking-water directly from the distribution mains, but from local water tanks and water towers elevated above the end-users. The final distribution to end-users through a local pipe network is often gravity-fed at lower and steadier pressure. The treated water in these tanks and towers is not under pressure and may therefore be more vulnerable. However, since they are in specific locations, tanks and towers are easier to protect.

To improve the security of water tanks and towers, they must be made difficult to access. This can be accomplished by securing the sites with strong fences, erecting multiple barriers to entry, and sealing entry points. These measures can be supplemented by intrusion detectors and silent alarms connected to the police and the water control room. If resources permit, monitoring of water quality parameters, closed-circuit television surveillance, or appropriate on-site security personnel can be used.

5.6 Local piped distribution systems

While systems for piped water pumped or gravity-fed to residential water tanks and taps or other end-users have many points that are vulnerable to deliberate contamination, this is not likely to affect large populations. However, since drinking-water in these distribution systems has already been treated and is not subject to significant dilution, the risk of injury and death among populations exposed to agents introduced at this point in the drinking-water system is high. Certain buildings and houses have their own community piped distribution systems, with water often received from tanks. This makes intrusion by terrorists much easier than in other parts of the water-supply system. Deliberate introduction of contamination in distribution systems could be used to target specific buildings or areas or various points in the overall water-supply system. Widespread public panic could result from the contamination of even a small part of a distribution system.

Both water suppliers and consumers should pay special attention to local distribution systems, and these should also be included in preparedness planning. In local distribution systems, such as those of office and apartment buildings, water lines and meters should be secured, e.g. by means of locked access covers and utility rooms. All suspicious activities, particularly if associated with unusual maintenance or repair work, should be immediately reported to the proper authorities.

The separation of individual parts of the water-distribution system improves control and permits the rapid isolation of suspect or contaminated parts of the system. This is a routine design feature in most modern water-distribution systems, and is used in dealing with conventional problems, such as pipe repair and replacement, and the removal of non-deliberate microbiological contamination.

In particularly sensitive facilities, such as hospitals, public health services, security services, and bottled water and food-processing plants, additional water-treatment processes can be considered.

5.7 Monitoring

Monitoring should be carried out as necessary to give time for an appropriate response. The ability of the quality-control system to detect the presence of contaminating agents will depend on the frequency and range of the analyses undertaken. However, it is impractical to carry out specific analyses for all of the potential chemical and biological agents that could be used. On-line monitors for certain parameters, such as conductivity and pH, may provide some nonspecific indication of a change in water quality and of potential problems. Instrumentation is available for in-line or rapid general screening of processed water for specific chemical contaminants, and is being developed for biological agents. Bioassays can be a low-technology component of monitoring programmes, and can sometimes give rapid results. A number of nonspecific in vivo and in vitro assays are useful in detecting contamination, particularly by chemicals, and simple immunoassay screening tests for certain bacteria and viruses can be used in response to specific threats.

Emergency-response plans must include specific instructions for an immediate response to abnormal values and for preventing contaminated drinking-water from entering the distribution system, since there will not be time to discuss how to handle a problem once it is detected. These instructions should include the immediate notification of the appropriate public health authorities. When there is evidence that a drinking-water system has been contaminated by toxic chemicals or pathogenic microbes, the temporary suspension of the water supply may be the only practical way to prevent serious public health problems. However, this may cause great social inconvenience. The decision-making process on such occasions should be carefully planned and modelled in advance so that such decisions can be reached very quickly.

6. Food

Safeguarding food supplies and food ingredients from the deliberate introduction of chemical, radioactive, and biological agents by terrorists is a major challenge in industrialized countries, and especially those with access to a wide range of raw and processed foods and other products from around the world. At the pre-farm stage, e.g. in feed ingredients, in farms, or in the case of meat products, in slaughterhouses, there are opportunities for chemical or microbiological contamination with a resulting spread of disease of considerable magnitude. The unintentional contamination of food at retail markets and in local catering sites such as restaurants, schools, hospitals, and other institutions, is quite common and much more difficult to prevent. The opportunities for post-processing contamination of packaged foods in bottles, jars, packets and cans have been reduced substantially by the widespread introduction of tamper-resistant containers. This has been in response to incidents of tampering with food and medicines aimed at extorting money from large companies and retailers. While contamination at the retail level is not likely to result in large-scale adverse health effects, coordinated contamination at a number of different locations could lead to widespread disruption. Although tamper-resistant and tamper-evident containers are not fail-safe, they can be cost-effective in reducing the opportunities for deliberate contamination.

The precautions that should be taken to safeguard food supplies should be considered systematically for each stage in the production process from farm to retail and by the consumer. The number of precautions required may be considerable in complex processing operations. With street vendors and restaurants, perhaps the most appropriate precaution that can be taken is to promote more careful observation by the workers concerned, particularly of any suspicious behaviour by individuals and any unusual appearance of the food. As with inadvertent contamination, individual food preparers and consumers must play their part in food safety.

Agricultural and other production problems that do not directly result in human illness include short- or long-term loss of use of tracts of land or water resources, the economic disruption of agriculture, food processing, or other economic sectors (e.g. by non-human pathogens in livestock, insect infestations or diseases of crops, and the contamination of food-processing facilities with agents that are difficult to remove) are not considered here.

A general food-production system includes the following stages:

- pre-farm;
- agricultural production and harvesting;
- storage and transport of the raw materials;
- processing;
- storage and transport of processed products;
- wholesale and retail distribution; and
- food service and individual home food preparation.

Such systems range from families who sell to nearby communities to organizations with global production and distribution systems. Many foods, such as fish, meat, poultry, fruit, and vegetables, undergo only minimal processing before consumption. Others, such as most cereal products, cooking oils, and sweeteners, have undergone considerable processing before reaching the consumer. The food-production systems and the specific steps vulnerable to attack may be different for each type of food. The interfaces between the components of the food-production system – where the food changes hands – are the most vulnerable parts. While food safety plans should include measures designed to ensure physical and personnel security, different methods for deciding whether contamination is deliberate or inadvertent may be required.

6.1 Agricultural pre-production, production and harvesting

6.1.1 Security of animal feeds

The contamination of animal feeds that resulted in the spread of bovine spongiform encephalopathy (BSE) and the contamination of poultry feed with dioxins demonstrate the impact that inadvertent contamination has had and that deliberate contamination could have on human health, consumer confidence, and the economy. Many animal feed ingredients are important commodities in the international marketplace, and safety-assurance systems should be included in the quality control of such ingredients. Security measures, such as control of access and tamper-resistant or tamper-evident systems, should be considered during manufacture, transport, and storage. Mechanisms for the recall of animal feeds and animal feed ingredients should be developed where feasible.

6.1.2 Security of agricultural production areas

Agricultural production areas range from those of small farms to very large commercial farms and feedlots. In general, priority has been given to production, and not to food safety *per se*. Recent programmes designed to promote good agricultural practices have also included food safety. Agricultural production areas can be vulnerable to deliberate contamination, such as with highly toxic pesticides and other chemicals. Irrigation water can be easily contaminated with chemical and biological agents. Subsequent processing may sometimes provide critical control points where inadvertent or deliberate contamination can be detected and controlled. Because fruits and vegetables are consumed directly without processing, there are limited opportunities for critical control points for the detection or removal of contamination. The large number of incidents of inadvertent contamination with pathogenic micro-organisms during the production of meat, fish, poultry, and milk products are clear indications of the vulnerability of these products.

The good agricultural practices (including the application of HACCP systems) that are being implemented in many areas, coupled with routine inspections, can greatly reduce the likelihood of inadvertent or deliberate contamination. The latter should be taken into account in the establishment and monitoring of critical control points. Certain harvesting practices, such as open-air drying, offer opportunities for deliberate contamination. Controlling access to and the surveillance of agricultural production areas should be considered, particularly in response to known or probable threats.

6.2 Storage and transport of raw materials

Although storage facilities for raw agricultural commodities range from the open air to large elevators, and means of transport range from human carriers to large ocean-going vessels, there are some precautions that are generally applicable. Physical measures, such as fencing and locks, can be used to secure and prevent unauthorized access to storage facilities and transport containers. These can be supplemented with on-site security personnel, intrusion detectors, and silent alarms linked to the appropriate authorities. If resources permit, remote-controlled television surveillance is another feature that can be introduced. Tamper-resistant or tamper-evident locks or seals on bulk containers should be used where feasible. These can be improvised from materials such as annotated tapes and waxes, which are widely available.

6.3 Processing

Precautions designed to prevent deliberate contamination should be included in food safety plans for processing operations, such as those where the HACCP system is used. Slaughterhouses are particularly vulnerable, especially when not covered by HACCP or comparable systems. The water used in food processing is also important, particularly for minimally processed foods such as fruits and vegetables, where washing is often the critical processing step. Precautions similar to those for drinking-water systems, including the analysis of the water used, should be taken. Air systems in processing plants can also be sources of inadvertent and deliberate contamination. In many food-processing systems, a heat-treatment step is often a critical control point for microbiological contaminants. If HACCP approaches are extended to cover deliberate contamination, normal time/temperature treatments at these control points might not necessarily be adequate for all the microbiological agents that could be used, and would have little or no effect in reducing contamination by toxic chemicals.

6.3.1   Security of processing areas

Access to all critical areas and equipment, including storage areas and water and air systems, should be controlled and monitored. Closed systems, which are often perceived to be less vulnerable and therefore subject to less surveillance, should also be considered. Personal items, such as lunch containers, should not be allowed in critical areas.

6.3.2   Analysis of raw materials and processed products

The introduction of raw materials into the processing stream is a critical control point in most processing operations. Sources of raw materials known to be secure should be used whenever possible. Since analysis for all possible threat agents is impossible, emphasis should be placed on deviations from normal characteristics. The possibility of deliberate contamination should always be taken into account in sampling and analysing the final processed products. All deviations from normal that may indicate contamination should be carefully investigated.

6.4   Storage and transport of processed products

Physical measures, such as fencing and locks, should be used to secure and prevent unauthorized access to storage facilities and transport containers. These can be supplemented with on-site security personnel, intrusion detectors, and silent alarms linked to the appropriate authorities. Remote-controlled television surveillance is another feature that can be introduced. Tamper-resistant and tamper-evident packaging for larger lots as well as for single packages should be considered. All returned products should be carefully examined before reshipment.

6.5   Wholesale and retail distribution

Wholesale establishments and retail markets are among the most vulnerable parts of the food-supply system.

While tamper-resistant and tamper-evident containers have proved to be extremely useful in reducing deliberate contamination, all such containers are vulnerable to individuals who know how to penetrate such protective measures. Controlled access and increased vigilance, including security cameras and other types of surveillance, may be needed. Stopping customers from bringing packages into retail markets can reduce the likelihood of contaminated products being placed on the shelves. Bulk foods in many markets are particularly vulnerable to deliberate contamination. More secure containers for bulk foods and the use of prepackaged materials may be required to prevent deliberate contamination. Wholesale and retail managers should use reliable suppliers. Substitution of substandard food products for products of perceived greater value (counterfeiting) occurs in most parts of the world, and has included the use of products with false labels and replaced ingredients, which have sometimes been contaminated. These same approaches could be used to distribute deliberately contaminated products. Buyers should be suspicious of food being sold under unusual circumstances, e.g. at much less than its normal price or from outside the normal distribution systems.

6.6   Food services and home food preparation

6.6.1   Security in food-service operations

Food services have already been the target of criminal attacks *(6).* Condiments in open containers in restaurants and institutions are vulnerable to deliberate contamination. Increased monitoring of salad bars and other communal food services may be necessary to deter deliberate contamination. Vending machines may constitute targets of opportunity since they are often unsupervised. Increased surveillance may be necessary and additional tamper-resistant and tamper-evident devices may be required.

6.6.2   General food safety in food preparation in individual homes

Consumer education programmes should include information on deliberate contamination. As with inadvertent contamination, washing and cooking food adequately before consumption should be emphasized. Careful attention should also be given to tamper-resistant or tamper-evident seals. Products for which the integrity of the seal or the container is in doubt or that do not meet the usual quality expectations, e.g. having an abnormal appearance, odour, or taste, should not be purchased or consumed. If tampering is suspected, the retailer or supplier and the appropriate public health and law-enforcement authorities should be informed.

7. Other products

A wide variety of manufactured products are used in everyday life, some of which come into contact with the human body and could therefore be exploited by terrorists to disperse chemical and biological agents. Among these consumer products, cosmetics, such as shampoos and lotions, and pharmaceuticals are especially important. In a well developed market economy where many competing products are available, deliberate contamination of a single product is unlikely to lead to widespread disease outbreaks. Similarly, it is unlikely that a terrorist would have the resources to contaminate simultaneously all brands of a particular product. However, the loss of public confidence in the safety of their environment might be far greater than would be justified by the actual extent of the incident. The economic impact on the company and the country producing the affected product might have repercussions that will affect human health. Much of what has been said about food production will also apply to other consumer products. To reduce the likelihood of deliberate contamination, measures such as the careful screening of employees, confirmation of the identity and safety of the raw materials, maintaining security during the manufacturing process, using tamper-resistant or tamper-evident containers, and providing security during transport and storage, and in retail premises may be considered.

In most countries, the manufacture and distribution of medicines are controlled to very high standards, and include the licensing of all those involved in the prescribing and direct dispensing of these products. However, these quality-control processes should be reviewed from the perspective of deliberate contamination. The analytical methods used in quality control may not always detect certain chemical contaminants and toxins. Security systems during storage and transport should also be reviewed for vulnerability to tampering and the substitution of products. International counterfeiting of certain drugs demonstrates the need for such precautions. As with retail food markets, the checking of all packages brought into the market can reduce the possibility that deliberately contaminated products may be placed on the shelves. The increasing international nature of the marketplace, and particularly the availability of many products via the Internet and mail order, has increased the vulnerability of medicines to deliberate contamination.

In addition, the deliberate inactivation of certain drugs and biological products by heat treatment could compromise their effectiveness.

Traditional medicines are often not controlled to the same standards as pharmaceuticals. There have been several recent reports of the inadvertent substitution of toxic plant materials for the intended medicinal plant in some of these preparations in international trade *(7)*. This is clear evidence of the vulnerability of this market to deliberate contamination. As a minimum, the same precautions as those taken in food production should also be taken with traditional medicines. These include the careful screening of employees, the confirmation of the identity and safety of the raw materials, maintaining security throughout the manufacturing process, using tamper-resistant or tamper-evident containers, and providing security during storage and transport and at the retail level. Recall of raw materials, if necessary, is essential, but may prove difficult, as some of these are harvested in the wild by individuals and sold to buyers who generally mix the individual lots together.

8. Conclusions

The possibility that terrorists may deliberately contaminate water supplies, foods, and other consumer products must be taken seriously. Reducing the risk of sabotage will require an unprecedented degree of cooperation among the public health and law-enforcement agencies of governments, utilities, commercial and other private sector organizations, and the public. WHO has developed guidelines on preventing terrorist threats to food to assist Member States *(8)*. Public health authorities must not only take the lead in disease surveillance and incident response, but also strongly support planning and preventative measures.

There are often security and legal difficulties in sharing sensitive intelligence information, particularly about nonspecific threats. Since the public availability of information on systems operations and vulnerability to threats can increase the danger of sabotage, direct partnerships between water-treatment systems and trade and other commercial private sector organizations should be used to share information necessary to improve security. Mechanisms should be developed and put in place to improve monitoring and surveillance.

Publicity given to threats can be as effective as an actual attack in destroying public confidence. In addition to the possibility of generating panic, such publicity often encourages hoaxes and "copycat" actions that can rapidly overwhelm emergency-response systems. National and local governments should consider their responsibilities and their ability to manage these situations and, in close cooperation with commercial, service, and other private sector organizations, draw up appropriate action plans and carry out training exercises. These plans must include provision for communication with the public to manage fear and avoid unfounded rumours.

The total elimination of all risk of inadvertent or deliberate contamination is impossible. The goal must be to reduce this risk to the greatest possible extent and to respond rapidly when contamination and disruption do occur. Safety-assurance systems should incorporate appropriate mechanisms to deter deliberate contamination. The resources allocated for dealing with threats and accidents should be appropriate to the magnitude of the risk. Consumers have an important part to play in preventing exposure, and need to be more aware of the risk. Threats and suspicious actions should be reported to the proper authorities. Consumer education should therefore be included in preparedness planning. Consumers must be aware of the possibility of deliberate contamination and how to respond appropriately. However, efforts to prevent such contamination should complement, not replace, other activities.

REFERENCES

1. Khan AS, Swerdlow DL, Juranek DD. Precautions against biological and chemical terrorism directed at food and water supplies. *Public Health Reports*, 2001, 116:3–14.

2. *HACCP: Introducing the Hazard Analysis and Critical Control Point System*. Geneva, World Health Organization, 1997 (document WHO/FOS/97.2; available at *http://whqlibdoc.who.int/hq/1997/WHO_FSF_FOS_97.2.pdf*).

3. Van Larebeke N et al. The Belgian PCB and dioxin incident of January–June 1999: exposure data and potential impact on health. *Environmental Health Perspectives*, 2001, 109:265–273.

4. MacKenzie WR. A massive outbreak in Milwaukee of *Cryptosporidium* infection transmitted through the public water supply. *New England Journal of Medicine*, 1994, 331:161–167.

5. Mermine JH et al. A massive epidemic of multidrug-resistant typhoid fever in Tajikistan associated with consumption of municipal water. *Journal of Infectious Diseases*, 1999, 179:1416–1422.

6. Torok TJ et al. A large community outbreak of salmonellosis caused by intentional contamination of restaurant salad bars. *Journal of the American Medical Association*, 1997, 278:389–395.

7. Slifman NR et al. Contamination of botanical dietary supplements by *Digitalis lanata*. *New England Journal of Medicine*, 1998, 139:806–811.

8. *Terrorist threats to food: guidance for establishing or strengthening prevention and response systems*. Geneva, World Health Organization, 2002 (document WHO/SDE/PHE/FOS; available at *http://who.int/fsf*).

ANNEX 6: INFORMATION RESOURCES

This report provides a broad overview of what may need to be taken into account in building public-health preparedness against deliberate releases of biological or chemical agents. The report does not seek to provide detailed guidance on any individual component of preparedness, nor is it meant as a design or operating manual. Readers who need more detailed or more specific information are referred to the sources identified below. All are open publications that, so far as can be ascertained, are not subject to international transfer controls.

The information resources are grouped into three categories. First, there are the major texts and general sources: authoritative books or monographs (often available online as well) each covering several aspects of preparedness. Next, there are task-specific information resources. The order in which these are presented broadly follows the sequence of tasks set out in Chapter 4: threat and hazard identification; hazard evaluation and planning for hazard management; and hazard reduction and control. There are subsections on resources specific to biological aspects and to chemical aspects. Agent-specific information sources are not included, for these can be found in the bibliographical sections at the end of Annexes 1, 2, and 3. Finally, there are references to major web sites that themselves host authoritative information about the component tasks and that are added to or updated frequently.

1. Major texts and general sources

Canada

Leonard B, ed. *Emergency response guidebook: a guidebook for first responders during the initial phase of a dangerous goods/hazardous materials incident*. Ottawa, ON, Diane Publishing Co., 2000 (available at *http://www.tc.gc.ca/canutec/erg_gmu/en/Table_of_contents.htm*).

France
Blanchet JM et al. *Les agressions chimiques.* [Chemical aggressions.] Paris, Éditions France-Sélection, 1997.

North Atlantic Treaty Organization
NATO handbook on the concept of medical support in NBC environments. AMedP-7(a).

NATO handbook on the medical aspects of NBC defensive operations. Part II-biological. AMedP-6(B). The USA edition is published as Army Field Manual 8-9, Navy Medical Publication 509, Air Force Joint Manual 44-151, Departments of the Army, the Navy and the Air Force, Washington, DC, 1 February 1996 (available at *http://www.fas.org/nuke/guide/usa/doctrine/dod/fm8-9/toc.htm*).

NATO handbook on the medical aspects of NBC defensive operations. Part III-chemical. AMedP-6(B).

Netherlands
Defence against bioterrorism. The Hague, Health Council of the Netherlands, 2001 (publication no. 2001/16).

Organisation for Economic Co-operation and Development
Guidance concerning health aspects of chemical accidents. For use in the establishment of programmes and policies related to prevention of, preparedness for, and response to accidents involving hazardous substances. Paris, Organisation for Economic Co-operation and Development, 1996. [To be read in conjunction with the OECD *Guiding Principles for Chemical Accident Prevention, Preparedness and Response*, OCDE/GD(96)104; available at *http://www.oecd.org/ehs/ehsmono/#ACCIDENT*.]

Health aspects of chemical accidents: guidance on chemical accident awareness, preparedness and response for health professionals and emergency responders. Paris, Organisation for Economic Co-operation and Development, OCDE/GD(94)1 [prepared as a joint publication with IPCS, UNEP-IE and WHO-ECEH]. (Environment Monograph, No. 81 (1994), UNEP IE/PQC Technical Report No. 19.)

Report of the OECD workshop on risk assessment and risk communication in the context of accident prevention, preparedness and response, No. 1, OCDE/GD(97)31 (1997) (available at *http://www.oecd.org/ehs/ehsmono/#ACCIDENT*).

Sweden

Ivarsson U, Nilsson H, Santesson J, eds. A *FOA briefing book on chemical weapons - threat, effects, and protection*, No. 16. Umeå, National Defence Research Establishment, 1992.

Norlander L et al., eds. *A FOA briefing book on biological weapons.* Umeå, National Defence Research Establishment, 1995.

Switzerland

Steffen R et al. Preparation for emergency relief after biological warfare. *Journal of Infection*, 1997, 34:127–132.

United Kingdom

Deliberate Release Homepage. London, Health Protection Agency, 2003 (available at *http://www.hpa.org.uk/infections/topics_az/deliberate_release/menu.htm*).

Measures for controlling the threat from biological weapons. London, Royal Society, 2000 (document 4/00; available at *http://www.royalsoc.ac.uk/files/statfiles/document-114.pdf*).

United States of America

Bartlett J et al., eds. *Bioterrorism and public health: an internet resource guide.* Montvale, NJ, Thomson Medical Economics, 2002.

Catlett C et al. *Training of clinicians for public health events relevant to bioterrorism preparedness.* Washington, DC, Department of Health and Human Services, Agency for Healthcare Research and Quality Evidence, Report Number 51, 2002. ["The purpose of this evidence report is to identify and review data on the most effective ways to train clinicians to respond to a bioterrorist attack".]

Chin J, ed. *Control of communicable diseases manual*, 17th ed. Washington, DC, American Public Health Association, 1999.

Defense against toxin weapons. Fort Detrick, MD, United States Army Medical Research Institute of Infectious Diseases, 1997 (available at *http://www.usamriid.army.mil/education/defensetox.html*).

Ellison DH. *Emergency action for chemical and biological warfare agents.* Boca Raton, FL, CRC Press, 1999.

Ellison DH. *Handbook of chemical and biological warfare agents.* Boca Raton, FL, CRC Press, 1999

Emergency Medicine – Chemical, Biological, Radiological, Nuclear and Explosives Articles (available at *http://www.emedicine.com/emerg/ WARFARE__CHEMICAL_BIOLOGICAL_RADIOLOGICAL_NUCLEAR_AND_EXPLOSIVES.htm*).

Fraser MR, Fisher VS. *Elements of effective bioterrorism preparedness: a planning primer for local public health agencies.* Washington, DC, National Association of County and City Health Officials, 2001.

Government publication on CD-ROM. *21st century complete guide to bioterrorism, biological and chemical weapons, germs and germ warfare, nuclear and radiation terrorism: military manuals and federal documents, with practical emergency plans, protective measures, medical treatment and survival information.*

Graves B, ed. *Chem–bio: frequently asked questions. Guide to better understanding Chem–Bio.* Alexandria, VA, Tempest Publishing, 1998.

Health and medical support plan for the federal response to acts of chemical/biological (C/B) terrorism: final interim plan. Washington, DC, Department of Health and Human Services, 1995.

Institute of Medicine and National Research Council. *Chemical and biological terrorism: research and development to improve civilian medical response,* Washington, DC, National Academy Press, 1999.

Jane's chemical–biological defense guidebook. Alexandria, VA, Jane's Information Group, 1999.

Khan AS, Levitt AM, Sage MJ. Recommendations and Reports. Biological and chemical terrorism: strategic plan for preparedness and response. Recommendations of the CDC Strategic Planning Workgroup. *Morbidity and Mortality Weekly Report,* 49 (RR-4), 21 April 2000 (available at *http://www.bt.cdc.gov/Documents/BTStratPlan.pdf*).

Khan AS, Morse S, Lillibridge S. Public-health preparedness for bioterrorism in the USA. *Lancet*, 2000, 356:1179–1182.

Mandell GL, Bennett JE, Dolin R, eds. *Mandell, Douglas, and Bennett's principles and practice of infectious diseases*, 5th ed. New York, NY, Churchill Livingstone, 2000.

Kortepeter M et al., eds. *USAMRIID's medical management of biological casualties handbook*, 4th ed. Fort Detrick, MD, United States Army Medical Research Institute of Infectious Diseases, 2001 (available at *http://www.nbc-med.org/SiteContent/HomePage/WhatsNew/MedManual/Feb01/handbook.htm*).

Medical management of chemical casualties handbook, 3rd ed. Aberdeen, MD, United States Army Medical Research Institute of Chemical Defense, 1999 (available at *http://ccc.apgea.army.mil/*).

Sidell FR, Patrick WC, Dashiell TR. *Jane's chem–bio handbook*. Alexandria, VA, Jane's Information Group, 1998.

Sifton D, ed. *PDR guide to biological and warfare response*. Montvale, NJ, Thomson/Physicians' Desk Reference, 2002.

Snyder JW, Check W. *Bioterrorism threats to our future. The role of the clinical microbiology laboratory in detection, identification, and confirmation of biological agents. A report from the American Academy of Microbiology and American College of Microbiology.* Washington, DC, American College of Microbiology, 2001 (available at *http://www.asmusa.org/acasrc/pdfs/bioterrorism.pdf*).

United States Army Chemical and Biological Defense Command, Domestic Preparedness Program, Defense Against Weapons of Mass Destruction. *Technician-hospital provided course manual.* Aberdeen, MD, US Army CBDCOM, Domestic Preparedness Office, 1997.

United States Department of Defense. *21st century terrorism, germs and germ weapons, nuclear, biological and chemical (NBC) warfare – army medical NBC battlebook.* Washington, DC, Department of Defense, 2001.

Venzke BN, ed. *First responder chem-bio handbook. Practical manual for first responders.* Alexandria, VA, Tempest Publishing, 1998.

Zajtchuk R, ed. *Medical aspects of chemical and biological warfare.* Washington, DC, Department of the Army, Office of the Surgeon General, 1997 (available at *http://www.nbc-med.org/SiteContent/HomePage/ WhatsNew/MedAspects/contents.html*).

World Health Organization
Community emergency preparedness: a manual for managers and policy-makers. Geneva, World Health Organization, 1999.

WHO recommended strategies for the prevention and control of communicable diseases. Geneva, World Health Organization, 2001 (document WHO/CDS/CPE/SMT/2001.113).

2. Task-specific sources

2.1 Hazard identification

Bean N, Martin S. Implementing a network for electronic surveillance reporting from public health reference laboratories: an international perspective. *Emerging Infectious Diseases*, 2001, 7:773–779.

Franz DR et al. Clinical recognition and management of patients exposed to biological warfare agents. *Journal of the American Medical Association*, 1997, 278:399–411.

Green M, Kaufman Z. Surveillance for early detection and monitoring of infectious disease outbreaks associated with bioterrorism. *Israel Medical Association Journal*, 2002, 4:503–506.

Jortani SA, Snyder JW, Valdes R. The role of the clinical laboratory in managing chemical or biological terrorism. *Clinical Chemistry*, 2000, 46:1883–1893.

Klietmann WF, Ruoff KL. Bioterrorism: implications for the clinical microbiologist. *Clinical Microbiology Reviews*, 2001, 14:364–381.

Olson JE, Relman DA. Biologic weapons: what infectious disease practitioners need to know. *Infections in Medicine*, 2000, 17:29–44.

Teutsch SM, Churchill RE, eds. *Principles and practice of public health surveillance*, 2nd ed. Oxford, Oxford University Press, 2000.

Worldwide chemical detection equipment handbook. Gunpowder, MD, Chemical and Biological Defense Information Analysis Center, 1995.

2.2 Evaluation and management

Cieslak TJ et al. A field-expedient algorithmic approach to the clinical management of chemical and biological casualties. *Military Medicine*, 2000, 165:659–662.

Fullerton CS, Ursano RJ. Behavioral and psychological responses to chemical and biological warfare. *Military Medicine*, 1990, 155:054–059. [About the longer-term consequences of acute and chronic exposure to nerve agents and others.]

How would you handle a terrorist act involving weapons of mass destruction? *ED Management*, 1999, 11:121–124 (available at *http://www. ahcpub.com/ahc_online/edm.html*).

2.2.1 Biological

Anderson RM. The application of mathematical models in infectious disease research. In: Layne SP et al., eds. *Firepower in the lab: automation in the fight against infectious diseases and bioterrorism.* Washington, DC, National Academic Press, 2000:31–46.

Association for Professionals in Infection Control and Epidemiology. APIC/CDC, *Bioterrorism readiness plan: a template for healthcare facilities.* APIC Bioterrorism Task Force (Judith F. English, Mae Y. Cundiff, John D. Malone and Jeanne Pfeiffer) and CDC Hospital Infections Program Bioterrorism Working Group (Michael Bell, Lynn Steele and Michael Miller), 13 April 1999 (available at *http://www.cdc.gov/ ncidod/hip/Bio/13apr99APIC-CDCBioterrorism.PDF* and at *www.apic.org*.

Bioterrorism preparedness and response: use of information technologies and decision support systems. File Inventory, Evidence Report/Technology Assessment Number 59. Rockville, MD, Agency for Healthcare Research and Quality, 2002 (AHRQ Publication No. 02-E028; available at *http://www.ahrq.gov/clinic/bioitinv.htm*).

Chemical–biological terrorism and its impact on children: a subject review. American Academy of Pediatrics, Committee on Environmental Health and Committee on Infectious Diseases. *Pediatrics*, 2000, 105:662–670. [A review of disaster planning in the event of a chemical or biological warfare act and the implications concerning the health of children.]

Dickinson Burrows W, Renner SE. Biological warfare agents as threats to potable water. *Environmental Health Perspectives*, 1999, 107:975–984.

Henderson DA. Bioterrorism as a public health threat. *Emerging Infectious Diseases*, 1998, 4:488–492.

Inglesby TV, O'Toole T, Henderson DA. Preventing the use of biological weapons: improving response should prevention fail. *Clinical Infectious Diseases*, 2000, 30:926–929. [This article "offers ways by which the infectious diseases professional community might address the challenges of biological weapons and bioterrorism". Emphasis on preparation to respond to BW use: awareness and education; laboratory diagnosis; systems for distributing therapeutics; hospital response and scientific research.]

2.2.2 Chemical

Guiding principles for chemical accident prevention, preparedness and response: guidance for public authorities, industry, labour and others for the establishment of programmes and policies related to prevention of, preparedness for, and response to accidents involving hazardous substances. [Under revision in 2000–2001.] Paris, Organisation for Economic Co-operation and Development, Environment, 1992 (Monograph, No. 51; available in English, French, Russian and Spanish at *http://www.oecd.org/ ehs/ehsmono/#ACCIDENT* ()).

International assistance activities related to chemical accident prevention, preparedness and response (follow-up to the joint OECD and UN-ECE workshop to promote assistance for the implementation of chemical accident programmes). Paris, Organisation for Economic Co-operation and Development, 1997 (No. 3, OCDE/GD(97)181; available at *http://www.oecd.org/ehs/ehsmono/ #ACCIDENT*).

Karalliedde L et al. Possible immediate and long-term health effects following exposure to chemical warfare agents. *Public Health*, 2000, 114:238–248.

Public health and chemical incidents guidance for national and regional policy makers in the public/environmental health roles. Cardiff, WHO Collaborating Centre for an International Clearing House for Major Chemical Incidents, University of Wales, 1999.

Report of the OECD workshop on human performance in chemical process safety: operating safety in the context of chemical accident prevention, preparedness and response. Paris, Organisation for Economic Co-operation and Development, 1999 (No. 4, ENV/JM/MONO(99)12; available at *http://www.oecd.org/ehs/ehsmono/#ACCIDENT*).

Report of the OECD workshop on new developments in chemical emergency preparedness and response. Lappeeranta, Finland, November 1998. Paris, Organisation for Economic Co-operation and Development, 2001 (No. 5, ENV/JM/MONO(2001)1; available at *http://www.oecd.org/ehs/ehsmono/#ACCIDENT*).

Reutter S. Hazards of chemical weapons release during war: new perspectives. *Environmental Health Perspectives*, 1999, 107:985–990.

Shapira Y et al. Outline of hospital organization for a chemical warfare attack. *Israeli Journal of Medical Sciences*, 1991, 27:616–622.

Report of the OECD workshop on pipelines (prevention of, preparedness for, and response to releases of hazardous substances). Paris, Organisation for Economic Co-operation and Development, 2001 (No. 2, OCDE/GD(97)180; available at *http://www.oecd.org/ehs/ehsmono/#ACCIDENT*).

2.3   Reduction and control

Ballantyne B, Schwabe PH, eds. *Respiratory protection: principles and applications.* London, Chapman & Hall, 1981.

Canadian Forces Operations NBC Defence (Book 1 of 2); NBC Defence Equipment (Book 2 of 2).

Colton CE et al. *Respiratory protection: a manual and guideline,* 2nd ed. Akron, OH, American Hygiene Association, 1991.

Dashiell TR et al. *Overview of US chemical and biological defensive equipment.* Alexandria, VA, Chemical and Biological Defense Information Analysis Centre, 1997.

Fullerton CS, Ursano RJ. Health care delivery in the high-stress environment of chemical and biological warfare. *Military Medicine*, 1994, 159:524–528.

Jane's Yearbooks (yearly). *Jane's NBC protection equipment*. Coulsdon, England, Jane's Information Group.

Kadivar H, Adams SC. Treatment of chemical and biological warfare injuries: insights derived from the 1984 Iraqi attack on Majnoon Island. *Military Medicine*, 1991, 156:171–177.

Macintyre AG et al. Weapons of mass destruction events with contaminated casualties. Effective planning for health care facilities. *Journal of the American Medical Association*, 2000, 283:242–249.

Revoir WH, Ching-Tsen B. *Respiratory protection handbook*. Boca Raton, FL, Lewis Publishers, 1997.

Sohns T, Voicu VA, eds. *NBC risks. Current capabilities and future perspectives for protection*. Dordrecht, Kluwer Academic Publishers, 1999.

Sullivan FR, Wand I, Jenouri I. Principles and protocols for prevention, evaluation, and management of exposure to hazardous materials. *Emergency Medicine Reports*, 1998, 19:21–32.

The selection, use and maintenance of respiratory protective equipment: a practical guide. London, Health and Safety Executive, 1988.

United States Army Soldier and Biological Chemical Command (SBCCOM). *Overview of the latest development of US chemical and biological defensive equipment. Detection, decontamination, and protective equipment* (available at *http://www.sbccom.army.mil/products/nbc.htm*).

Worldwide NBC mask handbook. Alexandria, VA, Chemical and Biological Defense Information Analysis Centre, 1992.

Yuan LL. Sheltering effects of buildings from biological weapons. *Science and Global Security*, 2000, 8:329–355.

2.3.1   *Biological*

Barbera J et al. Large-scale quarantine following biological terrorism in the United States: scientific examination, logistic and legal limits, and possible consequences. *Journal of the American Medical Association*, 2001, 286:2711–2717.

Casadevall A. Passive antibody administration (immediate immunity) as a specific defense against biological weapons. *Emerging Infectious Diseases*, 2002, 8:833–841 (available at *http://www.cdc.gov/ncidod/EID/vol8no8/pdf/01-0516.pdf*).

Cieslak TJ et al. Immunization against potential biological warfare agents. *Clinical Infectious Diseases*, 2000, 30:843–850.

Guidance document on the use of medicinal products for the treatment and prophylaxis of biological agents that might be used as weapons of bioterrorism. London, European Agency for the Evaluation of Medicinal Products, 2002 (document CPMP/4048/01; available at *http://www.emea.eu.int/pdfs/human/bioterror/404801.pdf*).

Richard P et al. *Guide to infection control in the hospital: an official publication of the International Society for Infectious Diseases.* Hamilton, ON, BC Decker, 1988.

Treatment of biological warfare agent casualties. Field Manual 8-284, NAVMED P-5042, Air Force Manual (Interservice) 44-156, Marine Corps MCRP 4-11.1C, Headquarters Departments of the Army, the Navy, and the Air Force, and Commandant Marine Corps, Washington, DC, 17 July 2000.

2.3.2   Chemical

Chemical accident contamination control. Field Manual 3–21 Headquarters Department of the Army, Washington, DC, 23 February 1978 (available at *http://155.217.58.58/cgi-bin/atdl.dll/fm/3-21/toc.htm*).

List of items to be stockpiled for Emergency and Humanitarian Assistance. The Hague, Organisation for the Prohibition of Chemical Weapons, 1998 (generic list of items for Assistance under Article X of the CWC; available at *http://www.opcw.org/html/global/c_series/csp1/ci_dec12.html*).

Lundy PM. Treatment of organophosphate nerve agents, current therapy and future prospectives. In: Sohns T, Voicu VA, eds. *NBC risks. Current capabilities and future perspectives for protection.* Dordrecht, Kluwer Academic Publishers, 1999:197–218.

Marrs TC, Sidell FR, Maynard R. *Chemical warfare agents: toxicology and treatment*. Chichester, Wiley, 1999.

Mashhadi H. Delivering assistance and protection. *OPCW Synthesis*, 2001:25–30.

Munro NB et al. The sources, fate, and toxicity of chemical warfare agent degradation products. *Environmental Health Perspectives*, 1999, 107:933–974 (available at *http://www.nbc-med.org/others/Default.html*).

Romano J, Hurst C, Newmark J. Supporting homeland defense: training for chemical casualty management. *Army Medical Department Journal*, 2002, PB 8-02-4/5/6:46–52.

Treatment of chemical agent casualties and conventional military chemical injuries. Field Manual 8-285, NAVMED P-5041, Air Force Joint Manual 44-149, Fleet Marine Force Manual 11.11, Headquarters Departments of the Army, the Navy, and the Air Force and Commandant Marine Corps, Washington, DC, 22 December 1995 (available at *http://www.nbc-med.org/others/Default.html* or *http://www.nbc-med.org/SiteContent/MedRef/OnlineRef/FieldManuals/FM8_285/new/toc.pdf*).

United States Army Soldier and Biological Chemical Command (SBCCOM). *Guidelines for mass casualty decontamination during a terrorist chemical agent incident*, January 2000 (available at *http://www2.sbccom.army.mil/hld/cwirp/cwirp_guidelines_mass_casualty_decon_download.htm*).

United States Army Soldier and Biological Chemical Command (SBCCOM). *Guidelines for mass fatality management during terrorist incidents involving chemical agents*, November 2001 (available at *http://www2.sbccom.army.mil/downloads/cwirp/guidelines_mass_fatality_mgmt.pdf*).

United States Army Medical Research Institute of Chemical Defense. *Field Management of Chemical Casualties Handbook*, 2nd ed., July 2000 (available at *http://ccc.apgea.army.mil/training/training_mat.asp*).

3. Resource-hosting web sites

Note: Readers should be aware of the transience of Internet links. All those listed here were alive in 2003.

Israel
Israel Defence Forces
http://www.idf.il/english/organization/homefront/index.stm

Organisation for the Prohibition of Chemical Weapons (OPCW)
http://www.opcw.org.

Singapore
Singapore Civil Defence Forces
http://www.mha.gov.sg/scdf/ready.html

United Kingdom
Home Office [information and links in regard to emergency planning and disaster management]
http://www.homeoffice.gov.uk/epd/publications/dwd.htm

Health Protection Agency
http://www.hpa.org.uk/

United States of America

Deputy Assistant to the Secretary of Defense for Counterproliferation/ Chemical and Biological Defense. [The home page of the DATSD (CP/CBD). Includes summary of activities of the Counterproliferation Support Program, the DoD Chemical and Biological Defense Program, and downloadable versions of reports.]
http://www.defenselink.mil/pubs/

Department of Defense, Defense Threat Reduction Agency, Chem-Bio Defense: *http://www.dtra.mil/cb/cb_index.html*

Department of Defense, Anthrax Vaccine Immunization Program Agency: *http://www.anthrax.osd.mil/*

Department of Defense, Chemical and Biological Defense Information Analysis Center. [CBIAC serves as the DoD focal point for CW/CBD technology. The CBIAC serves to collect, review, analyse, synthesize, appraise and summarize information pertaining to CW/CBD. It provides a searchable database for authorized users and links to many other CW/CBD related sites.] *http://www.cbiac.apgea.army.mil/*

Department of Health and Human Services, Centers for Disease Control and Prevention, CDC BioTerrorism Preparedness and Response: *http://www.bt.cdc.gov*

Department of Health & Human Services, Metropolitan Medical Response System (MMRS): *http://www.mmrs.hhs.gov*

Department of Health & Human Services, Office of Emergency Preparedness ["OEP has the Departmental responsibility for managing and coordinating Federal health, medical, and health related social services and recovery to major emergencies and Federally declared disasters including: Natural Disasters, Technological Disasters, Major Transportation Accidents, Terrorism"] *http://www.ndms.dhhs.gov*

Federal Emergency Management Agency: *http://www.fema.gov*

Federal Emergency Management Agency, Rapid Response Information System (RRIS). ["The Rapid Response Information System (RRIS) can be used as a reference guide, training aid, and an overall planning and training resource for response to a chemical, biological and/or nuclear terrorist incident. The RRIS is comprised of several databases, consisting of chemical and biological agents' and radiological materials' characteristics, first aid measures, Federal response capabilities, Help Line, Hotlines, and other Federal information sources concerning potential weapons of mass destruction."]

Johns Hopkins University. Center for Civilian Biodefense Studies: *http://www.hopkins-biodefense.org/*

Medical NBC Online Information Server: *http://www.nbc-med.org*

St Louis University School of Public Health Center for the study of Bioterrorism and Emerging Infections
http://www.slu.edu/colleges/sph/bioterrorism/

Tempest's Chem–Bio.com ["designed to help those on the front lines of countering today's chem-bio terrorism threat"] *http://www.chem-bio.com/*

US Army Medical Research Institute of Chemical Defense. [Mission: to develop medical countermeasures to chemical warfare agents and to train medical personnel in the medical management of chemical casualties. The USAMRICD home page provides data links to open literature for medical management of chemical casualties and assay techniques for chemical agents.] *http://chemdef.apgea.army.mil/*

US Army Medical Research Institute of Chemical Defense, Chemical Casualty Care Division: *http://ccc.apgea.army.mil*

US Army Medical Research Institute of Infectious Diseases *http://www.usamriid.army.mil*

US Army Soldier and Biological Chemical Command. [Information on chemical/biological defense equipment and chemical agents. Information about products, clothes, protection, detection, etc.] *http://www.sbccom.apgea.army.mil/*

US Army Soldier and Biological Chemical Command, Homeland Defense Business Unit. [Its mission is "to enhance the response capabilities of military, federal, state and local emergency responders to terrorist incidents involving weapons of mass destruction (WMD). The Homeland Defense Program integrates the critical elements of WMD Installation Preparedness, Improved Response and Technical Assistance upon the solidly proven foundation of the Domestic Preparedness Program."] *http://hld.sbccom.army.mil/*

ANNEX 7:
AFFILIATION OF WHO MEMBER STATES TO THE INTERNATIONAL TREATIES ON BIOLOGICAL AND CHEMICAL WEAPONS

The table below sets out which WHO Member States are (+) or are not (–) parties to the international treaties that afford protection against CBW attack or threat of attack, namely the *Protocol for the Prohibition of the Use in War of Asphyxiating, Poisonous or other Gases, and of Bacteriological Methods of Warfare*, signed at Geneva on 17 June 1925 ("the Geneva Protocol" (GP)), the *Convention on the Prohibition of the Development, Production and Stockpiling of Bacteriological (Biological) and Toxin Weapons and on Their Destruction*, signed at London, Moscow and Washington on 10 April 1972 ("the 1972 Biological and Toxin Weapons Convention" (BWC)), and the *Convention on the Prohibition of the Development, Production, Stockpiling and Use of Chemical Weapons and on their Destruction*, signed at Paris on 13 January 1993 ("the 1993 Chemical Weapons Convention" (CWC)). The table also shows (|) which Member States have signed a treaty but not yet ratified it. The information given is current as at 25 September 2002 with regard to the GP, 15 July 2004 with regard to the BWC, and 25 June 2004 with regard to the CWC.

WHO Member States	GP	BWC	CWC
Afghanistan	+	+	+
Albania	+	+	+
Algeria	+	+	+
Andorra	–	–	+
Angola	+	–	–
Antigua and Barbuda	+	+	–
Argentina	+	+	+
Armenia	–	+	+
Australia	+	+	+
Austria	+	+	+
Azerbaijan	–	–	+

WHO Member States	GP	BWC	CWC
Bahamas	–	+	|
Bahrain	+	+	+
Bangladesh	+	+	+
Barbados	+	+	–
Belarus	–	+	+
Belgium	+	+	+
Belize	–	+	+
Benin	+	+	+
Bhutan	+	+	|
Bolivia	+	+	+
Bosnia and Herzegovina	–	+	+
Botswana	–	+	+
Brazil	+	+	+
Brunei Darussalam	–	+	+
Bulgaria	+	+	+
Burkina Faso	+	+	+
Burundi	–	|	+
Cambodia	+	+	|
Cameroon	+	–	+
Canada	+	+	+
Cape Verde	+	+	+
Central African Republic	+	|	|
Chad	–	–	+
Chile	+	+	+
China	+	+	+
Colombia	–	+	+
Comoros	–	–	|
Congo	–	+	|
Cook Islands ⋎	–	–	+
Costa Rica	–	+	+
Côte d'Ivoire	+	|	+
Croatia	–	+	+
Cuba	+	+	+
Cyprus	+	+	+
Czech Republic	◆	+	+
Democratic People's Republic of Korea	+	+	–
Democratic Republic of the Congo	–	+	|
Denmark	+	+	+
Djibouti	–	–	|
Dominica	–	+	+
Dominican Republic	+	+	|

WHO Member States	GP	BWC	CWC
Ecuador	+	+	+
Egypt	+	|	−
El Salvador	|	+	+
Equatorial Guinea	+	+	+
Eritrea	−	−	+
Estonia	+	+	+
Ethiopia	+	+	+
Fiji	+	+	+
Finland	+	+	+
France	+	+	+
Gabon	−	|	+
Gambia	+	+	+
Georgia	−	+	+
Germany	+	+	+
Ghana	+	+	+
Greece	+	+	+
Grenada	+	+	|
Guatemala	+	+	+
Guinea	−	+	+
Guinea-Bissau	+	+	|
Guyana	−	|	+
Haiti	−	|	|
Honduras	−	+	|
Hungary	+	+	+
Iceland	+	+	+
India	+	+	+
Indonesia	+	+	+
Iran, Islamic Republic of	+	+	+
Iraq	+	+	−
Ireland	+	+	+
Israel	+	−	|
Italy	+	+	+
Jamaica	+	+	+
Japan	+	+	+
Jordan	+	+	+
Kazakhstan	−	−	+
Kenya	+	+	+
Kiribati	−	−	+
Kuwait	+	+	+
Kyrgyzstan	−	−	+
Lao People's Democratic Republic	+	+	+

WHO Member States	GP	BWC	CWC
Latvia	+	+	+
Lebanon	+	+	–
Lesotho	+	+	+
Liberia	+				
Libyan Arab Jamahiriya	+	+	+
Lithuania	+	+	+
Luxembourg	+	+	+
Madagascar	+				
Malawi	+			+
Malaysia	+	+	+
Maldives	+	+	+
Mali	–	+	+
Malta	+	+	+
Marshall Islands	–	–	+
Mauritania	–	–	+
Mauritius	+	+	+
Mexico	+	+	+
Micronesia, Federated States of	–	–	+
Monaco	+	+	+
Mongolia	+	+	+
Morocco	+	+	+
Mozambique	–	–	+
Myanmar	–				
Namibia	–	–	+
Nauru	–	–	+
Nepal	+			+
Netherlands	+	+	+
New Zealand	+	+	+
Nicaragua	+	+	+
Niger	+	+	+
Nigeria	+	+	+
Niue ϒ	–	–	–
Norway	+	+	+
Oman	–	+	+
Pakistan	+	+	+
Palau	–	+	+
Panama	+	+	+
Papua New Guinea	+	+	+
Paraguay	+	+	+
Peru	+	+	+
Philippines	+	+	+

WHO Member States	GP	BWC	CWC
Poland	+	+	+
Portugal	+	+	+
Qatar	+	+	+
Republic of Korea	+	+	+
Republic of Moldova	–	–	+
Romania	+	+	+
Russian Federation	+	+	+
Rwanda	+	+	+
Saint Kitts and Nevis	+	+	+
Saint Lucia	+	+	+
Saint Vincent and the Grenadines	+	+	+
Samoa	–	–	+
San Marino	–	+	+
Sao Tome and Principe	–	+	+
Saudi Arabia	+	+	+
Senegal	+	+	+
Seychelles	–	+	+
Sierra Leone	+	+	│
Singapore	–	+	+
Slovakia	+	+	+
Slovenia	–	+	+
Solomon Islands	+	+	–
Somalia	–	│	–
South Africa	+	+	+
Spain	+	+	+
Sri Lanka	+	+	+
Sudan	+	+	+
Suriname	–	+	+
Swaziland	+	+	+
Sweden	+	+	+
Switzerland	+	+	+
Syrian Arab Republic	+	│	–
Tajikistan	–	–	+
Thailand	+	+	+
The former Yugoslav Republic of Macedonia	–	+	+
Timor-Leste	–	+	+
Togo	+	+	+
Tonga	+	+	+
Trinidad and Tobago	+	–	+
Tunisia	+	+	+
Turkey	+	+	+

WHO Member States	GP	BWC	CWC
Turkmenistan	–	+	+
Tuvalu	–	–	+
Uganda	+	+	+
Ukraine	–	+	+
United Arab Emirates	–	|	+
United Kingdom of Great Britain & Northern Ireland	+	+	+
United Republic of Tanzania	+	|	+
United States of America	+	+	+
Uruguay	+	+	+
Uzbekistan	–	+	+
Vanuatu	–	+	–
Venezuela	+	+	+
Viet Nam	+	+	+
Yemen	+	+	+
Yugoslavia	◆	+	+
Zambia	–	–	+
Zimbabwe	–	+	+

◆ In regard to the Czech Republic and Slovakia, communication from the depositary of the Geneva Protocol, namely the Government of France, dated 30 October 2002, lists only Slovakia as a State Party to the Geneva Protocol. Previous communications from the depositary stated that the Czech Republic, Slovakia and Yugoslavia were States Parties to the Geneva Protocol, Yugoslavia having ratified the Protocol on 27 March 1929, and that both the Czech Republic and Slovakia had become States Parties in their own right through declarations of succession that took effect as of 1 January 1993. Currently only Slovakia is listed as a State Party.

The French Government's interpretation of the relevant international law is that state succession requires an express declaration by a new state for it to be bound by a treaty. The Vienna Convention on the Succession of States in Respect of Treaties 1978, which supports this interpretation of the law, entered into force on 6 November 1996. It currently has only 17 parties, including the Czech Republic, Slovakia, Croatia, Bosnia & Herzogovina, Slovenia, the former Yugoslav Republic of Macedonia and Yugoslavia [*sic*], but not France. There is no single definitive rule of customary international law on the question of state succession to treaties.

ϒ Member State of WHO but not a Member State of the United Nations.

Further notes

* The Holy See is neither a WHO member nor a United Nations member. It is a State Party to the Geneva Protocol, the BWC and the CWC.

* Liechtenstein is not a WHO member, but is a member of the United Nations. It is a State Party to the Geneva Protocol, the BWC and the CWC.

* Puerto Rico and Tokelau are WHO associate members but not United Nations members.

Sources

* *Geneva Protocol*: Communication dated 30 October 2002 received from the Government of France, which is the depositary of the treaty, transmitting a list of States Parties dated 25 September 2002.

* *Biological Weapons Convention*: Meeting of the States Parties to the Convention on the Prohibition of the Development, Production and Stockpiling of Bacteriological (Biological) and Toxin Weapons and on their Destruction, BWC/MSP/2004/MX/NF.4, dated 15 July 2004.

* *Chemical Weapons Convention*: OPCW Technical Secretariat (Office of the Legal Adviser), document S/432/2004 dated 25 June 2004.